PRAISE FOR
OUR BODIES, OURSELVES

T0046049

"A mother lode of information and resources for the client/consum
—*Journal of the American Medical Association*

"[T]he best women's health reference book I've ever seen."
—Julianne Moore, O, *The Oprah Magazine*

"*Our Bodies, Ourselves* is the bible for women's health. . . . It has served as a way for women, across ethnic, racial, religious, and geographical boundaries, to start examining their health from a perspective that will bring about change."
—Byllye Avery, Founder of the National Black Women's Health Project

"[A] trusted resource for sifting through bewildering medical developments . . . intended not to dispense advice from on high but to provide information that women themselves could analyze."
—*The Boston Globe*

"What has made each generation of women rejoice in discovering themselves in *Our Bodies, Ourselves* is that it still emanates from women's experiences as faithfully as ever."
—Helen Rodriguez-Trias, Former President of the American Public Health Association

"Within these pages, you will find the voice of a women's health movement that is based on shared experience. Listen to it—and add your own."
—Gloria Steinem

"More than a book, OBOS is a health movement that deserves a place on every woman's bookshelf."
—*Publishers Weekly*

"[T]his updated compendium is fresh, authoritative, and packed with information and insight. . . ."
—O, *The Oprah Magazine*

"[E]xceedingly readable, strikingly comprehensive, and thoroughly documented . . . remarkable and necessary."
—*Library Journal*

"It's almost impossible to imagine a world without *Our Bodies, Ourselves*. . . . The wealth of indispensable information . . . is all there."
—*Health*

"The newest version of *Our Bodies, Ourselves* . . . remains a wonderful reference. . . . Like Dr. Spock's book on child rearing, which seemed to stay in print for decades, *Our Bodies, Ourselves* keeps being updated because it has become a bible on health care for women."
—Chicago *Sun-Times*

PRAISE FOR
OUR BODIES, OURSELVES: MENOPAUSE

"Encouraging menopause advice from the authors of the bestselling women's health bible. . . . The go-to guide for women with menopause."
—*Kirkus Reviews*

"As a general reference on menopause, this volume will be embraced by a wide female audience."
—*Publishers Weekly*

"By furnishing tools for empowerment, this book goes beyond other fine guides. Highly recommended."
—*Library Journal*

"*Our Bodies, Ourselves: Menopause* is more than just another health reference book. Through accurate medical information and illustrative stories that value women's lives, it gives women the power to be advocates for their own health and well-being. Not only are women able to become more informed consumers, they are inspired to become involved socially and politically in creating a better future for women's health care."
—Mary Hayashi, founder of the National Asian Women's Health Organization

"Our Bodies Ourselves has done it again! After raising us from girlhood to womanhood and never shying from 'taboo' topics, our beloved guides to our own bodies are now here to lead us through menopause with this detailed, inclusive, and woman-centered book—a must-read for every woman in her middle years."
—Helen Zia, former executive editor of *Ms. Magazine*

OUR BODIES, OURSELVES:

Pregnancy and Birth

OTHER MAJOR BOOKS BY MEMBERS
OF THE BOSTON WOMEN'S HEALTH BOOK COLLECTIVE

Our Bodies, Ourselves: A New Edition for a New Era

Our Bodies, Ourselves: Menopause

Changing Bodies, Changing Lives

Ourselves and Our Children

The New Ourselves, Growing Older

OUR BODIES, OURSELVES:

Pregnancy and Birth

THE BOSTON WOMEN'S HEALTH BOOK COLLECTIVE

ATRIA PAPERBACK
New York   London   Toronto   Sydney   New Delhi

CLINIC DISCOUNT: *Our Bodies, Ourselves: Pregnancy and Birth* is available to clinics and other groups providing health-counseling services at 50 percent off the cover price plus shipping (a 55 percent discount is available for those who purchase more than 1,000 books). To place your order, download a book order form at http://www.ourbodiesourselves.org/uploads/pdf/clinicdiscounts.pdf and fax that to 212-698-2863. Orders must include payment (all major credit cards accepted) and a document verifying health service status and your IRS license number for tax exemption. The document must include a copy of a statement filed with a state or federal agency indicating health services or health education as a primary purpose of your group. Copies so purchased may not be offered for resale. Please contact Simon & Schuster Special Sales with any questions at 1-877-989-0009.

ATRIA
PAPERBACK

An Imprint of Simon & Schuster, Inc.
1230 Avenue of the Americas
New York, NY 10020

This Atria Paperback edition June 2021

ATRIA PAPERBACK and colophon are trademarks of Simon & Schuster, Inc.

For information about special discounts for bulk purchases,
please contact Simon & Schuster Special Sales at 1-866-506-1949
or business@simonandschuster.com.

The Simon & Schuster Speakers Bureau can bring authors to your live event.
For more information or to book an event, contact the Simon & Schuster
Speakers Bureau at 1-866-248-3049 or visit our website at www.simonspeakers.com.

Designed by Katy Riegel

Manufactured in the United States of America

20   19   18   17   16   15

Library of Congress Cataloging-in-Publication Data is available.

ISBN 978-0-7432-7486-9
ISBN 978-1-4165-6591-8 (ebook)

Acknowledgments

In producing this book, I have collaborated with a wide-ranging team of contributors, whose dedication and intelligence have been inspiring. I would like to thank the 150 or so women, and the few men, who wrote, reviewed, and revised sections of the manuscript, as well as the photographers and illustrators who brought the words to life in images. Each of the many contributors to the text is named individually, chapter by chapter, in the "Authorship and Acknowledgments" section, which starts on page 338; short biographical statements about the writers are on pages 343–346.

I also would like to thank the dozens of women who shared their own experiences for this book and the many women who attended brainstorming sessions that helped us get started. Although most of these women remain anonymous in these pages, we benefit from all their wisdom and insight.

Certain women deserve special mention. Kiki Zeldes, Our Bodies Ourselves website manager, took part in the many stages of planning for the book and served alongside me as editor. An essential group of advisors read every chapter of the manuscript and participated in the editorial process, from early meetings about the book's vision through final review of the text. These editorial advisers were Elana Hayasaka, an Our Bodies Ourselves staff member who also served as graphics editor for the book; Neda Joury-Penders, MPH, a board member of Our Bodies Ourselves; Tekoa King, CNM, MPH, a certified nurse-midwife and the editor-in-chief of the *Journal of Midwifery & Women's Health;* Lydia Mayer, MD, MPH, an obstetrician-gynecologist and medical ethicist; Judy Norsigian, executive director of Our Bodies Ourselves; and Cornelia van der Ziel, MD, an obstetrician-gynecologist and coauthor of *Big, Beautiful and Pregnant.* I thank them all.

Last, but certainly not least, I offer my gratitude to everyone who has contributed over the years to *Our Bodies, Ourselves* and to the organization that produces it, particularly the founders, staff, and volunteer board members, all of whom are listed on page 341. Without these many foremothers, this book would never have been born.

Heather Stephenson, executive editor

Contents

BECOMING A MOTHER

KNOWLEDGE IS POWER

Introduction

If you are newly pregnant, or are close to someone who is, we hope this book will serve as a friendly companion through the months to come. From the first weeks of pregnancy through the "fourth trimester," the months of early motherhood, *Our Bodies, Ourselves: Pregnancy and Birth* offers guidance to help you take care of yourself and make informed decisions. We hope that it will inspire you to feel more confident and comfortable about approaching motherhood.

Our primary goal in writing this book has been to offer guidance to women like you who are navigating the health care system at an exciting and somewhat vulnerable time. Like expectant mothers everywhere, you want the best for your own health and the health of your baby, but you most likely aren't a medical expert—and you don't have time to become one. That's where we can help. The pages that follow present the best available evidence about the advantages and disadvantages of a range of maternity care practices that you may be considering. They also include the important warning that some common procedures are not consistently helpful to women in good health and might better be avoided in some cases. Informing yourself about these standard practices and their alternatives is an essential step toward creating a better birth experience for yourself and your baby.

HOW WE GOT HERE

Pregnancy and birth have always been vital topics in *Our Bodies, Ourselves,* the groundbreaking women's health "bible." As we produced the thirty-fifth-anniversary edition of *Our Bodies, Ourselves,* our editorial team realized that several topics covered in a chapter or two were ripe for more in-depth treatment. We decided to create new books on those topics, starting with *Our Bodies, Ourselves:*

Menopause, which was published in 2006. *Our Bodies, Ourselves: Pregnancy and Birth* is the second new title to complement and expand on the work of our original book, which has been translated or adapted into twenty-one languages and has sold close to 4.5 million copies over the past four decades.

In this new book, we examine childbearing in greater depth than ever before—with up-to-date information about birth in the United States today. Like *Our Bodies, Ourselves,* this book features many women sharing personal experiences. It also combines trustworthy medical information with thoughtful analysis of the social, economic, and political forces affecting our health.

BEYOND SELF-HELP

Our Bodies, Ourselves: Pregnancy and Birth gives a reader like you tools to take care of yourself, from tips on eating well during pregnancy to strategies for coping with stress and depression. But this book is about more than self-help. It puts individual choices in cultural and political context. Many factors, from obstetricians' training to insurance restrictions to the lack of paid maternity leave, are beyond an individual's control. We can change these conditions only by advocating with others for policies and programs that protect the health of all mothers and babies.

FROM "I" TO "WE"

Throughout this book, women share their experiences of pregnancy, birth, and the "fourth trimester" of life as a new mother. Most of these first-person stories are told anonymously, set off in italicized passages in the text. Longer stories are set apart from the main text in boxes, each with the name and photograph of the woman telling her story.

Our Bodies, Ourselves: Pregnancy and Birth uses the pronoun "we" to refer to all women, whatever our racial, ethnic, and class backgrounds, countries of origin, sexual orientations, or gender identities. The choice to refer to women as "we" rather than "they" reflects the early decision of the Boston Women's Health Book Collective to change the title of its book (initially *Women and Their Bodies*) to *Our Bodies, Ourselves.* By speaking about women's bodies with the voice of personal experience, referring to "our bodies" rather than "their bodies," the book rejects the distancing voice of some medical texts and celebrates that this is a book written for, about, and primarily by women.

MORE ON THE WEB

For more information about pregnancy and childbirth, including links to other helpful resources, please visit the website of Our Bodies Ourselves at www.ourbodies ourselves.org. Our website also includes a blog featuring daily women's health news and analysis, extensive material about other aspects of women's health, and information about our organization and its work around the globe.

FROM US TO YOU

On behalf of all of the women and men who worked on this book, we offer you, our readers, our congratulations and good wishes as you embark on the journey toward becoming a mother. May our book be one helpmate along the way.

Judy Norsigian, executive director,
Heather Stephenson, executive editor,
and Kiki Zeldes, editor, for the Boston
Women's Health Book Collective
(also known as Our Bodies Ourselves)

The Journey
to Parenthood

CHAPTER 1

Approaching Birth
with Confidence

Congratulations! As a pregnant woman planning to bring a new life into this world, you are embarking on an amazing journey.

Pregnancy and birth are as ordinary and extraordinary as breathing, thinking, or loving. Whether you are pregnant for the first time or are already a mother, pregnancy will call on your creativity, flexibility, endurance, and humor. You will face many choices that will affect your pregnancy, birth experience, and life as a new mother. As you consider your options, you'll want to learn as much as you can about your developing pregnancy and various childbirth practices and think about the experiences you hope to have. What kind of care do you want to receive during pregnancy? Where do you wish to give birth? Who would you like to be with you when you are in labor?

Most pregnant women are bombarded with advice from well-meaning friends, relatives, and even strangers. Everyone seems to have an opinion on what you should or shouldn't do, and it's easy to feel overwhelmed by their conflicting recommendations.

This book will help you sort fact from fiction. By drawing on the most accurate research, the personal experiences of many individual women, and the advice of midwives, physicians, and other health care providers, it will give you the information you need to make wise decisions and approach birth with confidence.

CLIMATE OF CONFIDENCE, CLIMATE OF DOUBT

Pregnancy and birth are normal, healthy processes for most women, the vast majority of whom have healthy pregnancies and babies. But when was the last time you saw a newspaper article titled "3.5 Million American Women Had Normal

Labors and Healthy Babies This Year" or a TV episode that showed a healthy woman giving birth to a healthy newborn, without a sense of emergency or a heroic rescue?

The media's preference for portraying emergency situations, and doctors saving babies, sends the message that birth is fraught with danger. Other factors, including the way doctors are trained, financial incentives in the health care system, and a rushed, risk-averse society, also contribute to the popular perception that childbirth is an unbearably painful, risky process to be "managed" in a hospital with the use of many tests, drugs, and procedures. In such an environment, the high-tech medical care that is essential for a small proportion of women and babies has become the norm for almost everyone.

Some advocates for childbearing women describe this as a "climate of doubt" that increases women's anxiety and fear. In contrast, a climate of confidence focuses on our bodies' capacity to give birth. Such a climate reinforces women's strengths and abilities and minimizes fear. Some of the factors that nourish a climate of confidence include high-quality prenatal care; healthy food and time to rest and exercise;

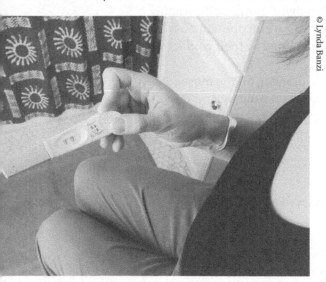
© Lynda Banzi

a safe work and home environment; childbearing leave; clear, accurate information about pregnancy and birth; encouragement, love, and support from those close to you; and skilled and compassionate health care providers. As your pregnancy develops, do what you can to seek out such resources.

When I found out I was pregnant, my blood pressure was a little on the high side. But I had a great doctor who helped me take care of myself and my baby. She knew all the details of my personal problems—being unmarried, and with a partner who had an addiction problem—and she treated me with nothing but respect. I think it made all the difference in having a healthy baby. In spite of my difficult circumstances and the stress, I actually had a very good pregnancy and had a lot of love and support.

My husband loved my pregnancy. He'd want to play jazz to my belly and sing to my belly. He'd rub cream on the stretch marks and tell the baby the play-by-play of the baseball game. He and our cat both seemed more protective of me and I felt very loved by my little family of two.

QUESTIONING HIGH-TECH BIRTH

The path to motherhood involves navigating through a health care system that can be complex and sometimes intimidating. While some aspects of maternity care are shaped by economic, social, and political forces that are beyond our individual control, there are things you can do to increase your chances of having a healthy and satisfying pregnancy, birth, and early postpartum period. The following chapters provide advice, support, and resources to guide you as you learn about your pregnancy, seek prenatal care, and face decisions about the kind of birth you want.

As you make these decisions, it's important to understand that some elements of the care most women receive during pregnancy and childbirth are not based on the most reliable research on what is safe and effective. Some high-tech procedures are overused in the United States, while other practices that have been shown to improve birth outcomes are not offered widely. Being aware of this can help you access the best care for your situation.

When used appropriately, maternity care interventions such as artificial inductions of labor (use of drugs or techniques to try to start labor), episiotomies (cutting to enlarge the vaginal opening), epidurals (a kind of anesthesia), and cesarean sections (surgical deliveries) can improve health outcomes and even save lives. Yet far too often, these interventions are used routinely on healthy women who are at low risk for medical complications, despite clear scientific evidence that they are unnecessary, ineffective, and/or can cause harm. The widespread routine use of medical interventions during labor and birth has failed to improve the safety of childbirth for low-risk women. In addition, these interventions can disrupt the natural rhythms of labor, undermine women's confidence in our capacity to give birth, and decrease our satisfaction with our birth experiences.

At the same time that such procedures are *overused,* practices that have been shown to improve birth outcomes—as well as increase women's satisfaction with the experience of giving birth—are widely *underused.* These practices include receiving continuous one-on-one support from a skilled, experienced caregiver during labor; being able to change positions, get out of bed, and walk during labor; and using comfort measures such as massage, warm baths, and birthing balls. (For more information on how and why U.S. health systems are not always providing the best care possible and about efforts to change this, see Chapter 17, "Advocating for Better Maternity Care.")

As much as possible, surround yourself

with the kinds of supportive practices that have been proven effective but are sometimes underused, and avoid unnecessary medical interventions. Choosing a health care provider and birth setting that make judicious, conservative use of interventions, learning about the advantages and disadvantages of different medical procedures and treatments that are offered to you, and declining those procedures and treatments that you do not need can help you have a safer, more satisfying birth experience.

My tips for pregnant women? Exercise. Eat healthy but splurge once in a while. Enjoy all of the attention. Wear comfortable shoes. Sleep every chance you get for as long as you can. Read and educate yourself about all of your choices regarding childbirth so you can feel in control and not like it is something that is happening to you. In addition, have an open mind [in case] things don't go how you planned.

It really helps to have someone there (if in a hospital) who can act as an advocate for the mother, like a doula [trained birth companion], mother, or good friend. . . . You also have to make very clear what you want, because hospitals have certain routines and procedures that they are used to, and unless you tell them otherwise, they will go ahead with their routines (examples: putting drops in the baby's eyes right away and giving the shot of vitamin K, giving the baby a bath). I would say to keep an open mind, learn what your options are, [and try] to be an active participant in the whole process.

PLANNING A BETTER BIRTH[2]

If you are healthy and have no medical complications that call for a "high-risk" approach to your care during labor and birth, you can increase your chances of having a safe and satis-

fying vaginal birth by trying the following strategies:

- **Find a doctor or midwife with low rates of intervention.**

  Some caregivers have much lower rates of intervention than others. While rates of intervention will vary depending on the population served (for example, women carrying multiple babies and women with high blood pressure are more likely to need interventions), they also vary by the type of provider and the practice style. Although there are many exceptions, family physicians tend to have lower rates of intervention than obstetricians, and midwives generally have the lowest rates of all. These differences are partly due to varying degrees of risk among the women who choose an obstetrician, family physician, or midwife (for example, a woman with pregnancy complications will likely choose an obstetrician), and partly due to the differences in practice styles between types of providers. (For more information, see Chapter 2, "Choosing Your Health Care Provider and Birth Setting," particularly the section "Models of Maternity Care," page 15.)

- **Choose a birth setting with low overall rates of intervention.**

  Some birth settings have far lower rates of intervention than others. Use of interventions is much lower in out-of-hospital birth centers and home births, compared with hospitals. However, the rates of intervention among different hospitals can also vary widely, depending on the practices and policies of the hospital as well as the health problems of the women it serves. (For more information, see "Birth Settings," page 22.)

- **Create your own birth plan and discuss it with your caregivers.**

  Writing down your values, preferences, and priorities can help you clarify your own thinking and feelings. Moreover, this type of birth plan helps prepare you to discuss these issues with your partner and your caregivers. Find out if your caregivers will work with you to meet your goals and preferences. If their response does not satisfy you and you have other options, seek a better match. (For more information, see "Birth Plans," page 37, and "Some Questions to Ask Midwives and Physicians," page 21.)

- **Arrange for continuous labor support from someone with experience.**

  Arrange for someone in addition to your partner to be with you throughout your labor and birth. You can work with a *doula* (a trained labor support companion) or ask a friend or family member who is experienced with birth and with whom you are comfortable. Women who receive continuous, one-on-one support have fewer complications, better health outcomes, and greater satisfaction with their birth experiences. (For more information, see "Your Birth Team," page 32.)

- **Explore your options for pain relief.**

  There are a wide range of medications and nondrug approaches to managing pain in childbirth. Learn about the advantages and disadvantages of all the options. (For more information, see "Planning for Pain Management," page 38, and Chapter 11, "Coping with Pain.")

- **Avoid continuous electronic fetal monitoring when possible.**

  Continuous electronic fetal monitoring (EFM) increases the likelihood of both cesarean sections and operative vaginal births (births in which forceps or a device known as a *vacuum extractor* are used to help pull the baby out of the birth canal). Continuous EFM does not offer clear benefit for babies when compared to monitoring the fetal heart rate intermittently during labor. Talk with your caregiver and check hospital policies to find out whether they are willing to check your baby's heart rhythm with a handheld device or occasional use of EFM instead of continuous EFM. With some types of intervention that involve increased risk (for example, epidurals for pain control), you will be required to use continuous EFM. (For more information, see "Fetal Monitoring," page 174.)

- **Avoid routine use of other medical interventions when possible.**

  Using medical interventions when there is no clear medical need offers no benefit to mothers while increasing the likelihood of harm. For example, labor augmentation (use of drugs to increase the speed and strength of your contractions) can increase the discomfort of contractions and lead to fetal heart patterns that cause concern. Some research links labor induction (use of drugs or techniques to try to start labor) with increased likelihood of cesarean section, especially in first-time mothers, or before full term, or when the cervix is not soft and ready to open. Avoid having a provider break your bag of waters (artificial rupture of membranes) before labor starts or in early labor, unless there is a clear medical reason to do so; early breaking of the bag of waters may increase the likelihood of a cesarean. It is also good to avoid arbitrary time limits for your labor. There is no need to turn to a cesarean if you and your baby are doing well. Talk with your caregivers about these practices and how to avoid them. (For more information about induction, see page 146. For information on rupture of membranes, see page 180.)

Being informed can help you negotiate the choices you face during pregnancy and childbirth. While you won't be able to control everything that happens in the months to come, you can clarify what is important to you. Excellent support can also help, so surround yourself with caregivers and others who understand your priorities and will advocate for you.

At first I was really scared of labor. I knew I wanted a birth as free of interventions as possible, but I thought this meant I had to be some kind of Amazon who squatted in the field, grunted out her baby, then stood up to pick the crops. Or else a superfit marathon runner who *had endless endurance and tolerance for pain. But the more I learned, the more I talked to other women, and the more support I got from my midwife, the more confident I felt. I took great comfort in the fact that women have been giving birth forever—every one of us had a mother who managed to birth us!*

NOTES

1. Adapted with permission from Great Starts Birth and Family Education, 2517 Eastlake Ave. E, Suite 102, Seattle, WA 98101; 206-789-0883; www.greatstarts.org.
2. Adapted from content produced by Childbirth Connection. The organization's website (www.childbirth connection.org) has information about the best available research on the safety and effectiveness of maternity care practices as well as extensive materials to help women and families make informed decisions during pregnancy, labor, and birth.

CHAPTER 2

Choosing Your Health Care Provider and Birth Setting

I had a long, intense labor at the hospital, and Annie, my doula (trained birth assistant), was great. She helped me in and out of the shower, got me on the birthing ball, pressed hard on my back during the worst of the contractions, told me I was doing a great job at birthing my baby. When I was about 9 centimeters dilated, the baby's heart rate dropped. The nurse had me change positions—roll on my side, get on all fours—to see if that would help. She paged the obstetrician on call, who came in immediately. He looked at the monitor results, tried a few more position changes, and came over to the side of my bed. He squatted down on the floor so that his eyes were level with mine, and told me that he was concerned that the baby wasn't getting enough oxygen, and that he thought I should have a C-section. I knew cesarean sections were frequently done unnecessarily and I wanted to avoid one if at all possible. He listened to my concerns, agreed with me that cesareans are overperformed—but also said that in his judgment this one was necessary. . . . While I wish the C-section hadn't been needed, I so appreciate how attentive and respectful all my providers were.

After talking with Jennifer (a midwife who attends home births), I knew I wanted her to be my provider. She told me about some of the births she had attended, and told me what I could expect. "You'll be in your own home," she said, "comfortable and secure, surrounded by people you love. You can labor as you need to, with all of our support, and when you're ready you can reach down and birth your baby." She presented a beautiful picture of what birth could be.

During my prenatal visits I would go to her house, sit on the couch in her living room, drink tea. While we talked she would do small checks on the baby, measure my belly, ask me how I felt. She was very organized and motherly, and provided all the appropriate medical care. . . . I always felt important, like she cared about me and really wanted me to have the kind of pregnancy and birth experience I wanted. And

I never felt like she had her hand on the door, waiting to go. . . . I loved being treated like a healthy pregnant woman, not like someone who is sick and needs treatment.

Where we give birth and who attends us throughout pregnancy, labor, and birth can powerfully affect both what happens to us and our feelings about our experiences. Because of this, it's important to take the time before becoming pregnant or early in our pregnancies to learn about our options and make thoughtful decisions.

An optimal provider and birth setting will offer you:

- care that is consistent with the best available research on safety and effectiveness
- an environment and treatments that enhance, rather than interfere with, the natural process of pregnancy and birth
- individualized care that takes into account your health needs (and those of your baby) as well as your personal preferences and values
- abundant support, comfort, and information[1]

A skilled and attuned provider helps each woman step into motherhood in the best physical, emotional, and spiritual condition possible for her. Identifying your priorities, learning about the differences among various approaches to childbirth, and finding out which options are available to you can help you make decisions that fit your circumstances and preferences. You can gather the information you need in numerous ways. You can talk with other women about their experiences and read birth stories and books about childbirth (see "Resources," page 325). You can learn how your choice of provider and birth setting are linked, as some providers practice only in certain birth settings. (Doctors, for example, rarely attend home births, while some midwives cannot supervise your care in a hospital.) You can learn what you can do if you experience or anticipate complications and may need specialized care. You can find out which specific types of caregivers and birth settings are available in your area, and what your health insurance, if you have any, will cover. You can interview potential caregivers and take tours of different birth settings.

In the United States today, women's options in maternity care are often limited by finances and by insurance or managed care requirements. If you are pregnant and cannot afford insurance, you may be able to receive Medicaid coverage, which is available to pregnant women in all fifty states. You may be eligible once you are pregnant even if you were refused previously, when not pregnant, because the eligibility requirements are different for pregnant women. In addition, a special program called Presumptive Eligibility pays for medical care for pregnant women whose applications have not yet been approved. Medicaid eligibility requirements vary from state to state. To learn about local services and find out if you are eligible for Medicaid or other government benefits, ask your health care provider for help, call your state Medicaid office, or look online at www.govbenefits.gov.

In the future, women's options for maternity care may narrow in the United States. Because of lifestyle and liability concerns, fewer young doctors are choosing to specialize in obstetrics. At the same time, certified nurse-midwife programs are closing, for a variety of reasons. We can work toward making a wider array of childbirth options available to all women by supporting organizations that advocate on behalf of these options. (For more information, see Chapter 18, "Advocating for Mothers and Families.")

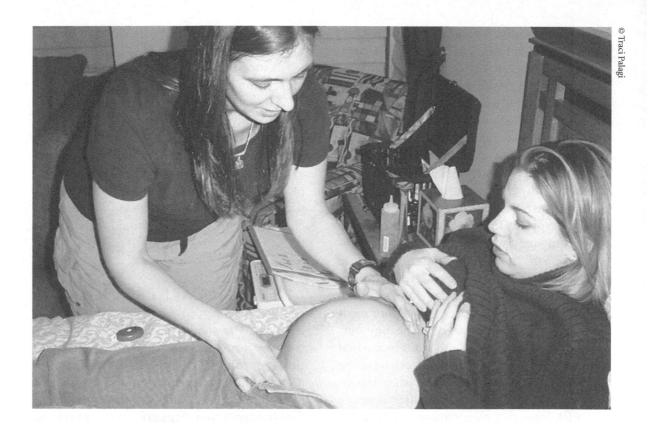

MODELS OF MATERNITY CARE

The care you receive during your pregnancy, labor, and childbirth will vary according to the type of provider and birth setting you choose. The different training that midwives and doctors receive prepares them to approach pregnancy and childbirth differently. In the United States, there are two main paradigms in maternity care training, described as the *midwifery model* and the *medical model.**

The classic **midwifery model** is based on the

---

* These terms derive from the kinds of care physicians and midwives have historically provided. However, their use is not meant to imply that all midwives follow a midwifery model or that all physicians follow a medical model. Some people believe it is more accurate to refer to the different models of care as a *physiologic model* (that is, care in accord with the normal functioning of a woman's body) versus an *interventionist* or *pathology-driven model.*

assumption that most pregnancies, labors, and births are normal biological processes that result in healthy outcomes for both mothers and babies. It focuses on maximizing the health and wellness of a woman and her baby, identifying and managing medical problems early on, and attending to the emotional, social, and spiritual aspects of pregnancy and birth. Midwifery care seeks to protect, support, and avoid interfering with the unique rhythm, character, and timing of each woman's labor. Midwives are trained to be vigilant in identifying women with serious complications. Medical expertise and interventions are sought when necessary, but are not used routinely. In most parts of the world, midwives are the primary caregivers for women with uncomplicated pregnancies. (For more information, see "The Midwifery Model of Care" at www.ourbodiesourselves.org/childbirth.)

A strict *medical model* of care focuses on preventing, diagnosing, and treating the complications that can occur during pregnancy, labor, and birth. Making use of medical expertise is essential for women who have particular conditions or illnesses, and the drugs and interventions used to manage such complications are invaluable and even lifesaving at times. However, interventions can also interfere with the normal rhythms of birth and actually create problems. Training in the medical model does not typically focus on developing skills to support the natural progression of an uncomplicated birth. In addition, under the medical model, care generally follows a certain routine. This standardization reduces individualized care, but it can protect women from poor medical care and increase safety and healthy outcomes overall. Providers who work in medical settings (including nurse-midwives) are often constrained by hospital protocols (such as policies forbidding vaginal births after cesarean sections), insurance requirements, and liability concerns. The medical model of birth is prevalent in the United States today.

The midwifery model of care and the medical model of care are linked to certain birth outcomes. Healthy women (with healthy infants) working with midwives generally have fewer interventions than those working with physicians, and comparable (sometimes even better) outcomes.[2] This is also true for women in challenging social circumstances (for example, low-income or teenage mothers). Women who are experiencing complicated pregnancies can also benefit greatly from many traditional midwifery approaches while also working with a medical specialist.

Although it is crucial to understand the differing philosophies and training among practitioners, it is also important to note that the letters after someone's name do not tell you much about her or him as an individual. Some doctors have attitudes, styles, and approaches that fit the midwifery model, and some midwives incorporate the medical model that is more common for doctors.

The vast majority of us enter pregnancy as healthy women, with no major medical problems. If this is true for you, you can choose from the full range of providers and birth settings available in your area. If you have a serious medical condition or are at risk for developing such a condition, an obstetrician or maternal-fetal medicine specialist should be on your team.

HEALTH CARE PROVIDERS

If you have a choice of maternity caregivers, compare providers and find out how much time they can spend with you. Assess their willingness to share information and involve you in decision making, and learn their preferences for (and how often they perform) various types of intervention. In addition, pay attention to how you feel in the presence of the provider. Are you being treated as an equal? Do you have good communication? Are your concerns being taken seriously? Are you happy with her or his attitudes toward such things as age, ethnic background, sexual orientation, marital status, and disability?

Many providers are part of group practices, which means that you will be attended at birth by whichever provider is on call at that time. In addition, the provider on call will respond if you have any concerns during pregnancy that come up outside of regular office hours. This can be frustrating if you have a good relationship with a particular provider. On the positive side, working in such teams can give midwives and doctors more predictable, limited work hours; this entails less fatigue and can reduce medical error. If you will be working with a

THE LANGUAGE OF BIRTH

The language used to describe pregnancy and childbirth reflects assumptions about women that set the stage for different styles of maternity care. Woman-centered terminology portrays women as active, healthy, and powerful, and labor as "natural" and "normal." In this view, associated traditionally with the midwifery model, providers "attend" women, "assist" at births, and "catch" babies. In contrast, some medical language depicts women as passive subjects, putting doctors in the role of "managing labor" and "delivering babies." Medical terms such as "failure to progress," "inadequate pelvis," and "incompetent cervix" imply that something is wrong with a woman's body. This influences how we see ourselves, how providers see us, and how the media portray birth.

group practice and have a choice, look for one in which all members have comparable education, training, experience, and philosophies of care. Some practices host events to introduce all the providers. When scheduling a prenatal visit, some ob-gyns and midwives can provide a longer session by booking a double session, but this may be difficult to arrange.

Some doctors and certified nurse-midwives follow a model for group prenatal visits called Centering Pregnancy. At each prenatal visit, the provider facilitates learning and discussion among a group of pregnant women. In addition, the provider gives individualized private care to each woman at every meeting. Special Centering Pregnancy groups cater to the needs of pregnant teens. One study of the program's work with teens suggests that it is associated with low rates of preterm birth, few low-birth-weight infants, and satisfaction with prenatal care experiences.[3]

MIDWIVES

I had always used an MD for my gynecological needs until I got pregnant and did some research. Between lots of reading and a friend who is a

doula, I decided to use a midwife and birth center for my first pregnancy. I went to the [local midwifery practice] and had a wonderful experience. I felt listened to and honored and my pregnancy was treated as a natural part of life instead of as a medical disorder. Everything was low-key and low-stress. They provided extra services such as a

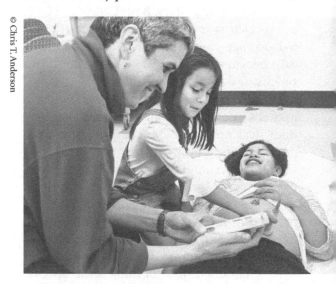

© Chris T. Anderson

A girl listens to the heartbeat of her sibling-to-be during a group prenatal care session that follows the Centering Pregnancy model. Centering Pregnancy groups provide education and support for women.

nutritionist and lots of birth classes. Information was available to make whatever choices felt right for me. They even provided a doula free of charge!

Midwives have been attending and supporting women during pregnancy and childbirth, and teaching other women to do so, for centuries. All midwives are trained to provide women with prenatal care, care during labor and birth, and follow-up care after the baby is born. In the United States today, midwives attend approximately one in ten vaginal births, primarily in hospitals. They most commonly have the kinds of education and training described in the sections that follow.

Certified Nurse-Midwives and Certified Midwives

Certified nurse-midwives (CNMs) are educated in the two disciplines of nursing and midwifery. Certified midwives (CMs) are educated only in midwifery. Both CNMs and CMs are specialists in both natural childbirth and well-woman care, which includes gynecological checkups, pelvic and breast exams, Pap smears, and family planning services.

CNMs are registered nurses who earn a master's degree in an accredited nurse-midwifery program. CMs complete an accredited midwifery program that also provides a master's degree and pass the same national certifying exam. Most midwives are CNMs.

CNMs and CMs work in their own private practices, the private practices of physicians, freestanding birth centers, hospitals, health departments, and homes. Both CNMs and CMs have established relationships with specific doctors and will consult with them, collaborate with them, and refer to them as needed.

Certified nurse-midwives and certified midwives are able to attend births in any setting, and they have established access to resources and backup. Their services are often covered by health insurance policies. They usually practice within the medical system, where their ability to offer you full individualized care may be constrained by insurance protocols, standard hospital procedures, and financial concerns.

Because I had conceived through in vitro fertilization and had previously had a miscarriage, I was worried about my pregnancy. The reproductive endocrinologist I worked with frowned on any birth setting but a hospital. In addition, I had a serious gastroesophageal complication and wanted my providers to be on equal footing with each other. All this led me to choose an obstetrician. But when she announced she was leaving the practice (in my sixth month), I took the opportunity to reexamine my situation.

Not only had my OB and my gastroenterologist never communicated with each other, they gave me contradictory advice. I met with the other members of the obstetric practice and was uncomfortable with how they discussed epidurals and C-sections. I realized that no matter how I had conceived, I now had a normal pregnancy. Well into my third trimester, I switched to a midwifery practice and was able to have a natural childbirth like I wanted.

Direct-Entry Midwives

Direct-entry midwives—sometimes called "independent," "lay," or "community" midwives—specialize in healthy pregnancy and natural childbirth, and primarily attend home births. They learn their profession through apprenticeship to other midwives (or sometimes physicians), and through reading and study. Some attend freestanding midwifery schools. Some direct-entry midwives are certified professional midwives (CPMs), who have nationally recognized credentials. The licensing of direct-entry midwives varies from state to state, and in some states this type of midwifery is still illegal. (To learn more about your state's rules, check www.cfmidwifery.org/states.)

Direct-entry midwives may or may not have established relationships with individual physicians and/or emergency rooms. It is important to carefully explore the issues of medical backup and emergency care with your provider, because you may need to arrange for physician or hospital backup yourself. (For information on who is a good candidate for home birth, see "Birth Settings," page 22.)

Insurance coverage of home births differs from state to state and insurer to insurer. It is more common where home-birth midwives are certified. For more information about direct-entry midwives, consult the Midwives Alliance of North America (see "Resources").

PHYSICIANS

In the United States today, physicians attend more than 90 percent of all births.[4] Increasingly, obstetrician-gynecologists are replacing family practice doctors in providing maternity care.

Family Physicians

A family physician (FP) is a primary care doctor trained in family medicine. She or he can provide basic, comprehensive care to people of all ages. Some family physicians practice obstetrics and have delivery room privileges in community hospitals. A few are trained to perform cesarean sections. These doctors often know the whole family, which can enhance planning for a woman's care. Studies have shown that family physicians' usage of common interventions such as episiotomy, cesar-

ean, and labor induction tends to fall between that of midwives and that of obstetrician-gynecologists.[5]

Obstetrician-Gynecologists

Obstetrician-gynecologists (ob-gyns) are physicians who have completed a four-year surgical residency program in obstetrics and gynecology after four years of medical school. They provide gynecological care, preventive, medical, and surgical care to women during pregnancy and childbirth, and care for women of all ages with reproductive tract problems. Because ob-gyns are trained to diagnose and manage complications of pregnancy and birth, they are especially appropriate providers for women or babies who have serious medical conditions. (For examples of these conditions, see "Hospital," page 23.) Women with such health problems often can work with a midwife, too. Ob-gyns also provide care for childbearing women without specific medical concerns who either prefer to work with an ob-gyn or must do so because of limited options.

The majority of ob-gyns work in hospitals and private practices. Their services are normally covered by insurance policies. Ob-gyns commonly provide prenatal checkups and oversee labor, but rarely stay with you throughout labor and may be present only at the time of birth. (During labor, your hands-on care is generally left to labor and delivery nurses, whom you may not know in advance.)

Maternal-Fetal Medicine Physicians

Maternal-fetal medicine physicians (MFMs) are subspecialists in the ob-gyn field. After completing medical school and the standard four-year ob-gyn residency training, MFMs get an additional three years of training in compli-

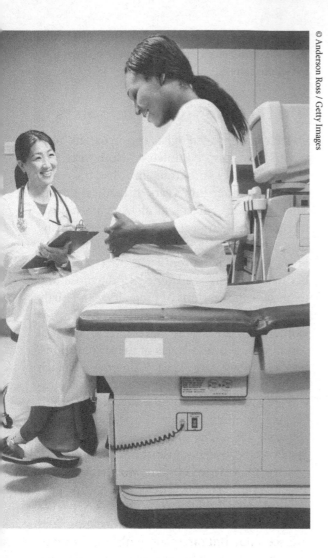

woman's midwife or physician in her home community.

FINDING A PROVIDER

As you look for a provider, your options depend on various factors, including your location, health insurance coverage, income, and medical history. You may have to strike a balance between the kind of practitioner you want to work with and the kind available to you. To get names of practitioners, you can ask your family and friends for referrals, contact professional organizations that represent maternity care providers, and find out which providers and services your health insurance covers (if you have insurance). Then, interview the people who you think are most likely to be a good fit for you. (Some insurers will cover an interview visit, and some practices will not charge for the interview; this varies.) Or, you can choose your birth setting first, and select a provider from those who attend births in that location. If you are not happy with the care you receive, you have the right to change providers at any time.

As you consider a particular provider, try to assess the person's training, competence, safety record, and standard methods of care. Seek publicly available data about your provider and birth site but understand that numbers do not tell the whole story. Check to see how the provider presents choices in a given situation, from the most to the least invasive or risky interventions to "doing nothing." Can the provider discuss—in plain language—the risks and benefits of each choice as it relates to you? Does the provider articulate her or his own views while demonstrating interest in your opinions, or does the provider come across as inflexible? Can the provider discuss C-section rates in her or his practice and hospital in depth and with explanations? (There is a big differ-

cated obstetrics. They are experts regarding how certain medical conditions affect pregnancy and birth and often assume care of women with serious conditions such as diabetes or heart disease. These doctors usually practice in large academic medical centers or urban areas and see women only on referral from a physician or midwife. Many perform ultrasound and prenatal testing procedures and have expertise in the field of genetics. Frequently, they devise a plan of care that can be carried out in collaboration with a pregnant

SOME QUESTIONS TO ASK MIDWIVES AND PHYSICIANS

- Are you covered by my insurance? Will I pay for any portion of my care?
- What is your training and how long have you been practicing?
- For how many births have you been the primary attendant in the past few years?
- What is your philosophy of childbirth, and who practices with you? Do the other providers in your group practice share your views, and how do you handle disagreements over care and treatment?
- How can I reach you? How can I have my questions answered between visits?
- Would you or someone you work with stay with me throughout labor? If not, do you allow or encourage the presence of doulas, labor assistants, and family and friends? What do you see as their role?
- Do you support moving around during labor, changing positions, and eating and drinking?
- What are your policies on continuous fetal monitoring, cutting the umbilical cord, and episiotomy?
- Under what circumstances would you transfer my care to an OB or MFM? (This is a question for midwives and family physicians.)
- Under what circumstances do you recommend inducing labor? About what proportion of your patients have labor induced?

ADDITIONAL QUESTIONS FOR MIDWIVES AND PHYSICIANS IN HOSPITALS

- What are your policies regarding monitoring the baby's heart rate in labor, using IVs, breaking the mother's bag of waters, using epidurals, and performing episiotomies?
- What are your reasons to do a cesarean? How often do you find it necessary? How do you try to avoid the need for a cesarean?

ADDITIONAL QUESTIONS FOR HOME-BIRTH MIDWIVES

- What are your medical backup and emergency care arrangements?
- What problems are you able to deal with at home and which ones require transfer to a hospital?
- What is your role if I transfer to a hospital?
- Do you have statistics from your practice? May I see them?
- What is your plan if another client is in labor when I am?
- Where will I go for any lab work?
- What is your experience with methods for inducing labor?
- What equipment and medications do you bring to the birth?
- What methods do you suggest for alleviating pain?
- Are you currently certified in neonatal resuscitation?
- Can you provide references?

BIRTH ASSISTANTS

In addition to receiving care from a doctor or midwife, many women are supported through labor and birth by doulas, who are trained birth companions. For more information about doulas and the importance of continuous care during labor, see pages 32–34.

ence between sites with similar C-section rates if one performs elective cesarean "on demand" without medical reason and the other delivers many twins or triplets by cesarean because it is associated with an in vitro fertilization program.)

BIRTH SETTINGS

The birthplace that you choose can shape your birth experience. The environment and any procedures and requirements it routinely involves can affect the process of labor and birth. Your birth setting will also affect the kinds of pain management techniques that are available to you. If you give birth in a hospital, you will have access to a range of pain medications, but you may have less support or help with methods of pain management other than medication. (If you don't have a doula or other knowledgeable support person, assistance with nondrug pain management will depend largely on the skill and availability of the labor and delivery nurses.) If you give birth at home or in a freestanding birth center, you will likely have access to many comfort measures and pain relief techniques, but you will not have access to certain medications, including epidurals, unless you transfer to a hospital.

As with selecting a practitioner, you may have to strike a balance between your ideal environment and what is available to you. Bear in mind that some providers practice only in one setting. In order to make an informed choice, gather information and carefully consider the possible benefits and downsides of each situation. You may want to consult with your health care providers about what setting is best for you, especially if you have specific preferences or medical concerns.

I had been seeing an ob-gyn throughout most of my pregnancy. My visits were always extremely short and impersonal. I felt like if I had seen her outside of the office, she wouldn't have known who I was. . . . When I mentioned to her that I didn't want an epidural like I had with Madison, my four-year-old, she still made me feel pressured for one. I told her how after I had the epidural I ended up with a major complication (a spinal headache), but she just reassured me that they had great anesthesiologists there. I didn't feel supported.

So, at 36 weeks pregnant, I called a local midwife to set up a consultation meeting. As soon as Gabe and I met her we loved her. . . . I showed up at her office with a list of questions about the safety of home birth. The idea of it appealed to me, but I was still nervous that it wasn't safe, or that I was taking "risks" by having my baby at home. . . . I learned of all her extensive training . . . and all the equipment [she would] bring in case of emergency . . . and felt safe with her.

HOSPITAL

A hospital is the standard setting for many women who prefer to be close to medical care while giving birth. It is also the setting of choice for women and babies who have medical conditions that increase the chances of needing special care. Hospital care is considered safest for women with hypertensive disorders, diabetes, or seizure disorders; women carrying multiple babies; women who are more than two weeks beyond their due date; and women whose babies are not in a head-down position or have problems that have been identified during the pregnancy. If you have one of these conditions, look for practitioners and facilities with experience treating your medical condition.

In addition to specialized medical care, hospitals provide pain medication and epidural anesthesia, consultations with other specialists, and immediate access to emergency care. (For more information on deciding what kind of pain management you want to have available, see Chapter 11, "Coping with Pain.")

Usually women stay longer in a hospital than in a birth center after giving birth. Under federal law, all insurers must cover a minimum hospital stay of two days after a vaginal birth and four days after a cesarean birth if medically necessary. If either you or your child needs significant recovery time, this can be particularly welcome.

For some women, there are disadvantages to giving birth in a hospital. Hospital maternity care places more emphasis on standardized than on individualized care and relies more on technology than on the body's normal processes. Hospital routines are set up to promote efficiency and to facilitate emergency medical treatment. The routines are sometimes not flexible enough to accomodate an individual woman's needs.

A hospital is the environment most likely to lead to what has become known as "a cascade of interventions." This is a situation in which an intervention given routinely (whether needed or not) leads directly to other interventions. For example, many hospitals use equipment that restricts a woman's movement, which in turn can result in a slower, more difficult labor, and may trigger the use of interventions that would otherwise be unnecessary.

In addition, some hospitals limit the number of companions you can have with you dur-

MOTHER-FRIENDLY CARE

Hospitals vary widely in their routine procedures and their use of interventions, including cesarean sections. They also vary in the types of labor support they offer. In an attempt to make it easier for women and families to understand and find high-quality maternity care, the Coalition for Improving Maternity Services (CIMS) has created a "gold standard" model of maternity care. Hospitals, birth centers, and home birth services that follow the evidence-based standards, called the Ten Steps of the Mother-Friendly Childbirth Initiative, earn the designation "Mother-Friendly." There is also a version designed to be taken with you when you tour a facility; it is called "Having a Baby—Ten Questions to Ask." For more information, see www.motherfriendly.org.

SOME QUESTIONS TO ASK WHEN SELECTING A HOSPITAL

If you are considering giving birth in a particular hospital, look at its website and/or go on a tour to find answers to these questions:

- What kind of anesthesiology and pediatric coverage does the hospital offer? Does it have a blood bank available?
- What is its registered-nurse-to-patient ratio? What is it in active labor?
- What percentage of births at the hospital are cesarean deliveries? What percentage of women who are admitted for VBAC deliver vaginally?
- What are the routine policies for laboring women? How does the hospital deal with requests for nonroutine practices?
- What percentage of women have an epidural for labor?
- Are showers, tubs, or whirlpool baths available for laboring women?
- Can I labor, give birth, and recover in the same room?
- Are there restrictions on the number of people allowed in the labor and delivery room at once? Under what circumstances would I be separated from my companions?
- What is the rooming-in policy for babies, and under what circumstances would my baby be separated from me?
- What are the routine newborn care policies? Does the hospital mandate certain shots for all newborns? What if I don't want my child to have them?
- What assistance is available for breast-feeding mothers? Is this hospital certified as "Baby-Friendly"?
- Are private or semiprivate rooms available? Is there an additional charge?

ing labor and birth, and many hospitals do not have adequate staffing to provide continuous physical, emotional, and informational support during labor and birth. While some labor and delivery nurses are experts at providing such support, other demands on their time often make providing continuous support difficult. This can influence maternal satisfaction and birth outcomes, as well as the early postpartum experience. Hospitals also have a range of policies on issues affecting postpartum women and newborns, such as allowing mothers and babies to stay in the same room and providing support for breast-feeding.

I almost never hear of the totally natural, completely positive hospital birth experience, and that's why I'd like to share our story. . . . We chose the hospital we did because of the fact that there were many nurse-midwives on staff that I hoped would be supportive of my desire to have a natural birth. I . . . felt very supported by my husband's medical knowledge and he knew how strongly I wanted to do it drug free—he would be my advocate. He also shared a very empowering piece of advice with our birth class: that should you be in a hospital and not comfortable with the plan, you are entitled to say that you understand the risks and benefits of a procedure and [you] can refuse it. That is your right.

When my contractions had not kicked in . . . twelve hours after my water broke and the usual time they give before they start to induce, we said we wanted to wait a bit. We walked, delaying the Pitocin, but [later] . . . negotiated half the normal dosage. . . . By that time, my husband looked at the monitor and noticed the contractions were getting stronger and more frequent without being induced. Despite the suggestion to continue as planned, we decided to go natural, asserting our right. The doula arrived, and after four hours of intense labor . . . I reached a point where I said that I couldn't go on. She said to me, "No, . . . you are there. Let's get ready to start pushing!"

Like a set change in a play, there was a whole new team, the bed changed position, and we started to push. Our incredible nurse-midwife was on her knees for the entire two hours while I pushed, holding a warm compress to my perineum so I wouldn't tear—which I didn't. At 5:40 P.M., Sadie was born. It was the single most incredible moment of my life. We feel very blessed to have had the seemingly elusive wonderful, natural hospital birth.

BIRTH CENTER

Freestanding Birth Centers

Birth centers provide comprehensive family-centered care for women during pregnancy, childbirth, and the time immediately following birth. In the birth center philosophy, pregnancy and birth are normal and healthy processes, to be interfered with as little as possible.

Usually birth centers are homelike places, in contrast to the institutional setting of hospitals, and personalized care is provided by midwives. They provide continuous care to the laboring woman and have resources such as birth tubs and birthing balls to provide comfort and relieve pain. Birth centers have systems in place to deal with any complications during labor and birth and to transfer you to a hospital if necessary.

As with home birth (see "Home," page 28),

SOME QUESTIONS TO ASK WHEN SELECTING A BIRTH CENTER

If you are considering giving birth in a particular birth center, look at its website, call for information, and/or go on a tour to find answers to these questions:

- Is the center licensed by the state and accredited by the Commission for the Accreditation of Birth Centers?
- What are the requirements for admission?
- Are there birthing tubs? What kind?
- What are the backup arrangements if I have a complication or want pain medication?
- When and why are women advised or required to go into the hospital?
- What percentages of clients transfer to a hospital before, during, and after labor?

at a birth center you can expect greater reliance on your own physiology than on technology, a focus on individualized care, and staff available to give you continuous support. Usually you get admitted into a birth center once your labor is fully established. Once you are there, the focus is on allowing your labor to unfold at your individual pace and on responding to your needs and preferences.

Birth centers vary in their rates of using tests and procedures, in their policies and restrictions, and in their medical backup arrangements. There are certain situations in which you may be required to switch to hospital care before or during labor, either as a precaution due to complications or in the rare event of an emergency. Often women are discharged between six and twelve hours after giving birth.

Not all women are eligible to give birth at a birth center, and each place has its own screening guidelines. Most commonly, this affects women seeking vaginal births after cesarean sections. (For more information about VBACs, see page 233.) You can find out if there is a birth center in your area through the American Association of Birth Centers (www.birth centers.org).

Birth Centers in Hospitals

A birth center that is located in a hospital may have a philosophy and practice anywhere on a continuum between that of a typical freestanding center and that of a hospital. Emergency care will be available in the same building. It is important to learn if the care offered at a particular center differs from the care offered at the affiliated hospital. The availability of midwives, continuous support during labor, and various options for pain relief (both natural and medical/pharmacological) will be an indication. You can also find out about restrictions placed on laboring women, such as on eating and drinking; freedom of movement during labor; and routine care including electronic fetal monitoring and procedures regarding newborns. (For more information, see "Mother-Friendly Care," page 23.)

My plan was to labor and give birth at the Birth Center . . . in their lovely Victorian house and big Jacuzzi tubs. Although it was my first labor, when the day came I felt reasonably confident and in control. The HypnoBirthing worked very well for me. Not that the labor was painless, but I never felt like I was out of control. I experienced the contractions like a strenuous hike up and down mountain peaks. I labored in the tub for most of the time and my husband says he couldn't even tell when I was having a contraction (although I definitely could feel them). My labor really was exactly how I wanted it. My husband prepared wonderful music to play and we dimmed the lights and got rid of the clock.

MYTH OR REALITY?

Hospital births are the safest for everyone.
- Myth. In fact, for healthy women with uncomplicated pregnancies, there is no evidence that giving birth in a hospital is safer than doing so at home or in a birth center.[6]

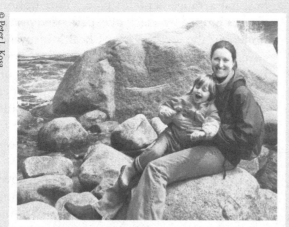

© Peter L. Kosa

"Respect the normal physiological process of birth."

Jessica Lang Kosa

My first labor stalled soon after I got to the hospital. I had an epidural and Pitocin drip to augment my labor, which worked, but wasn't optimal for my son's health or mine.

When I later read studies showing that home births—for low-risk mothers attended by an experienced midwife—have fewer interventions and complications and are as safe as hospital births, it made sense to me. My body is wired like [those of] other mammals, who instinctively seek a safe, secluded spot to give birth. I liked the idea of being in my own space, with only familiar and trusted people around, allowing my body to work at its own pace. So for my second baby, I decided on home birth. That approach seemed to respect the normal physiological process of birth.

When my second labor started, I ate, slept, and walked as I liked, with my husband and midwives taking care of me. A rented hot tub and a deep relaxation technique called HypnoBirthing kept the pain completely manageable. My daughter was born underwater and [seemed to sleep] right through the whole process. My husband and son cut the cord together.

The midwives cleaned us up and tucked the whole family into my own bed. We watched the fire in the fireplace and the snow falling outside. My daughter was busy at my breast. My son was too excited to sleep. My husband got out a box of chocolates and we ate them together. Soft baby flesh, all four of us together, and chocolate: This is joy. I couldn't ask for a healthier or sweeter birth.

The doula and midwife (and my husband) were very supportive.

I labored without any interventions until my baby was stuck sideways under my pubic bone. I pushed for many hours without much progress. At this point, the midwife recommended that we move to the hospital (across the street) because she recommended we use Pitocin to strengthen my contractions. We all discussed the options and I felt like I made the best decision at the time. We moved to the hospital, tried the Pitocin and more pushing, to no avail. My lovely daughter was born by C-section in the hospital. I was given a spinal just before the surgery and this was the first medical intervention I had. It was not the birth that I had envisioned or planned for, but I definitely felt like my wishes had been respected and that I had been in control of the decisions all along the way.

HOME

Some women prefer to labor and give birth in the comfortable, known environment of home. Most women will at least start labor at home. The benefit of being at home is that labor can unfold naturally and at its own individual pace and rhythm, without restrictions.

Healthy, low-risk women who have planned home births attended by a skilled provider have excellent outcomes. One recent prospective study of 5,418 women in North America found that women who had planned home births attended by skilled midwives had comparable health outcomes and fewer medical interventions such as cesarean sections, episiotomies, and vacuum extractions or forceps deliveries than healthy women having uncomplicated births in hospitals.[7]

Home birth is a good option for healthy women who have uncomplicated pregnancies, a safe and supportive home environment, and easy access to backup medical care. Two critical characteristics of home birth are that you rely on your body's natural processes, not on technology, and that you can receive continuous support (because you are the only one in labor) from attendants of your own choosing.

A disadvantage of giving birth at home is that if complications arise or you need to use pain medication, you have to transfer to a hospital. In a small number of circumstances, immediate medical attention might be needed before you could reach a hospital. In the study mentioned above, three in twenty-five women transferred to a hospital at some point during labor or after birth.

Home birth requires more preparation time and effort on your part than giving birth in a hospital or birth center. The first step is selecting a care provider (usually a midwife) who is skilled and experienced in attending home births, including having backup medical and hospital arrangements in place. Your options may be limited by a lack of experienced practitioners in the area, a lack of health insurance coverage for this kind of birth, or the distance between your home and a hospital. It is important to learn about your midwife's experience, skill, policies, and arrangements regarding situations where you would be shifted to hospital care (see "Some Questions to Ask Midwives and Physicians," page 21).

If you have insurance but it does not cover home birth, you may be able to persuade your insurer to authorize an exception for you. You might make a case that the care you request is more cost-effective than what your standard plan provides (home birth can be cheaper than hospital birth). You may have to pay out of pocket, or come up with another solution, such as asking for a sliding scale, raising money in your community or within your family, or making a bartering arrangement with your midwife.

When I was first pregnant with [my] son Cole, I thought women who gave birth at home were a bit crazy—why would someone deny [herself] the miracle of modern medicine, or at least the option to get the drugs when the going got rough? I had a great OB whom I liked, and [I] knew that we'd give birth at a nice, small regional hospital. . . . But as the pregnancy went on, my views on the standard American birth began to change. . . . I had thought I'd want the option of the epidural. . . . But the more I read about the possible complications, and the more I read about the millions of women that had had babies without drugs, the more convinced I was that I could do it. . . .

Next birth, I'd definitely consider laboring at home—this wasn't anything I couldn't handle, and I know that I'd find great caregivers in case a problem did come up.

THOUGHTFUL CHOICES

Taking the time early in your pregnancy to find a trustworthy provider and a safe, comfortable birth setting is a worthwhile endeavor. By making thoughtful choices, by learning to trust the birth process, and by surrounding yourself with people who support your vision, you are better able to let the process unfold.

NOTES

1. Childbirth Connection, "Choosing a Caregiver," accessed at www.childbirthconnection.org/article.asp?Clickedlink=247&ck=10158&area=27 on July 18, 2006.
2. Childbirth Connection, "Choosing a Caregiver: Best Evidence: Caregiver," accessed at www.childbirthconnection.org/article.asp?ck=10155 on July 18, 2006.
3. Mary Alice Grady and Kathaleen C. Bloom, "Pregnancy Outcomes of Adolescents Enrolled in a Centering Pregnancy Program," *Journal of Midwifery & Women's Health* 49, no. 5 (2004): 412–420.
4. Childbirth Connection, "Choosing a Caregiver: Options: Caregiver," accessed at www.childbirthconnection.org/article.asp?ck=10163 on July 18, 2006.
5. Childbirth Connection, "Choosing a Caregiver: Best Evidence: Caregiver," accessed at www.childbirthconnection.org/article.asp?ck=10155&Clickedlink=247&area=27 on July 18, 2006.
6. Childbirth Connection, "Choosing a Birth Setting: Best Evidence: Birth Setting," accessed at www.childbirthconnection.org/article.asp?ck=10142&Clickedlink=252&area=27 on July 18, 2006.
7. K. C. Johnson and B. A. Daviss, "Outcomes of Planned Home Births with Certified Professional Midwives: Large Prospective Study in North America," *BMJ* 330 (June 18, 2005): 1416. Another study demonstrating the safety of home birth for low-risk women is J. P. Rooks, N. L. Weatherby, E. K. Ernst, S. Stapleton, D. Rosen, and A. Rosenfield, "Outcomes of Care in Birth Centers: The National Birth Center Study," *New England Journal of Medicine* 321 (December 28, 1989): 1,804–1,811.

CHAPTER 3

Preparing for Childbirth

No two births are exactly alike, and no woman can prepare completely for the new and challenging experience of giving birth. We each have our own unique experiences before and during pregnancy, our own individual health and medical histories, and varying access to different types of health care and support. As you prepare to give birth, consider your own desires, hopes, and fears. What factors are within your influence? For many of us, a safe and satisfying birth experience is one in which we are cared for with respect, participate in decisions regarding our care, and have knowledgeable support from others. This chapter will help you understand various ways of preparing for your own labor and birth experiences.

The decisions you make during your pregnancy, labor, and birth may affect whether you have a vaginal or cesarean delivery, how long it takes for you and your baby to recover, how successful breast-feeding is, and how you feel about the birth. Learning about the safety and effectiveness of various labor and birth practices and exploring your options for pain relief can help you make decisions that are right for you. Of course, your options may be limited by your insurance or other financial concerns, a caregiver or birth setting's standard practices, or health issues that affect the pregnancy.

While our choices can affect what happens, it's good to remember that planning does not equal total control. There are many paths to a positive birth experience. Learning about the options available, identifying our goals and desires, working with care providers we trust, and maintaining a flexible attitude can strengthen our ability to weigh our options during the process of labor and birth and help us cope with whatever occurs.

"There's so much you can do."

Keiko Inoue

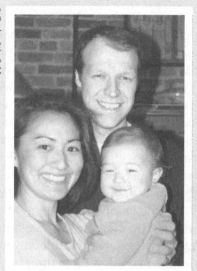

© Corina Warfield

What was striking to me about getting ready for birth was that there's so much you can do, from nutrition to yoga (which was very important to me) to just asking a lot of questions.

My husband and I started off wanting home birth but our insurance wouldn't cover it. Our second choice was a birth center, but it was far away. We ended up with our third choice, the hospital, and at the time we weren't thrilled about it, especially after the hospital tour.

I chose my obstetric practice based on its proximity (we have no car) and because it had midwives. A lot of my yoga instructors were also doulas and highly recommended midwives.

We did a lot of reading. . . . We wrote a birth plan and kept it to a page by deciding what really was most important to us. It had a lot of caveats that said, "Assuming everything is normal, . . . " We understood that we had to be flexible if something unexpected came up, and felt it was important for us to go into the birth with that mind-set. Our doula did tell us to go in with a sense of control, though, and not to apologize for our birth plan. We realized then there were certain basic things about our birth that we didn't want to let go, and so we wrote them down.

But our birth didn't go according to plan. The two things that strayed from our plan were getting the water broken manually and getting an episiotomy. Those things were offered after I had been pushing a long time, and I declined both of them at first. I tried to push longer. We never felt like *we* were being pushed, though—just offered options. In the end it was my decision to say yes to those interventions, and because of my reading, I knew what they were and what the risks were. If the midwife hadn't given us a choice, we might have walked out of the birth with a bitter taste, but that didn't happen. Nikolai was also born with a cleft lip, which was a surprise. The midwife and hospital we chose treated our family respectfully. We felt like we could ask them anything—that made a big difference to us.

The birth of our son was such a culmination of learning for us. One obstetrician said to us at one point, "Too much information can harm you," and I completely disagree. This would have been a very different story had we not had the opportunity to learn as much as we did before the birth.

YOUR BIRTH TEAM

Having continuous, high-quality, supportive care from others during labor and birth is one of the best ways you can ensure a satisfying experience. Many of us count on and receive excellent support from our partners or our health care providers. Yet our partners may be inexperienced at birth and need their own support, especially in long labors, and midwives, doctors, and nurses in hospitals may not be able to provide continuous care because of the many different demands on their time. (Midwives who attend women at home or in a birth center typically do provide continuous support.) For these reasons, some women choose to be accompanied by a doula (a trained labor support person) or a relative or friend who is knowledgeable and comfortable around birth and who can stay through the whole process.

WHY CONTINUOUS SUPPORT?

Continuous support in labor improves health outcomes and increases women's satisfaction with our birth experiences. A recent review of high-quality scientific studies found that women who received continuous, one-on-one support in labor had fewer complications, better health outcomes, and greater satisfaction with their birth experiences than women who did not.[1] Women who had such support had fewer cesarean sections and fewer vacuum extractions and forceps deliveries. They used pain medications or anesthesia less often and felt more positive about their birth experience. Support that started early in labor seemed to be particularly helpful in improving outcomes.

FAMILY AND FRIENDS

Depending on your family and cultural background, it may seem that either everybody or hardly anybody wants to be in your labor room. Before your labor starts, think about who you want to have with you. Choose a person or people around whom you feel comfortable expressing your needs and feelings, and whom you trust to advocate for you if you need help communicating with your care providers. While most settings permit you to have anyone you like with you, at times a particular setting may limit the number of people allowed in your labor room. For example, in a cesarean birth, the anesthesiologist may permit only one support person, or may allow up to three.

My entire family came with me. My grand-mamma got the chair and everybody else was either standing around me or sitting on the floor. The midwife and the doctor were both laughing when they came in; they already knew a lot of my cousins on that floor.

The person or people who plan to provide labor support for you can get ready in different ways. Many midwives devote at least one prenatal visit to talking about plans for labor support, and family members and friends may learn a lot from coming with you to this visit, if you are comfortable with this. If you are reading pregnancy books, share what you learn with your support people. Let them know your thoughts about pain management. A birth experience can bring out the best and the worst in our relationships, and old family issues and patterns can follow us into the birth room. Your loved ones may be scared to see you in pain, may feel the need to protect you, or may feel confused at seeing a "caregiver" in the "cared for" role. Try to get comfortable talking with them about your needs and plans before the birth.

DOULAS

In addition to getting support from partners, relatives, or friends, some women turn to doulas for help. Doulas are childbirth support professionals who have basic training and experience accompanying women (and our partners and other companions) during labor and birth. Doula care is not covered by most insurance policies, so most doulas are hired directly by pregnant women as an out-of-pocket expense. Some hospitals and birthing centers include doula services free of charge; you may want to ask about this as you consider birth settings.

Doulas can provide emotional support and reassurance, as well as assistance in increasing physical comfort and relieving pain during childbirth. They focus on expectant mothers' needs and wishes around the birth experience, and help women and our partners understand when and how to advocate for the type of care we would like from doctors, nurses, and midwives.

Doulas can also offer support to partners, family members, or other companions. Many relatives and friends, particularly those with little or no direct, hands-on experience with birth, find it helpful to be accompanied by an experienced doula. Because doulas are not

SUGGESTED QUESTIONS TO ASK WHEN CHOOSING A DOULA

- What are your background, training, and experience with regard to doing labor support? Are you certified by a doula training program?
- What is your birth philosophy?
- How often will we meet and what will prenatal visits entail?
- What conflicts have you had with midwives, doctors, or nurses, and how did you resolve them?
- How many births have you attended?
- How do you see your role at the birth?
- When and where will you come to meet me (as soon as I feel I'm in labor, or once I arrive at the hospital)?
- How long will you stay after the birth?
- What services do you offer?
- What do you charge?
- What are your backup arrangements? May I meet or speak with your backup?
- How many clients do you take a month? Do you have anyone else close to my due date?
- Are you affiliated with any particular hospitals, birth centers, physicians, or midwives?
- Will I see you after I go home?
- Can you provide references?

trained to do physical assessments or provide medical care, their work complements nursing, midwifery, and medical care.

My husband was my only labor support. If I could change anything . . . I would have definitely hired a doula, and had women for support, not only for myself but for my husband. He was so tired himself. . . . It would have been nice to have an extra person or two to support me, massage me, cheer me on.

You can find names of doulas through word of mouth or through professional organizations such as DONA International, the Association of Labor Assistants & Childbirth Educators (ALACE), the Childbirth and Postpartum Professional Association (CAPPA), and Birth Works. As with any care provider, interview prospective doulas to find someone who is experienced, capable, and a good match for you.

People who are not trained specifically as doulas can still fulfill the role.

I worked very closely with my OB to determine my comfort levels with birthing options, and ultimately decided on contracting privately with a veteran labor and delivery nurse at the hospital where I delivered my first daughter in 2003 and my second in 2005. I arranged for her to provide labor support for me while she was off duty.

The nurse I chose had forty years' experience in L&D and was a wonderful advocate for me, my husband, and my children. We met about three months before my first daughter's birth, and she gave my husband and me a tour of the L&D ward, explaining the equipment to us, how it was used, including the circumstances under which it would be used. Her calming presence and knowledge put me at ease right away, and I knew right at that moment I had made the choice that would make me feel the most comfortable and confident about the birth process.

CHALLENGES IN FINDING SUPPORT

Some of us have difficulty finding a support person for labor and birth. We may not feel comfortable asking anyone we know and we may not have the money to hire a doula. If this is true for you, tell your prenatal care provider about your situation; your provider may be able to help. If possible, find a midwife whose workload allows one-on-one attention to you. Some hospitals and health insurance plans offer free doula care; ask about this. You can also contact doula organizations to get referrals to doulas in your area who are in training or doulas who are willing to provide free or reduced-fee or bartered care. People at parenting centers and childbirth education classes in your community may know of other options.

If you have no support person for labor and birth because you are currently in a situation without a partner or friends, seek out community resources for single mothers, as your need for support will likely increase after your baby is born. Your prenatal care provider may also be able to refer you to a social worker or community health worker, who will likely have information on resources for single moms. Another good place to start is your local public library, where a librarian may be able to assist you in connecting to local resources through the Internet.

My baby's father was out of the picture for a while. His mom was telling everybody that the baby wasn't his. I really needed help then, and Julie [the community health educator] was so good to me.

CHILDBIRTH CLASSES

Today, many types of childbirth classes are available. Taking a class can be a good way to learn more about birth and create a support network with other expectant parents. If you want to incorporate classes into your preparation, consider your own goals for both the class experience and the birth. You may be referred to classes by your prenatal care provider, but you can also look for other options in your community. Classes vary in theoretical perspective, purpose, qualifications of instructors, number and length of classes, population served, and cost. Some are offered online or on video. When learning about different philosophies of childbirth education, ask yourself if they match your goals and objectives. Be wary of instructors who make guarantees about birth outcomes, encourage automatic compliance with routines, or avoid answering challenging questions about an institution or philosophy with which they are affiliated.

Look for a class that teaches communication skills and how to be an informed consumer. Many good childbirth classes teach some aspect of "BRANCH" (Benefits, Risks, Alternatives, doing Nothing, making your CHoice) decision making, which may help you advocate for your health care and eventually for your baby. Some insurance plans, including some types of Medicaid (sometimes called Medical Assistance or another name, depending on your area), will pay for childbirth classes. Many classes have a reduced fee for those who qualify.

Below are descriptions of various styles of childbirth preparation classes.

HOSPITAL-BASED CLASSES

Most hospitals where women deliver babies offer childbirth classes. Instruction in both small and large settings varies widely in content and quality. Instructors may be nurses or not. Typical content includes the anatomy of pregnancy, information about stages of labor, pain management options, possible complications and medical interventions, and a tour of the delivery unit. Classes generally prepare women for a standard hospital birth with routine medical interventions such as epidurals, but many instructors also cover relaxation practice and self-help/comfort techniques.

These classes can help women learn basic birth physiology, hospital routines, and the expected role of a partner. Some women have felt out of place at them, though, because the classes did not address a range of preferences or welcome "nontraditional" labor support people.

To get more out of hospital-based classes, remember that you are there as a consumer, and that actively voicing questions and concerns can help more people have their diverse needs addressed by the hospital. Don't be afraid to ask—chances are that you are not the only one who needs an answer.

LAMAZE

To many people, "Lamaze" is synonymous with specific breathing techniques, the "hee hee, hoo hoo" of their past approach to helping women focus on external cues to manage pain. Today, Lamaze introduces a variety of breathing techniques and offers a wide range of strategies to help women cope with labor. In the past few years, Lamaze has based its approach on evidence from scientific studies, highlighting six care practices that are most beneficial to women and babies. These include labor starting on its own and women being free to eat, drink, and move around in labor. The primary goal for Lamaze instructors is to increase women's confidence in birthing. Certified Lamaze instructors teach students that women have the right to give birth without routine medical interventions and that birth in most circumstances can occur safely in a home, birth center, or hospital.

BRADLEY METHOD

The Bradley Method historically has taught "husband-coached" childbirth as part of a series of twelve classes. Bradley instructors tend to have a strongly held belief in the benefits of unmedicated birth. The roles of good nutrition, advocacy, and confidence in labor are important parts of this philosophy. Classes tend to be smaller than those in hospitals, and they are often taught in instructors' homes, are informal, and provide extensive opportunities for questions and answers. A great deal of time is spent practicing prenatal exercises, such as pelvic tilts, and relaxation techniques, such as guided visualization and progressive relaxation. This method may not work as well for you if you are looking for classes later in pregnancy or you want interventions such as epidurals.

BIRTHING FROM WITHIN

This approach aims to prepare mothers to give birth "in awareness" rather than to achieve specific birth outcomes. Birthing from Within "mentors" encourage students to view labor pain as inevitable, but something that need not become helpless suffering. Birth is treated as a rite of passage that can be prepared for but not controlled, because unexpected events may happen during labor. Birth physiology is covered, but not given more weight than creative self-expression, including birth art, as a way to address feelings, fears, and expectations surrounding birth.

HYPNOBIRTHING

HypnoBirthing is a specific method of hypnosis and awareness practice for birth. Many proponents cite painless yet conscious (not trance-like) labors, while others are critical of the method, claiming it is not effective. (For more information about hypnosis, see page 200.)

MINDFULNESS-BASED

Mindfulness-based childbirth and parenting education is a mind-body approach to preparing for childbirth rooted in the practice of mindfulness meditation. Some women find that developing the practice of mindfulness—paying attention in the present moment—can enhance physical and mental health and well-being and help with birthing as well. This approach holds that there is no one right way to have a baby and that learning ways to cultivate balance, calm, and wisdom is helpful during pregnancy and childbirth, and throughout our lives.

BIRTH WORKS

Birth Works is a nonprofit organization of childbirth teachers and doulas who emphasize the spiritual aspects of birthing. Birth Works classes aim to develop a woman's self-confidence and faith in her ability to give birth. Birth Works instructors believe that women are born with the knowledge of how to have babies, and that it is essential for the mind, body, and spirit to work together in the birth process.

CERTIFYING ORGANIZATIONS (ICEA, ALACE, CAPPA)

Your childbirth educator may be certified by an organization, which means that she or he has met certain standards pertaining to training, examinations, and hours of teaching experience. Many certifying organizations exist.

The International Childbirth Education Association (ICEA) is a professional organization that supports childbirth educators and other health care providers who believe in freedom of choice based on knowledge of alternatives in family-centered maternity and newborn care. ALACE, the Association of Labor Assistants & Childbirth Educators, trains doulas and educators in a holistic and woman-focused approach to childbirth education that was developed by a midwife. The ALACE model teaches relaxation and coping tools to work with pain and discomfort, rather than to avoid the way that labor feels. The Childbirth and Postpartum Professional Association (CAPPA) certifies teachers and doulas to help empower women in pregnancy and birth through confidence building and information that is based on scientific evidence.

VBAC

Another growing model is classes specifically for women who want a vaginal birth after cesarean (VBAC; for more information, see page 233). These classes review risks and benefits as well as provide specific advocacy and labor education designed to improve women's chances for VBAC. To learn more about VBAC and community resources, contact your local chapter of the International Cesarean Awareness Network (www.ican-online.org).

BIRTH PLANS

A birth plan is a document that a woman provides to her birth attendants that describes how she would like her labor to be managed. It is not a contract and does not dictate the provid-

ers' actions. Birth plans often mention aspects of the birth setting, such as low lighting; wishes related to pain management, like wanting or not wanting to be offered an epidural; or particular parts of newborn care, such as a desire to delay application of eye ointment so that mother and baby can look into each other's eyes more clearly during the first feeding.

With appropriate expectations, a birth plan can be a valuable communication tool. Keep in mind that even attendants who are highly receptive to birth plans cannot guarantee that all of your requests will be granted. Many cite the unpredictable nature of birth, the rare possibility of emergency, hospital constraints, or changing wishes in labor as reasons that birth plans cannot be followed like scripts.

The value of a birth plan lies mostly in the exercise of thinking through what seems most important to you in labor, birth, and the early hours with your baby. This can then be a starting point for conversation with your prenatal care provider about the feasibility of your desires and the best way they can be achieved. Occasionally, a birth plan outlining wishes for natural birth, added to the chart, will guide staff to assign a woman to a particular nurse who enjoys providing one-on-one labor support. Birth plans may also alert hospital staff to alter routine practices to accommodate special wishes, cultural differences, or the need for an interpreter.

My husband and I wanted the name of Allah to be the first word our baby heard. Our midwife knew, but we wrote it down to make sure the hospital knew, too, in case things happened fast and we didn't have time to tell anyone.

There is no guarantee that birth attendants or other staff (such as nurses or pediatricians) will read or respect what you write in a birth plan. Because of this, a birth plan should not replace other efforts at effective and satisfying communication with your prenatal care providers and the staff at your birth setting.

PLANNING FOR PAIN MANAGEMENT

It is common to worry about labor pain. Thinking through the advantages and disadvantages of different options for managing pain before you go into labor can help you enter labor more confidently, with well-informed, realistic expectations.

STRATEGIES FOR PAIN RELIEF

Having good support is the foundation for coping with labor, whether we use comfort measures such as walking or being submerged in a birthing tub, mental strategies such as focused breathing, and/or medications such as narcotics or epidurals. The Pain Medications Preference Scale, developed by childbirth educator and author Penny Simkin, may help you clarify your feelings about pain management in labor (see page 196). Your choice of birth setting and provider can affect your options for pain management.

Because it is often challenging to make specific decisions about pain relief before labor, and because all pain-relieving medications can have adverse effects, it is generally best to approach normal labor with the idea of using no-risk or very low-risk strategies first, and then proceeding to the next-higher level of intervention if needed. (For more information on coping strategies and the risks and benefits of pain medicine, see Chapter 11, "Coping with Pain.")

PHYSICAL PREPARATION

Pelvic floor exercises and perineal massage may make your labor and birth experience easier. In addition, regular physical exercise in pregnancy (like walking and yoga) and special exercises such as pelvic tilts and squats have many benefits. (For more information on exercising while pregnant, see "Staying Active," page 73.)

PELVIC FLOOR EXERCISES

Pelvic floor muscle training, or Kegel exercises, has been shown to reduce urinary incontinence (the involuntary loss of urine) in women.[2] Further research on these exercises done during pregnancy has suggested that Kegels may prevent, improve, or cure urinary incontinence after giving birth.[3] Researchers found that an intensive program of exercises appears to produce better results than one that is less intensive; women who did Kegels regularly were less likely to be incontinent three months after delivery. Some care providers also believe that pelvic floor exercises done in pregnancy may help women push effectively in the second stage of labor, although research to provide evidence for or against this viewpoint hasn't yet been done or completed.

I found out that Kegels work only if I keep up with them. If I slack off and don't do them for a while, the leaking comes back! But if I do them consistently, I don't have to worry that I'll leak every time I sneeze, which is what started happening after I had my daughter.

PERINEAL MASSAGE

The perineum is the area between your vaginal opening and your rectum. This area stretches a

HOW TO DO PELVIC FLOOR (KEGEL) EXERCISES

Pelvic floor exercises can be done while standing, sitting, or lying down. The first step is to contract your pelvic floor muscles. To do this, mimic what you would do to try to stop the flow of urine. (Don't do this while actually peeing or with a full bladder.) Or you can insert a finger into your vagina and try to grip the finger with your vagina. Think of pulling upward and inward. Try to relax your abdominal muscles and buttocks, because if you are using those muscles, you're not exercising the pelvic floor. To confirm that you are using the right muscles, you can place a hand on your lower abdomen while contracting the pelvic floor muscles—your hand and belly should stay perfectly still. Remember to keep breathing.

Try to hold the contraction for 10 seconds, followed by a 20-second release. (You may want to start with smaller increments—a 5-second hold, a 10-second release—and build up to 10 seconds of holding the contraction.) Repeat for several minutes. To really train these muscles, try to work through a cycle of 30 to 35 contractions, or 10 to 15 minutes of the 10-second hold, 20-second release pattern.

Once you've learned how to do Kegels, you can do them almost anytime— waiting for the bus, watching TV, doing the dishes, or talking on the phone.

lot during childbirth and often tears, especially in women giving birth for the first time. It is the area that is cut in an episiotomy, to make the opening of the birth canal bigger.

Some research shows that perineal massage done in the final weeks of pregnancy may reduce the chance of tears requiring stitches and the chance of having an episiotomy for women who have never before given birth vaginally.[4] A different benefit was shown for women who previously had given birth vaginally: When they used perineal massage, they seemed to have less pain at three months postpartum.

You or your partner can do the perineal massage. Start six weeks before your due date and massage your perineal area slowly for 10 minutes daily. To do the massage, relax in a private place with your knees bent. Some women like to lean on pillows for back support.

If you are doing the message yourself, make sure that your hands are clean and your fingernails are short. Lubricate your thumbs and the perineal tissues with vitamin E oil, almond oil, a vegetable oil such as olive oil, a water-soluble jelly such as K-Y jelly, or your body's natural vaginal lubricant. Do not use baby oil, mineral oil, body lotion, or petroleum jelly. Place your thumbs 1 to $1\frac{1}{2}$ inches inside your vagina (see illustration, page 40). Press down toward the anus and to the sides until you feel a slight burning, stretching sensation. Hold the position for 1 or 2 minutes. With your thumbs, slowly massage the lower half of the vagina using a U-shaped movement. Relax your muscles and breathe slowly and deeply.

If your partner is doing the massage, he or she should use index fingers rather than thumbs, and follow the same basic instructions.

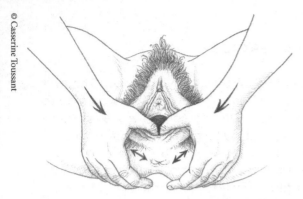

Perineal massage done in the final weeks of pregnancy may reduce the chance of tears requiring stitches and the likelihood of having an episiotomy (cutting to enlarge the vaginal opening).

Be sure to tell your partner if you have too much pain or burning.[5]

LOGISTICAL PREPARATION

HOME BIRTH

Home birth requires special preparation in your home. Your home birth care provider will give you the "homework" of assembling equipment at least three to four weeks before your due date. This may involve gathering phone numbers, sheets, towels, food, and other supplies, and making arrangements such as having a labor tub set up in your home. If you have other children, arrange for special companions to be with them, whether they will be at the birth or not. You may also find it useful to consult websites and books about home birth for tips that other families have found helpful. (See "Resources," especially the section "Birth Companions and Birth Preparation Techniques," page 328).

HOSPITAL OR BIRTH CENTER

If you are giving birth in a hospital or birth center, you may want to bring the following:

- a battery-operated radio or CD player and music, or an MP3 player, with batteries
- extra clothing, including two nursing bras, and, if you wish, your own clothing to wear during labor. (Your partner should bring a swimsuit if you both plan to use the tub or shower during labor.)
- a variety of easily digestible snacks for you (Your support team should bring snacks, too, and perhaps a change of clothes and toiletries for themselves.)
- lip balm in case your lips get chapped while you are in labor, and any other special toiletry items
- a tennis ball for applying back pressure in case of back labor, along with massage lotion, and photos or other objects to focus your gaze on during labor
- telephone numbers of family and friends
- a going-home outfit for baby (including clothes with separate legs to accommodate a car seat strap) and blanket if it's cold
- an infant car seat

EXTRA HELP AT HOME

As you approach the time of labor, try to delegate any caregiving responsibilities that you can, such as taking care of your other children or feeding your pets. This is also a good time to line up extra support for after the birth, for example by asking friends to bring you dinners.

While most labors last less than twenty-four hours, the typical length of stay in a hospital is two nights for a vaginal birth, three or four nights for a cesarean. You will most likely also need or want time for recovery at home. It is important to ask for help and take care of yourself during this time.

CORD-BLOOD BANKING

Some families choose to save their newborns' cord blood for the potential future use of that child or another family member. Cord blood contains stem cells that have potential for treating certain diseases, such as leukemia, and some immune disorders. It can be collected from your baby's umbilical cord and placenta in a short, painless procedure after birth. Several private companies will "bank" the blood for an initial and yearly fee. The cost is usually not covered by insurance.

Banking cord blood privately is controversial. The American Academy of Pediatrics (AAP) encourages families to donate their newborns' cord blood to *public* cord blood banks (if available in their area) for use by other individuals in need. According to the AAP, the chances of a child's needing her or his own cord-blood stem cells in the future range from 1 in 1,000 to 1 in 200,000.[6] The AAP does not recommend private banking of cord blood for the use of other relatives, unless the newborn has an older sibling with a condition that could potentially benefit from transplantation, such as genetic immunodeficiency.

Even if cord blood is saved, there is no guarantee that other family members would be a good genetic match for banked cells if they needed them for treatment. In addition, a baby's cord blood currently would not be recommended for use as a stem cell source for treatment if that baby developed leukemia later

MATERNAL REQUEST OF CESAREAN DELIVERY

One factor often cited as contributing to the rising rate of cesarean sections is maternal request. But is it true that increasing numbers of women are choosing to have cesareans for nonmedical reasons?

Although some studies describe an increase in caesareans without any medical indication, the authors of these studies are clear that these may not represent real "maternal request." The studies, based on birth certificates or hospital billing records, have no way of documenting whether the caesarean was initially sought by the mother, whether it was based on physician advice or pressure, or whether there was simply poor record keeping.

Moreover, there has been only one representative national study, entitled *Listening to Mothers,* that directly surveyed mothers about their birth experiences. The second phase of the study included mothers who gave birth in U.S. hospitals in 2005. It found that fewer than 1 in every 250 mothers who had a first cesarean had requested it and planned it in advance, with the understanding that there was no medical reason for it.[7] Thus, although there are undoubtedly some women who do seek elective cesareans, they are hardly enough to increase the number of cesareans by four hundred thousand nationally between 1996 and 2005.

in life, because genetic abnormalities might have been present at the time of birth.

Some have argued in favor of private cord-blood banking for ethnic minority women whose children may be less likely to find a match for bone marrow transplant in the National Marrow Donor Program. But others argue that using public cord-blood banks linked to the matching services of the National Marrow Donor Program may be more helpful to more minority families.

If you are considering cord-blood banking, talk with your prenatal care or pediatric provider about the possible costs, risks, and benefits for your family's situation. Don't rely on marketing materials from private cord-blood banks for information.

If you decide to bank your baby's cord blood either privately or publicly, contact a cord-blood bank in advance, ideally several months before your expected due date. Talk with your birth attendant, too, as there may be an extra collection fee, and not all doctors and midwives will participate in cord-blood collection. Keep in mind that even if you plan to collect and bank your baby's cord blood, sometimes it cannot be done due to complications in the birth.

ELECTIVE CESAREAN

Elective cesareans (the term used for cesarean sections done without a medical need) are increasingly presented by doctors and the media as an option for healthy pregnant women. So far, elective cesareans make up only a small portion of all cesarean sections, but the numbers are growing.

Some people argue that elective cesareans can be as safe as vaginal births and/or that a woman should have the right to choose her mode of birth. But while little research has focused on the safety exclusively of elective cesareans, evidence from research on all kinds of cesareans suggests that elective cesareans expose women and babies to unnecessary and potentially serious risks. Women who undergo surgical births are more likely than women who have vaginal births to experience severe bleeding, infection, painful scarring, blood clots, bowel obstruction, readmission to the hospital, and longer-lasting pain. In addition, having a cesarean birth increases a woman's chances of having future reproductive problems, including decreased fertility and an increased rate of placenta problems.[8] Babies who are born by cesarean section are more likely than babies born vaginally to have mostly temporary and mild respiratory problems that nevertheless require intensive care in the first few days after birth. While most women and babies are healthy after a cesarean, it is best to avoid major abdominal surgery if it is not necessary.

If you are offered a cesarean without a clear medical reason, or are considering asking for one, it would be wise to learn about all the possible risks before making a final decision. (To learn more about cesareans, see Chapter 13, "Cesarean Births.")

VALUING PREPARATION

Many childbirth educators believe that accurate information decreases fear in labor, and that knowledge helps break the fear-tension-pain cycle. Many women find this to be true. However, others among us look back on our experience of childbirth preparation with feelings of disappointment, having expected that classes or a birth plan would be enough to enable us to have a particular kind of labor or birth experience. No consistent benefits of childbirth classes have been proven scientifically. But planning to have a doula or other knowledgeable support person with us continuously throughout labor and birth does have a proven benefit.

A woman can "do everything right" and have the so-called best preparation but not have the birth outcome that she expected or wanted. Similarly, a woman can go into labor without having taken childbirth classes or done any reading, sometimes with only limited labor support, and sail beautifully through it. Clearly, preparation does not guarantee a certain outcome. But it may give us an increased sense of knowledge, self-awareness, and confidence in our ability to have a healthy and satisfying birth.

NOTES

1. E. D. Hodnett, S. Gates, G. J. Hofmeyr, and C. Sakala, "Continuous Support for Women During Childbirth," *Cochrane Database of Systematic Reviews* 2003, Issue 3. Art. No.: CD003766, DOI 10.1002/14651858. CD003766.pub2.
2. E.J.C. Hay-Smith and C. Dumoulin, "Pelvic Floor Muscle Training Versus No Treatment, or Inactive Control Treatments, for Urinary Incontinence in Women," *Cochrane Database of Systematic Reviews* 2006, Issue 1. Art. No.: CD005654 DOI 10.1002/14651858.CD005654.
3. S. Morkved, K. Bo, B. Schei, and K. A. Salvesen, "Pelvic Floor Muscle Training During Pregnancy to Prevent Urinary Incontinence: A Single-Blind Randomized Controlled Trial," *Obstetrics & Gynecology* 101, no. 2 (February 2003): 313–319.
4. M. M. Beckmann and A. J. Garrett, "Antenatal Perineal Massage for Reducing Perineal Trauma," *Cochrane Database of Systematic Reviews* 2006, Issue 1. Art. No.: CD005123, DOI: 10.1002/14651858.CD005123.pub2.
5. Adapted with permission from "Share with Women: Perineal Massage in Pregnancy," *Journal of Midwifery & Women's Health* 50, no. 1 (January–February 2005): 63–64.
6. Bertram H. Lubin, William T. Shearer, Joanne Kurtzberg, and Mitchell S. Cairo, "Cord Blood Banking for Potential Future Transplantation," *Pediatrics* 119, no. 1 (January 2007): 165–170, accessed at http://pediatrics.aappublications.org/cgi/content/full/119/1/165#T1 on January 29, 2007.
7. Eugene R. Declerq, Carol Sakala, Maureen P. Corry, and Sandra Applebaum, *Listening to Mothers II: Report of the Second National U.S. Survey of Women's Childbearing Experiences* (New York: Childbirth Connection, 2006).
8. Childbirth Connection. *What Every Pregnant Woman Needs to Know about Cesarean Section,* 2nd rev. ed. New York: Childbirth Connection, December 2006.

Your Pregnancy

CHAPTER 4

Your Developing Pregnancy and Prenatal Care

Pregnancy is a normal, natural process. One of its amazing aspects is that a new life develops inside you without any conscious work on your part. Cells divide, brain synapses develop, a new heart starts to beat.

You will notice many changes as your body supports your growing baby and prepares to give birth. These physical and emotional changes are experienced differently by different women.

Pregnancy was the most amazing time in my life. Never before did I appreciate and love my body like I did during those nine months. I wasn't just growing in pant sizes; I was growing a life inside of me. I honored my body like never before. It was amazing to me that my body knew exactly what to do to keep my child safe and growing strong.

Pregnancy was vaguely unpleasant, nothing physically painful, I just kept feeling like, When is this going to be over? I never fell in love with being pregnant, which made me feel guilty, since so many other pregnant women seem to have that glow.

This chapter describes the physical changes of pregnancy, how your baby develops, and what to expect from your prenatal visits.

YOUR DUE DATE

A full-term pregnancy lasts approximately 40 weeks, or three trimesters of 13 to 14 weeks each. Because not all pregnancies are equal in duration, it is impossible to predict the precise day on which your baby will be born. Pregnancies usually range from 37 weeks to 43 weeks, with most women giving birth between 39 weeks and 41 weeks after conception. Your due date is merely the middle of this fourteen-day window.

There are several ways to calculate your due date. If you know the exact date of conception, your due date will be 38 weeks from that date. If you know the first day of your last menstrual period, and you have regular cycles of twenty-eight to thirty days, your due date will be 40 weeks from that day.

If you have irregular cycles and don't know the date of conception, or if you cannot remember when your last period started, your provider will suggest getting an early ultrasound, which will measure the size of your baby. The due date determined by an early ul-trasound is as accurate as a due date determined by counting days from when your last period started. (For more information about ultrasound, see pages 116–119.)

FIRST TRIMESTER

WHAT'S HAPPENING IN YOUR BODY

Your body has begun to nurture a new life. During the coming nine months, you will experience enormous physical changes as the embryo grows from a single fertilized cell into a fully developed baby.

PREPARING FOR PREGNANCY: PRECONCEPTION CARE

If possible, it's good to have an appointment with your health care provider or a maternity care provider before you become pregnant. A preconception visit can help you learn about how to best prepare for a pregnancy. If you are able to have a preconception visit, your health care provider will do the following:

1. Learn about your past pregnancies and births, take a family history, and examine you to assess for potential problems during pregnancy.
2. Identify ways to help you manage any current medical conditions and avoid pregnancy complications.
3. Review all medications you are taking and recommend changes if necessary.
4. Learn whether you are a good candidate for genetic screening tests.
5. Offer any immunizations you need that cannot be given during pregnancy.
6. Recommend that you start taking folic acid supplements (400 mcg per day for most women) a few months before you start trying to conceive.
7. Offer support and help for substance abuse such as smoking cessation and/or alcohol or narcotic abuse.
8. Identify any environmental exposures you can eliminate that are not safe during pregnancy.

If you are pregnant now and you did not see your health care provider before you got pregnant, this list can be reviewed at your first prenatal visit.

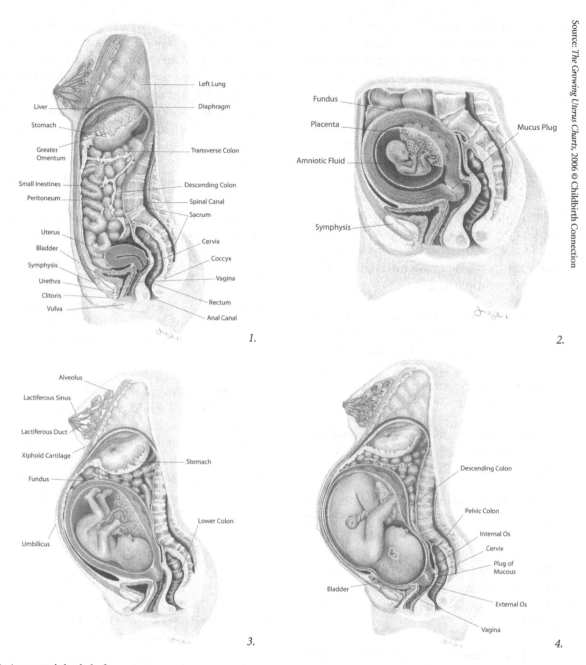

Source: The Growing Uterus Charts, 2006 © Childbirth Connection

1.

Left Lung
Liver
Stomach
Diaphragm
Greater Omentum
Transverse Colon
Small Inestines
Descending Colon
Peritoneum
Spinal Canal
Sacrum
Uterus
Cervix
Bladder
Symphysis
Coccyx
Urethra
Vagina
Clitoris
Rectum
Vulva
Anal Canal

2.

Fundus
Placenta
Mucus Plug
Amniotic Fluid
Symphysis

3.

Alveolus
Lactiferous Sinus
Lactiferous Duct
Xiphoid Cartilage
Stomach
Fundus
Lower Colon
Umbilicus

4.

Descending Colon
Pelvic Colon
Internal Os
Cervix
Plug of Mucous
Bladder
External Os
Vagina

1. A woman's body before pregnancy.

2. At 12 weeks. Although your body may not show your pregnancy during the first trimester, it will begin to go through tremendous physical changes.

3. At 28 weeks. As the fetus grows larger, so will your belly and breasts.

4. At full term. As your uterus continues to expand, it will press up against your other internal organs, such as your bladder. This may cause some discomfort and more trips to the bathroom!

I loved, loved being pregnant. I was taking the best care of myself in all my thirty years, in terms of food, lifestyle, sleep, exercise, and alone time. I felt as if my intuition and all my senses were heightened.

Despite the excitement of being pregnant, the first trimester can be particularly challenging. You may experience fatigue, constipation, decreased sex drive, increased urge to urinate, tender or sore breasts, increased vaginal secretion, and nausea or increased appetite. Moreover, the nausea or vomiting commonly referred to as "morning sickness" is clearly misnamed because women who have nausea often feel sick throughout the day.

My morning sickness seemed to increase as the day went on. I was unable to eat much and unable to stomach certain foods. I am vegetarian and used to eat soy products, but my body wouldn't have anything to do with that. I craved fruit and liked everything cold!

You may experience moments when you need to eat something immediately but, for the life of you, cannot figure out what.

I remember sitting cooling my cheek on the bathroom floor with my partner standing over me telling me to eat the crackers he was handing me, which I did not want to do, and then feeling immediately better once I did. I also remember standing in the kitchen with a lost look on my face saying, "You need to put some food in front of me right now."

(For more information about getting through nausea, see page 71.)

During the first trimester, your breasts may become larger, full and tender, and your areola, the area around your nipple, may begin to darken. Exhaustion is also common during the first trimester.

I didn't realize how all-encompassing the lack of energy could be. I used to take catnaps in an empty patient room during my twelve-hour shift. My charge nurse for the shift would call them "smoke breaks," since all the nurses who were smokers were allowed to relinquish care of their patients for 15 minutes to go smoke. I would do the same to sleep.

Not all women experience all of these changes. The absence of any of these first-trimester experiences is *not* an indication that something is wrong with your pregnancy.

To Tell or Not to Tell

Many of us discover we are pregnant as soon as, or soon after, we miss a period. Some women choose to wait before telling others about the pregnancy.

I was pregnant three times before I gave birth to our baby. I had three miscarriages, two at three months and one at 5 weeks. We had told our friends and family about the other pregnancies, but this time we didn't talk about it to anyone. I felt that I had this incredibly precious treasure inside me and I had to guard it as safely as I could.

Others tell immediately.

I've never been good about keeping secrets. I also wanted to tell my work because I am a laboratory technician and I didn't want to perform any experiments with dangerous chemicals.

I was so excited to be pregnant at forty-five that I couldn't keep the lid on!

I told right away. I figured, If I lose the baby, I'm going to need to get support and process that with the people I'm telling.

PRENATAL VISITS

Prenatal care consists of three interrelated elements: regular visits with your midwife or doctor, the care you give yourself, and the care you receive from friends, family, or other support people. This chapter concentrates on prenatal visits with your care provider; for information on other aspects of prenatal care, see Chapter 5, "Taking Care of Yourself," and Chapter 6, "Relationships, Sex, and Emotional Support."

A woman with a normally progressing pregnancy and no complications usually visits her health care provider every four to six weeks during weeks 4 to 28, every two to three weeks from weeks 28 to 36, and every one to two weeks in the last month before her due date. The style of care you receive and the quality of your interactions can affect not only your physical experience of birth but your emotional experience. (For more information about choosing a provider, see Chapter 2.)

Your First Prenatal Visit

Your first prenatal visit will be longer and more involved than the others. During your initial visit, you and your provider will calculate your due date and, ideally, begin to discuss your ideas, thoughts, hopes, and plans for your pregnancy. Your provider may confirm your pregnancy through a blood or urine test, and will also obtain a thorough health history of you, your family, and the baby's father. She or he will likely ask you about aspects of your life that may affect your pregnancy and your baby's health. The questions will cover, among other things, your past and present use of drugs (including prescription medicines), cigarettes, and alcohol; your diet (including any vitamins, other supplements, or herbs you may take); your level of physical activity; your occupation and hobbies; whether you have pets; and how much emotional support you have available.

In addition, your provider will give you a

THE FETUS IN THE FIRST TRIMESTER

During your first trimester, the fetus grows from a microscopic cluster of cells to nearly 3 inches long. The fetus develops a head, neck, legs, and arms, as well as toes and fingers (complete with nails and fingerprint lines).

By the end of 12 weeks, the fetus has eyes, ears, a nose, and a mouth, and the beginning of hair fuzz. At this stage, fetuses can move their hands and kick their feet. The brain is developing rapidly and the head will make up nearly half of the fetus's entire length.

The sucking reflex also develops in the first trimester and the fetus forms tiny taste buds and teeth. The intestines are forming, and the fetus can push substances through them and out into the amniotic fluid. (Your body refreshes the fluid about every three hours, keeping the uterine environment clean.) The genitalia also begin to form in the first trimester.

The fetus's heart begins to beat around week 6, and by the end of the first trimester you will probably be able to hear the heartbeat with the Doppler ultrasound stethoscope.

thorough physical examination that includes checking your heart and lungs, breasts, abdomen, blood pressure, and weight. She or he may also perform a pelvic exam to measure the size of your uterus (and growing fetus) and to obtain a Pap smear to screen for cervical cancer and infections. A urine sample will be taken in order to check for urinary tract infections and test for sugar in the urine (to detect potential problems with diabetes) or protein that might be a sign of kidney problems.

Tests During Pregnancy

You will be offered a variety of tests during your prenatal care. Some of them will be offered only once, while others (for example, a blood pressure check) will be done at each visit. Some are primarily tests of *your* health (those discussed in this chapter), while others give you information about *your baby's* characteristics (see Chapter 7, "Prenatal Testing").

At your first prenatal visit, you will have a complete blood count (CBC) as well as blood tests to determine your blood type, Rh status (see the discussion of the Rhesus status test, page 52), and rubella antibody status and to check for syphilis and hepatitis B. It is also recommended that all pregnant women have a blood test for HIV. If you find out that you are HIV-positive, there are treatments to keep you as healthy as possible and to help protect your developing baby from being infected. (For more information, see page 141.) In addition, your provider will collect a culture from your cervix to test for gonorrhea and chlamydia.

The CBC will also screen for anemia, or low red-blood-cell count. If you are anemic, you may feel even more tired than you would otherwise. If you are of African-American, Mediterranean, or Southeast Asian descent, you may be anemic secondary to a genetic mutation that causes sickle-cell trait or thalassemia. If this first blood test does show that you are anemic, additional blood tests will be done to determine what type of anemia you have. If you are anemic from iron deficiency, eating foods that have a lot of iron and/or taking iron supplements can increase your red-blood-cell count. (For more information, see "Iron," page 65.)

One of the initial tests at your first visit is a *Rhesus status test* (also known as Rh screening testing). This determines whether your blood is Rh-negative (you do not have Rh protein on your red blood cells) or Rh-positive. If the initial Rhesus status test shows that your blood is Rh-negative, a second blood test will be done when you are 26 to 28 weeks pregnant (see page 56). But if your blood is Rh-positive, there is no need for follow-up.

Your first prenatal visit is a good time to think about and discuss with your provider the possibility of screening for Down syndrome or other genetic impairments of the fetus via screening blood tests and ultrasounds, chorionic villus sampling (CVS), or amniocentesis (amnio). (For more information, see Chapter 7, "Prenatal Testing.")

SECOND TRIMESTER

WHAT'S HAPPENING IN YOUR BODY

For many women, the second trimester brings about several welcome changes. Nausea tends to subside or disappear entirely and your breasts become less tender. You will probably have increased energy and appetite. Perhaps the most exciting thing is that most women begin to feel the baby move at about 18 to 22 weeks. These first sensations, referred to as *quickening,* often feel like little fluttery movements or gas. Quickening, combined with the visual sign of a growing belly, may help make the pregnancy seem more real.

Month/ Weeks	Your Provider Will Likely:
Months 1–2 (Weeks 1–8)	• Confirm your pregnancy (with a blood test or urine test) • Take a thorough medical history • Conduct a physical exam and a pelvic exam (including a Pap smear) • Perform urine and blood tests • Talk with you about diet, exercise, drug use, emotional support, occupational exposures, etc. • Discuss your options for a hospital, birth center, or other setting in which he or she can attend your birth • Schedule future visits • Offer you an ultrasound/sonogram if needed to determine your due date
Month 3 (Weeks 9–13)	• Conduct a routine check (see page 55) • Listen for the fetal heartbeat • Offer you a sonogram/ultrasound if you choose one for Down syndrome screening at 11–14 weeks (see pages 116–120) • Discuss the possibility of screening for Down syndrome or genetic impairments of the fetus via chorionic villus sampling or amniocentesis (see Chapter 7, "Prenatal Testing")
Month 4 (Weeks 13–17)	• Conduct a routine check (see page 55) • Offer you maternal blood test screenings for Down syndrome and spinal cord defects in the fetus (sometimes called *multiple marker screening;* see page 117) if earlier Down syndrome screening or integrated screening has not been done
Month 5 (Weeks 18–22)	• Conduct a routine check (see page 55) • Offer you an ultrasound/sonogram (to do a careful survey of the fetus's vital organs and spinal cord, to check fetal growth, and to check for multiple fetuses) • Discuss childbirth classes

(continued on next page)

Month/ Weeks	Your Provider Will Likely: *(Continued)*
Month 6 (Weeks 23–27)	• Conduct a routine check (see page 55) • Teach you to recognize the signs and symptoms of preterm labor • Discuss when and whom you should call after you begin to show signs of labor • Offer tests for gestational diabetes, anemia, and, if you are Rh-negative, check if you have developed antibodies to the Rh factor • Discuss preparation for breastfeeding and signs of postpartum depression
Month 7 (Weeks 28–31)	• Conduct a routine check (see page 55) • Offer RhoGAM if needed (Rh-negative women only)
Month 8 (Weeks 32–35)	• Conduct a routine check (see page 55) • Assess cervix (if this check is needed)
Month 9 (Weeks 36–40)	• Offer a test to check for infections, particularly Group B streptococcus (GBS) At some point in this period, you may be visiting your provider weekly, or even more frequently. Aside from routine checks, the exams will probably focus on: • Size and position of the baby • Assessing cervix and descent of baby You may also want to discuss ways to induce labor if that should become necessary.
Beyond Week 40	Many pregnancies extend beyond 40 weeks. As long as you and the baby are healthy, there usually is no need to worry. Your provider may recommend routine checks of your cervix and the position/location of the baby and, past 41 weeks, tests to assess the health of the baby. (For more information, see "The Long Pregnancy," page 146.)

I had been feeling the baby move for a while but it didn't really sink in that the fluttering I felt was the little person inside me. One afternoon my husband had his hand on my belly and the baby kicked really hard. It was the first time I really knew that I had been feeling the baby kick. We were so excited!

As the baby grows, so will your belly. At 12 weeks, your uterus is at the level of your pubic bone. Around 20 weeks, the top of your uterus (the *fundus*) may reach your navel, and by the end of the second trimester, it reaches even higher, so it is right under your ribs. Women have tremendously varied responses to the changing shapes of our bodies.

I was excited to have my body change. It was nice to be recognized as pregnant and not just fat. We called the first few months my "beer belly stage" because I didn't look pregnant. It was just a wonder. My partner was so excited—I think she made it more real for both of us.

I'm fascinated with myself as a pregnant woman. I keep on staring at myself in the mirror in complete awe of the way my body is changing. Last night I just stared at my stomach for the longest time because the baby was kicking a lot and the way my stomach moved about was entrancing. It all feels so alien to me. I look so alien to me. Yet I really like the way I look pregnant. I'm more aware of my body, but not in a vain way.

As I got really big, sadly, I felt like a beached whale and didn't feel good mentally or physically. I realize it sounds shallow, but my psychological scars run deep. My partner said I looked incredibly beautiful, but I thought he was just patronizing me.

Women often feel ambivalent as a result of the value our culture places on being thin.

Many women try to live up to this cultural ideal, even while pregnant, with negative consequences. Unfortunately, images of big, powerful birthing mothers are largely absent from our culture. Recently, popular media have celebrated pregnancy as sexy, but only for celebrities with otherwise "perfect" bodies. Imagine if we were surrounded by images that embraced our roundness instead. Try not to allow narrow cultural lenses to rob you of the right to feel happy and proud of your pregnant body.

Another physical change that may happen during the second trimester is the appearance of a *linea nigra,* a dark line that extends from your navel to your pubic bone. It will last for your whole pregnancy.

Toward the end of the second trimester, you may also begin to experience *Braxton-Hicks contractions,* small, nonpainful contractions in which your uterus becomes hard for a moment and then releases. Braxton-Hicks contractions are different from labor contractions because they are usually not crampy at this stage and do not develop a rhythm. You can think of them as warm-up or practice contractions to prepare your uterus for labor.

Some women experience intense or unusual food cravings (see "Cravings," page 72). Others develop a heightened sense of openness to the world, and feel sensitive and emotional. You may begin to have interesting dreams and remember them more than usual. If this happens to you, consider keeping a journal by your bed to track them.

You may also want to seek out other women's pregnancy and childbirth stories. Sharing stories is an ancient and powerful way to build community, learn about the many different ways women birth, and prepare yourself for the choices you may be faced with in your own labor.

Sometimes the stories we hear are negative, scary, or disempowering.

Always around the lunch table at work somebody had a cousin or a friend who experienced some really traumatic birth, whose story they felt compelled to share. Many times, I could recognize the detrimental effect of snowballing medical interventions. I just tried to focus on my own goals for birth.

We tend to hear more from friends and the media about problem births than about typical births. Despite the reality that most births are safe and healthy, we are often given the message that birth is unsafe, and it's easy to have the perception that birth is more risky than it really is. Try to find people and resources to nourish your confidence so that you can trust that birth is a normal, healthy process. (Childbirth Connection is one such resource; for others, see "Resources," at the back of this book.)

YOUR PRENATAL VISITS

Every visit until you give birth will include a *routine check*. This routine check will likely include checking in with you about any concerns you may have; checking your weight gain; listening to the baby's heartbeat (using Doppler if you so choose); assessing the baby's growth (fundal height) and vital signs, as well as her or his position; collecting a urine sample to screen for diabetes, pre-eclampsia (protein in urine), or infections; and conducting a *physical exam*, which includes taking your blood pressure to check for gestational hypertension and checking your hands and feet for swelling and your legs for varicose veins. If you have not yet done so, the second trimester is a good time to discuss your birth preferences with your provider.

Some providers suggest that women conduct some of these physical assessments (such as weighing ourselves and checking urine) for ourselves. Many women appreciate the opportunity to participate in our own health care.

One of the purposes of testing your urine is to determine whether you have *pre-eclampsia*, a syndrome whose symptoms include high

YOUR BABY IN THE SECOND TRIMESTER

By the end of the second trimester, your baby will probably be a lot more active. She or he will have grown to about a foot in length and two pounds in weight. At this stage, babies' hands may grasp the umbilical cord, and their feet may kick at the uterus or may pedal in a walking motion. Some babies are capable of acrobatic feats, such as flips and somersaults in the amniotic fluid. Babies may also begin exercising their facial expressions, grimacing and smiling. All this movement helps babies grow and develop their muscles.

Your baby may also begin to react to the outside world and may respond to touches and pokes to your belly. During the second trimester, she or he will begin detecting and recognizing sounds. Loud noises may startle your baby into movement.

The digestive system becomes more developed during this period. The baby will swallow amniotic fluid and urinate.

REASONS TO CALL YOUR PROVIDER

If you experience any of the following, call your health care provider:

- blood or other fluid leaking from the vagina
- severe menstrual-like cramping or backache
- continuous pain, particularly abdominal pain
- persistent vomiting
- chills and fever, particularly a temperature of 101°F or higher
- burning with urination
- continuous headache
- blurry vision
- sudden swelling of hands or face
- five or more uterine contractions in one hour
- decreased fetal movement at 24 weeks or more (It is normal for babies to be quiet for short periods of time, and sometimes the movements are smaller in the last month or so of pregnancy, when the baby is bigger and not able to stretch out well. If you feel the baby is moving less often than usual, sit in a quiet place and monitor movements. Call your health care provider if the baby does not move four times in the hour that you are monitoring.)

blood pressure; generalized swelling of hands, feet, and face (edema); sudden weight gain; and protein in the urine. Pre-eclampsia has the potential to lead to serious problems during pregnancy. (For more information, see page 140.)

Toward the end of the second trimester, you will be offered another blood test to screen for anemia and gestational diabetes. (For information about anemia, see "Iron," page 66. For information about gestational diabetes, see page 138.)

The test for *gestational diabetes,* offered at about 26 to 28 weeks, is the glucose challenge test. During this test, you drink a glass of glucose solution (sugar solution, or sugar drink). Some providers offer the option of eating a specific high-carbohydrate meal, rather than drinking the sugar solution (which makes some

women feel sick). After a one-hour wait, a blood sample is drawn and the blood sugar (glucose) level is tested.

If you have high levels of sugar in your blood one hour after drinking the glucose solution, a more conclusive test, the glucose tolerance test, will be done. It will show how well you process sugar over time. On an empty stomach, you drink a more concentrated glass of the glucose solution. Over the next three hours, blood samples are taken and the blood sugar level is tested. The results tell if your response to the sugar is normal or if you have developed diabetes during pregnancy.

If the initial Rhesus status test showed that your blood is Rh-negative, an additional test will be done at this time. The test determines whether you have developed antibodies that

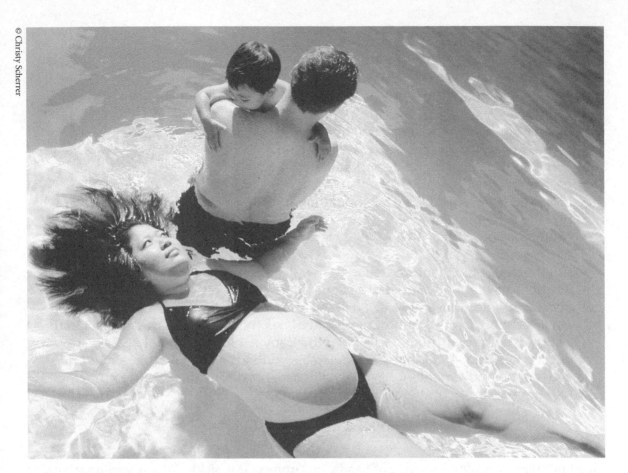
© Christy Scherrer

could cross the placenta and harm your baby if the baby is Rh-positive. If the test shows that you are not making antibodies against Rh-positive blood, you will be offered an injection of $Rh_0(D)$ immune globulin (RhoGAM). The RhoGAM prevents your immune system from making antibodies that can cause anemia in your baby if the baby is Rh-positive.

THIRD TRIMESTER

WHAT'S HAPPENING IN YOUR BODY

In the third trimester, your baby is growing a tremendous amount. Your belly—and for some

of us, other body parts, too—will be getting very big.

I had a big tummy and a big butt to match. Even though I was huge, it was okay with me. My big belly made everything make sense. I really was pregnant! I really was going to be a mother! I really did have every right to be shopping for baby clothes and to be treated with special care!

Your growing belly may elicit comments from well-meaning others who have opinions about your size relative to other pregnant women.

Sometimes I'd hear, "Oh, you're so small" and "Are you having twins?" in the same day. The comments were so mixed I learned to just laugh and brush them aside. This might not have been the case if I'd constantly heard the same thing—I might have started to believe it.

Many people like to touch big pregnant bellies, and sometimes they do so without asking permission. Most of the time, people's intentions are loving and they are reaching out toward your belly because seeing it has brought them joy. However, it is your body and you have the right to decide who can touch it. Women have very different feelings about this.

I usually didn't mind it much, except when they were complete strangers who'd strike up a conversation about my pending due date and feel like they needed to touch it, like you'd pet a dog if you were talking to its owner.

Your baby's movements become stronger as well. You may feel full-body movements as opposed to the flutters of the second trimester. You may also be able to distinguish body parts. Your partner or others will be able to feel the baby move if they can catch the right moment.

We were in England for my husband's grandmother's funeral, and late at night he felt [the baby] move for the first time. What a welcome moment of life in the midst of grief.

As she grew bigger and more active, I described the feeling as an alien invasion. I would often feel as though she could potentially kick her way out!

You may also notice the baby responding to sounds in the environment.

The most amusing movements were when listening to various types of music in later pregnancy and wondering if the increased movements were because the baby liked or hated what we were listening to.

The increased size and weight of the baby can bring about other changes as well. You may feel the baby's head on your pubic bone or bladder (leading to increased frequency of urination). As your ligaments loosen in preparation for birth, you may also experience backaches and pain with walking.

It became uncomfortable to sit for long periods. It was also hard to find a comfortable position to sleep. I stopped being able to hike long distances. One little muscle in my butt was controlling my life.

Your fundus, which is the top of the uterus, will be high up in your abdomen, and this can lead to heartburn, inability to eat large meals, and shortness of breath. The pressure from the baby's weight may create hemorrhoids or other varicosities (for example, dark veins in your legs).

Toward the end of pregnancy, you will begin to produce colostrum, a protein-rich fluid your breasts make before mature breast milk comes in. Your breasts begin to fill up with colostrum and may leak some of this fluid. Some women notice swelling in the ankles, as well as increased body heat and perspiration. You may also experience lighter sleep with lots of interruptions (often to use the bathroom).

Many women remain active until the end of pregnancy. You may find that even if you continue to participate in your regular activities, diminishing energy causes you to cut back and slow down a bit.

During the third trimester, many women experience increased Braxton-Hicks contractions. As birth draws near, the contractions may begin to change, becoming more frequent and even feeling a little crampy. Sometimes several contractions will come in a short period of time, and you may think that you are in labor.

Then the contractions stop and you go about your day (or night). These contractions begin to soften your cervix, helping to get it ready for labor.

At approximately 36 weeks or beyond, some babies will move down into the pelvis. This is known as *engagement,* or "lightening." If your baby moves down in this way, you may feel pressure on your bottom, as if a grapefruit is sitting in your pelvis. You may be able to eat a bit more and breathe more easily.

The Last Few Weeks of Pregnancy

During the last few weeks before the birth, your body will begin to prepare for labor. You may notice nonpainful tightening in your uterus, and the baby may drop lower, so you breathe easier but have to urinate more often. The mucous plug that rests in the cervical canal may come out as your cervix gets soft and ready to open. (Most women notice this as an increased amount of vaginal discharge, which may be blood-tinged, for a few days.) You may find your focus shifting away from the outside world and moving inward toward the baby. You may experience a strong desire to nest, to get everything into place at home. You might just feel done with being pregnant.

I really wanted to get it over with. I wanted to meet my little baby. The weather was hot and muggy and this added to my discomfort and high blood pressure. On the other hand, I knew those would be my last days as a free woman and my life would never be the same so I was okay with waiting it out.

YOUR BABY IN THE THIRD TRIMESTER

During the final months of your pregnancy, your baby's internal organs and systems will become mature enough for the baby to be able to survive outside your uterus. Much of the baby's growth will be in building muscle and fat, up to an ounce a day. The rolls of baby fat help babies regulate their body temperature once they leave their mother's body. Added muscle and fat make babies' faces plump and round and help give them the strength to breast-feed when they are born. By the end of the pregnancy, the average baby weighs about seven pounds.

As the fit in the uterus gets tighter, babies make fewer big movements and will eventually tuck themselves into one position. By late in your pregnancy, your baby may have only enough room for small wiggles. Hiccups are also common at this stage of a baby's development. You will probably be able to feel these tiny spasms inside you. From your baby's activities, you may notice definite periods of time when she or he is awake or asleep.

Brain growth and development continue in the third trimester. Grooves and ridges begin to form in the baby's brain as nerve cells rapidly increase. By the end of a full-term pregnancy, your baby's organs and systems will be able to function on their own, and she or he is ready to be born.

I [was] soooo tired of being pregnant. The baby had spent the last two to three months with his butt up under my left ribs. It felt like they were bruised, which in all actuality they were. I was miserable. . . . We had tried sex a couple nights before to stimulate labor, but it didn't work too well. I had heard that nipple stimulation can help to start labor, so I gave it a shot. I [immediately got] very, very hard contractions one right after the other, but they weren't regular and they seemed to taper off quickly after stopping the nipple stimulation. I decided to just accept the fact that I would be pregnant forever.

As your due date approaches, or even passes, it can be challenging to stay present and positive. This is normal, particularly if well-meaning family and friends begin calling and asking, "So, is anything happening yet?"

My dad was the worst. I kept telling him, "Oh shoot, that's right, we had the baby and I totally forgot to tell you!"

Anticipating your child's birth may bring up many emotions, such as anxiety, excitement, and impatience. Remember that your baby will come when she or he is ready and your body is ready for labor. If you are still pregnant on your due date, your care provider might begin to discuss testing that can help determine if your baby is continuing to thrive, problems that can occur if you don't go into labor spontaneously, and induction of labor. You may be tired of being pregnant, but your due date is just the middle of the time period in which labor is expected to start. Although induction is sometimes necessary, in general, you and your baby are not at risk for any complications until a week or more after your due date has passed.

(For more information about induction, see page 146).

YOUR PRENATAL VISITS

Prenatal care in the third trimester is focused on preparing for labor and birth as well as continuing to monitor the well-being of you and your baby. Your visits will become more frequent and, in addition to routine checks, your provider should begin to help you solidify your birth preferences and talk in more depth with you about how you are feeling about labor, birth, and the transition to motherhood.

Around 36 weeks, you will be advised to have a test to determine whether you have Group B streptococcus (GBS), a bacterium that may be living harmlessly in your vagina or rectum. About one in four pregnant women has the bacteria present. The test is performed by swabbing the vagina and the entrance to the rectum. Although harmless when you are pregnant, GBS can cause serious infections in newborns right after birth, and in rare cases in women. If you are a GBS carrier, the chance that your baby will get an infection from GBS is somewhat higher if you are in labor before 37 weeks, you have ruptured membranes for more than eighteen hours, or you have a fever during labor. To protect the baby, the Centers for Disease Control and Prevention (CDC) recommends giving antibiotics during labor to all women who have tested positive for GBS, as well as to women whose GBS status is unknown when preterm rupture of membranes or preterm labor occurs. Just one or two doses of penicillin during labor will decrease the amount of GBS in your vagina at birth. If you are a carrier of GBS, your baby will not be exposed to this bacterium until your membranes have ruptured or you are in labor.

CHAPTER 5

Taking Care of Yourself

Prenatal care isn't only about visiting your health care provider. It's also about taking care of yourself. This chapter focuses on what you can do—from eating nourishing food and being active to avoiding harmful substances—to help yourself and your developing baby to be healthy.

As a pregnant woman, it's easy to feel overwhelmed by the amount of advice and precautions you may hear. While it is wise to make healthy choices when you are able, it's important to maintain a sense of perspective.

When I got pregnant with my first baby, it was the first grandchild in both our families, and everyone suddenly became crazily focused on my health and well-being. My mother—a.k.a. the food police—would heap food on my plate. "She's eating for two!" She was ecstatic. My mother-in-law—the worrier—monitored my every move. "Should you be riding a bicycle?" "You look tired. Sit down. Put your feet up." "I don't think you should be out in the garden." "You two should stay over at our house while they are painting your living room." It was kind of unnerving. Everything went just fine, but I hardly knew what to do with myself. By the time my second pregnancy came around, the whole family was much more relaxed. I walked, rode my bike, worked in my garden, and ate normally right up until I delivered. Amazingly, even without all that attention, I had another healthy baby!

EATING WELL

Eating well during your pregnancy supports your health and the many developing systems in your baby.

GUIDELINES FOR HEALTHY EATING

We have some special nutritional needs while we are pregnant, but the basic principles for healthy eating remain the same throughout our lives:

- **Eat whole grains.** As much as possible, eat your grains in minimally processed whole-grain form. Try eating more whole grains such as brown rice, oats, or barley, and foods made with whole grains, such as whole-wheat pasta or whole-grain breads. Limit highly processed grains such as white bread, white pasta, and refined cereals. Check the labels on packaged foods and choose foods that list a whole grain as the first ingredient.
- **Eat plenty of vegetables and fruit.** Choose vegetables and fruits in a variety of colors—from the deep blue and purple of blueberries and eggplants to the dark green of spinach and broccoli to the bright red of tomatoes and strawberries—to ensure that you get adequate fiber and a wide range of vitamins, minerals, and phytochemicals. Try to eat at least one vitamin C–rich fruit or vegetable (orange, grapefruit, strawberries, papaya, sweet pepper, mustard greens, or tomato) and one vitamin A–rich food (dark, leafy greens; sweet potato; carrots; mango; cantaloupe; dried apricots) each day.
- **Choose healthy fats.** Different kinds of fat affect our bodies in differing ways. Unsaturated fats—the kind in olives, nuts, avocados, fish, and vegetable oils—are "good" fats that help our bodies absorb the nutrients in our foods. Saturated fats—found in foods such as whole milk, butter, cheese, red meats, and coconut—are considered less healthy and may contribute to a range of health problems. Trans fats—found in many commer-

cially prepared baked goods, margarines, snack foods, and processed foods—are "bad" fats that should be eliminated from our diet wherever possible. Foods whose labels list "hydrogenerated oil" or "partially hydrogenated oil" contain trans fats and should be avoided.

- **Choose healthy protein sources.** Choose nuts, beans, tofu and other soy-based products, eggs, fish, chicken, and lean cuts of red meat to meet your body's need for protein. These foods are high in protein and other nutrients but low in saturated fats.
- **Stay hydrated.** Drink plenty of water to keep your body hydrated and cool.
- **Cut down on highly processed food and "empty calories."** Avoid eating highly processed foods (especially those that contain trans fats) and drinking sodas and sugary sports drinks. These foods and drinks contain lots of calories but few, if any, nutrients; they also contribute to a variety of health problems.
- **Balance your food intake and activity levels to meet your body's needs.** During pregnancy, you may need to take in a slightly different amount of calories and your usual portion sizes may change. At some times, especially during the first trimester, you may be able to eat only small amounts throughout the day, while at other times you may want to eat more than you would when not pregnant.

Eating well during pregnancy, as during other times in our lives, can be challenging. Many factors, including nausea, finances, and our families' eating habits, can interfere with our good intentions.

My husband and I are Latino—from Michoacán in Mexico. We eat refried beans and a lot of fried foods. We were both kind of overweight, and when I got pregnant they said I was maybe getting diabetes. So I started trying to make our regular food in more healthy ways. I cooked beans without lard. I steamed and baked food instead of frying. My husband didn't like it too much at first. He still really likes fried stuff. But we both got healthier.

Millions of women eating a wide range of diets give birth to healthy babies all the time. While it is important to eat well during preg-

A VEGETARIAN PREGNANCY

With a little careful planning, vegetarian diets can supply all the nutrients you need during pregnancy. The primary nutrients that may take extra work to get enough of are protein, iron, essential fatty acids, vitamin B_{12}, and vitamin D. If you are a vegan (someone who eats no meat, fish, eggs, or dairy products), you may also need to increase your consumption of foods that contain calcium.

- **Protein.** Healthy vegetarian sources of protein are legumes, tofu, nuts, milk, cheese, and eggs. Try to eat a variety of these foods, as different protein foods have different amounts of essential amino acids and essential fatty acids.
- **Iron.** The type of iron in meat is easier to absorb than the type of iron in vegetables. Still, dark green, leafy vegetables; nuts; dried fruits; and whole-grain cereals and whole-grain breads that are fortified with iron are good sources of iron. (For more information, see "Iron," page 66.)
- **Essential fatty acids (omega-3 and omega-6 fatty acids).** These necessary acids are found in large amounts in eggs. Omega-6 fatty acids are also easily available in vegetable oils, soy foods, seeds, and nuts. If you do not eat eggs, it is important to have other sources of omega-3s, to maintain a beneficial balance of these two types of fatty acids. Excellent sources of omega-3 fatty acids are flaxseeds and flaxseed oil. Omega-3 fatty acids can be found in smaller quantities in other seeds and in nuts, canola oil, and soy products, as well as in beans, vegetables, and whole grains. (For more information, see "Essential Fatty Acids," page 67.)
- **Vitamin B_{12}.** This B vitamin, which is abundant in meat and dairy products, is essential for the development of nerve cells, DNA, and red blood cells. Because vitamin B_{12} is not found in plant foods, deficiency can occur in women who are vegans. If you do not eat eggs, milk, or cheese, you can get adequate amounts of vitamin B_{12} by eating fortified cereals or taking a supplement.
- **Calcium and vitamin D.** If you eat dairy products, you can easily meet your need for calcium and vitamin D. Vegans can get enough calcium and vitamin D in broccoli, kale, tofu, "soy nuts," calcium-fortified cereals or crackers, and calcium-fortified orange juice. Some women prefer taking a calcium supplement. (For more information, see "Calcium and Vitamin D," page 66.)

HELP GETTING FOOD

If you are having a hard time paying for enough food for yourself and your family, help is available when you are pregnant. One program available everywhere in the United States is the Special Supplemental Program for Women, Infants, and Children (WIC), a federal food program. WIC provides milk, fruit, cereal, juice, cheese, peanut butter, dried beans or peas, carrots, tuna fish, and eggs, and offers some prenatal and breast-feeding education to women who meet certain income requirements. Information about the WIC program is available at www.fns.usda.gov/wic. The website lists toll-free numbers for WIC agencies in each state. Your health care provider or your county health department (listed in the blue pages of the telephone directory) will be able to direct you to the WIC office nearest you.

Many communities also have food banks that can provide fresh or canned foods. America's Second Harvest can direct you to local food banks, soup kitchens, food pantries, or shelters. You can contact them at www.secondharvest.org or 1-800-771-2303.

nancy, try not to lose the pleasure of eating by worrying over every bite.

SPECIAL NUTRITIONAL NEEDS DURING PREGNANCY

During pregnancy, we need more protein, iron, and calcium, and larger amounts of some vitamins. Often you can get these nutrients from eating a well-balanced diet, but taking a vitamin supplement may be helpful. (For more on prenatal vitamins, see page 67.)

Folate / Folic Acid

Folate is an essential vitamin that your baby needs in order to grow. Consuming enough folate at the very beginning of pregnancy can prevent 50 to 70 percent of neural tube defects, which cause birth impairments such as spina bifida.[1]

Folate, which is a B vitamin, is sometimes called the "foliage" vitamin, because it is found in most dark green, leafy vegetables. Folate is also found in foods such as dried peas, beans, and lentils; liver; and beef. In addition, many ready-to-eat breakfast cereals, breads, and pastas are fortified with folic acid, the synthetic form of folate.

Many women do not get enough folate from the food we eat. Therefore, it is generally recommended that women who plan on becoming pregnant begin taking 400 micrograms of folic acid several months before trying to conceive and continue taking it through the first three months of pregnancy. Most prenatal vitamins include the full amount of folic acid needed per day during pregnancy.

If you are taking medication for a seizure disorder or if you have a family history of, or have had a previous pregnancy affected by, a neural-tube defect, it is recommended that you take 4 milligrams of folic acid.

Iron

Our bodies—and our babies—use huge amounts of iron while we are pregnant. During pregnancy, your baby uses iron to make red blood cells and absorbs all the iron she or he will get for the first six months of life. If you don't get enough iron in your diet, you may become anemic and the baby may have less stored iron after birth. To prevent this, it is recommended that we each get 27 milligrams of iron every day during pregnancy.[2] Getting this much iron is pretty easy. Just eat a portion or two a day of iron-rich foods, like meat, seafood, eggs, soy beans, lentils, black-eyed peas, greens, beets, sweet potatoes, dried fruits like raisins and prunes, molasses, and iron-fortified breakfast cereals. Cooking foods in cast-iron pans can add iron to the foods.

It is normal to be slightly anemic during the second trimester of pregnancy; our bodies can handle this without difficulty. But if you start pregnancy with too few iron stores, the demands of pregnancy can worsen anemia to the point that it becomes a problem for you and your growing baby. If you become clinically anemic, you may need to take an iron supplement. Here are some tips if you do:

- Some women who take iron supplements become constipated. If this happens to you, check out the strategies for managing constipation on page 72.
- Vitamin C helps our bodies absorb iron. Taking your iron with a glass of orange juice will help you get more from the supplement.
- Caffeine makes it hard for our bodies to absorb iron. Taking your iron several hours before or after consuming caffeine will help you get more from the supplement. (For more information about caffeine, see page 83.)
- Some women become nauseated from taking iron and prenatal vitamins. If this happens to

you, try taking your iron just before you go to bed. You may sleep through the immediate upset-stomach effects. (For more strategies for coping with nausea, see page 71.)
- Iron can be lost in cooking, especially if you cook foods for too long in too much water. If you cook meat or vegetables in water, try to use the cooking water in a soup to get the iron and other vitamins that have soaked out.
- There are three types of iron supplements: ferrous gluconate, ferrous sulfate, and ferrous fumarate. Each type has a different amount of elemental iron. Read the label to see how much elemental iron is in each tablet. If you want guidance on selecting a supplement, discuss the options with your health care provider.

Calcium and Vitamin D

Calcium and vitamin D are needed throughout pregnancy. There is some controversy over exactly how much calcium women need. The National Academy of Sciences recommends that pregnant women get about 1,000 milligrams of calcium every day (if you are under age nineteen, the recommendation is 1,300). This is the amount found in four cups of yogurt or milk. Calcium can also be found in dark green, leafy vegetables; broccoli; sardines or canned salmon; tofu; and calcium-fortified orange juice or soy milk. Women's bodies absorb calcium efficiently during pregnancy, and babies have mechanisms for getting all they need. Extra calcium in the form of more dairy products or other dietary sources is recommended only for women whose diets are significantly low in calcium. If you are lactose intolerant or have a diet that is low in calcium, you can get the recommended 1,000 milligrams by taking calcium supplements, which can be found in any drugstore. Antacids like Tums that are made of calcium carbonate are a good source of elemental calcium and may be better tolerated than other forms of calcium. Vitamin D helps us absorb calcium; if you do not get enough vitamin D through eating fish, milk, and fortified foods, or being exposed to the sun, you may want to take a supplement that contains both calcium and vitamin D. Women with dark skin and women who live at higher latitudes are more likely to need supplemental vitamin D.

Protein

If you eat a variety of foods rich in protein—such as meats, seafood, soy products, beans, and grains—you will easily meet your increased need for protein. If you are a vegetarian or vegan, you may need to plan more carefully to ensure that you get the protein you need. (For more information, see "A Vegetarian Pregnancy," page 64.)

Essential Fatty Acids

Essential fatty acids are needed during pregnancy, but the extra amount needed has not been established. The two essential fatty acids that cannot be made by your body and need to be obtained via diet are linoleic acid (LA), an omega-6 fat, and alpha-linolenic acid (ALA), an omega-3 fat. These essential acids are important for brain and eye development. Both are found in large amounts in fish and eggs. (If you do not eat fish or eggs, see "A Vegetarian Pregnancy," page 64.)

Prenatal Vitamins

Some recent research suggests that taking a multivitamin supplement before conception and in the early months of pregnancy may reduce the risk of miscarriage and prevent some impairments, such as cleft lip and palate, in the

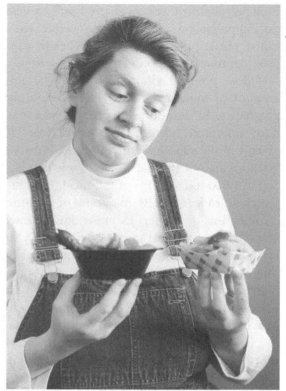

Being pregnant can make us feel as if we are being judged for every decision we make.

developing baby.[3] Taking a multivitamin supplement regularly for three months before conception and during the first trimester of pregnancy also may reduce a mother's risk of developing a complication known as *pre-eclampsia*.[4] Folic acid helps prevent neural-tube defects in the developing baby.

If you are eating a well-rounded diet, you may not need to take prenatal vitamins, except for folic acid supplements, which are recommended for all pregnant women. But many women find it easy to take one prenatal multivitamin supplement daily, to ensure that we are getting enough nutrients. Prenatal vitamins don't take the place of food; even if you take them, it's still important to eat a healthy diet.

Prenatal vitamins are considered safe to take during pregnancy, and they are available without a prescription, though your health care provider may have specific recommendations.

Most prenatal vitamins include the full amount of folic acid needed per day during pregnancy. In addition, all prenatal vitamins have some iron, calcium, and smaller doses of several other vitamins and minerals. Prenatal vitamins are not all alike. Look for one that has 600 to 1,000 micrograms of folic acid, 27 milligrams of iron, 70 to 250 milligrams of calcium, 2 milligrams of copper, 15 milligrams of zinc, 400 IUs (international units) of vitamin D, 50 milligrams of vitamin C, 2 milligrams of vitamin B_6, and 2 micrograms of vitamin B_{12}. Some prenatal vitamins contain fluoride. It is not clear whether taking fluoride during pregnancy will benefit the fetus, but doing so is considered safe.

In deciding whether to take prenatal vitamins, you may want to consider the following questions:

- **Are you a vegetarian who eats little or no dairy or eggs?** If so, you may want to take a prenatal multivitamin supplement that contains B vitamins, since these are often lacking in a vegan diet.
- **Are you feeling nauseous?** Prenatal vitamins may make your nausea worse. If you are having a hard time with nausea, try taking your prenatal vitamin before bed so that the side effects will not be as noticeable. You may also want to experiment with different kinds of vitamins. Some women find that liquid vitamins or chewable vitamins are easier on the stomach. If this does not help, you may want to hold off on the prenatal multivitamins supplement but continue taking a folic acid supplement until the first trimester has passed and you feel better.

There is no current evidence that taking high doses of any vitamin (more than the amounts in prenatal vitamins) is helpful during pregnancy. Taking too much of some vitamins can be dangerous. This is especially true of the fat-soluble vitamins, such as A, D, and E. If you take high doses of fat-soluble vitamins, they can build up to harmful levels in your body or in the body of your developing baby.

WEIGHT GAIN

The amounts of weight that women gain during pregnancy vary widely. When you eat well, your weight will take care of itself. Pregnancy is not a time to diet. In fact, it is important that you gain enough weight so that your baby can grow to a healthy weight.

I was a gymnast and a long-distance runner all through high school and college. I'm five feet tall and never weighed more than a hundred pounds. In my first pregnancy, I started out trying to maintain my running schedule. But I was ravenous all the time. I just couldn't seem to get enough to eat. I gained fifty-five pounds—more than half my prepregnancy body weight. That kind of put a stop to my running. It was just too hard to move around. Anyway, I had a very healthy daughter, and I'm back to a healthy weight and running regularly again, too. I think women need to [worry less about] how much they gain in pregnancy [and] focus on eating healthy and staying active.

Women who enter pregnancy at an average weight usually gain between twenty and thirty-five pounds. If you are underweight, you may gain more; if heavier, you may gain less. To help maintain your own healthy weight, balance the amount of food you eat with your activity levels and your body's needs.

FOODS TO WATCH OUT FOR

During pregnancy, the basic guideline is to eat a well-rounded diet rich in fresh, unprocessed foods. However, particularly in the early months of pregnancy, certain kinds of fish, meat, milk, and cheese should be avoided, as they can increase your risk of getting food poisoning or pose potential dangers to your developing baby.

Shark, Swordfish, King Mackerel, and Tilefish

Fish is rich in protein and healthy fats, including omega-3 fatty acids that are thought to help fetal brain development. Unfortunately, the water that fish swim in has become polluted with dangerous toxins such as mercury. Some fish absorb these chemicals when they eat plants or other fish, and the chemicals may become highly concentrated in the fishes' bodies. Eating too much fish with high mercury levels may cause mercury to build up in your body, too, and may harm your baby's developing brain. It is best to avoid eating shark, swordfish, king mackerel, and tilefish (also known as golden bass), as these large fish are more likely to be contaminated with mercury.

While it is important to avoid these four fish species, it is safe and even beneficial to eat a variety of other types of fish in moderation. Eating two servings or so a week of fish or other seafood that is generally low in mercury, such as sardines, cod, halibut, shrimp, canned light tuna, catfish, salmon, pollock, and trout, will provide healthy omega-3s to you and your growing baby. (Eggs, flaxseed oil, and walnuts also provide omega-3s.) If you want to eat canned tuna, stick to "light" tuna rather than albacore. Albacore tuna generally has higher levels of mercury.[5]

Soft Cheeses and Unpasteurized Milk

Soft cheeses and unpasteurized milk sometimes contain bacteria that cause an illness known as *listeriosis*. Listeriosis is a minor illness for most adults—like the flu—but when you are pregnant, it may lead to miscarriage, stillbirth, or serious health problems for your developing baby. By avoiding soft cheeses such as feta, Brie, and Camembert; blue-veined cheeses; and Mexican-style queso blanco fresco (or queso fresco) and by drinking only pasteurized milk, you will greatly reduce your risk of getting listeriosis.

Certain Meats

In general, the meat that is available in the United States and Canada is safe to eat during pregnancy. However, meat that has not been kept cold or that has not been prepared properly may have bacteria or parasites that could harm you or your baby. Cook all meats all the way through; you should not see any pink inside the flesh. After cutting up raw meat, clean the cutting surface with bleach, soap, and hot water before cutting any raw fruit or vegetables. Processed meats such as hot dogs or deli meats should be heated until piping hot before you eat them.

Alcohol

Heavy use of alcohol during pregnancy is harmful to the growing baby and may result in a group of birth impairments known as *fetal alcohol syndrome*. (For more information, see "Alcohol," page 82.)

EATING SAFELY DURING PREGNANCY: FISH, MEAT, MILK, AND CHEESE

Food	Recommendations
Fresh Fish Shark, swordfish, king mackerel, tilefish Farmed salmon Albacore tuna ("white" tuna) Wild-caught salmon Shrimp, canned light tuna, canned wild salmon, pollock, and catfish	Do not eat Eat no more than 1 meal a month Eat no more than 1 meal a week Eat no more than 2 meals a week Eat no more than 3 meals a week
Deli Meats and Smoked Fish Deli meat spread (pâtés) Deli hot dogs or sausages, sliced (or airtight plastic–packaged) deli meat, deli smoked fish Canned or smoked fish or meat spread	Do not eat Do not eat unless you reheat to steaming hot Eat no more than 2 meals a week
Meat—Beef, Chicken, Pork Any meat that is rotten, raw, or undercooked	Do not eat
Milk and Cheese Unpasteurized milk, feta cheese, Brie cheese, Camembert cheese, blue-veined cheeses, Mexican-style queso blanco fresco Hard cheeses, semisoft cheeses like mozzarella, processed cheese slices, cream cheese, cottage cheese, yogurt made with pasteurized milk Skim or 1% pasteurized milk	Do not eat or drink Eat all you want Drink all you want

Reproduced with permission from the *Journal of Midwifery & Women's Health* 49, no. 4 (July–August 2004): 374.

SPECIAL ISSUES IN PREGNANCY

Coping with Nausea

A few lucky women have neither nausea nor vomiting during pregnancy, but about half of us have both nausea and vomiting during the first months of pregnancy. Mild to moderate nausea and vomiting may make you feel awful, but it will not hurt you or your baby. Generally, nausea goes away or diminishes greatly by the beginning of the second trimester.

The first steps in coping with nausea or vomiting in pregnancy are lifestyle and diet changes. Sometimes making these changes is all it takes to feel better. Nausea during pregnancy is worse if you are dehydrated or if the level of sugar in your blood is low from not eating often enough. Here are some strategies for managing nausea:

- Eat plain saltine crackers or dry toast in the morning before getting out of bed and anytime during the day when you feel nauseous.
- Eat small meals every two to three hours instead of three large meals.
- Avoid foods that have strong odors.
- Try eating foods that are high in carbohydrates, such as potatoes, noodles, or bread.
- Wait for 30 minutes after eating to drink liquids.
- Try sucking on a slice of lemon or lime.
- Do not lie down right after eating.
- Try sipping room-temperature carbonated drinks that do not contain sugar throughout the day.
- Try eating foods with ginger, such as ginger ale, ginger snaps, and ginger candies. Ginger is a proven remedy for nausea.[6]
- Try eating yogurt. Dairy products may make nausea and vomiting worse, but some women say yogurt is helpful.

- Avoid foods that are greasy, fried, spicy, or very hot.
- Try wearing an acupressure band. These wristbands have a "nugget" that is placed on the presure point inside of your wrist. They are often used for motion sickness. Although significant research studies have not been done on these, some women find them helpful for nausea, and they are safe.
- If taking your prenatal vitamins makes nausea worse, check with your health care provider about stopping the vitamins and taking only a folic acid supplement until the nausea goes away.

I was nauseous a lot of the time. Mostly I just wanted to eat comfort foods like macaroni and cheese. To handle the nausea, I tried a lot of things that my midwife or my friends recommended: extra B₆, ginger, acupressure bracelets, yoga poses, saltine crackers. . . . In the end, what worked the best was to eat all the time. I would eat something the minute I woke up, eat three meals, and eat a snack almost every hour. My husband made me smoothies in the morning, and I packed a bag of healthy snacks for work. In my case, they had to be filling—granola bars, hard-boiled eggs, trail mix—rather than the typical saltine crackers. The other thing that helped was to sip mint tea, hot or cold. By the middle of my second trimester, the nausea was mostly gone, and I was able to go back to eating many of the foods that I liked before I was pregnant.

If your nausea or vomiting is severe, there are several different medications that may help. Let your health care provider know if you have nausea that keeps you from eating or drinking enough or keeps you from being able to carry out your normal activities. Call your health care provider right away if you are not able to keep any food or fluids down for twenty-four hours.

My second pregnancy was different from the first in every way possible. It was planned this time around, and I knew from the very beginning that I was pregnant based on the symptoms my body expressed. I was faced with significant morning sickness again, only this time [a prescription medicine] was a lifesaver for me. It had a stronger, longer-lasting effect for me than lemons.

Coping with Constipation

During pregnancy, our blood volume increases and removes a lot of water from our digestive system. The hormones of pregnancy slow down the digestive system, and many women become constipated. It is usually easy to relieve constipation in pregnancy with diet and exercise. Here are some tips:

- Increase the amount of water you drink. Try to drink at least eight big glasses of water every day.
- Munch on dried fruit—prunes, apricots, or raisins—as a daily snack.
- Add whole grains and bran to your diet. Cooked brown rice is excellent for this, as are oat and wheat bran.
- Increase your intake of fresh fruits and vegetables.
- Try eating yogurt. Some women find that it stimulates digestion and eases constipation. It is easy to digest and is also a good source of calcium.
- Get some exercise every day. (For more information, see the "Staying Active" section of this chapter, beginning on the facing page.)
- Give yourself time. Taking a walk in the morning, drinking a warm cup of mint or ginger tea, and waiting for your body to signal you that it is time to have a bowel movement may be all you need to stay regular.

If diet and exercise don't relieve your constipation, check with your health care pro- vider. Some over-the-counter stool softeners and fiber supplements or medications may be helpful.

Cravings

Many women have food cravings during pregnancy. For some of us, a craving is a signal from the body that something is missing in the diet, but most of the time, cravings are just cravings. This is usually not a problem if what you crave provides nutrients and is not dangerous.

During my third pregnancy I had such intense cravings. I wanted cantaloupe and root beer. It wasn't a big problem—'cause cantaloupe was in season, fortunately—and I was able to eat lots of other foods. I just wanted that cantaloupe and root beer. No, not together!

Sometimes women crave things that are not food—like ice chips, clay, or dirt. This is known as *pica*. The desire to eat nonfood items may be related to your sociocultural background and may be associated with diets that are historically deficient in certain nutrients. Pica can be a problem, as nonfood items have no nutritional value and may contain toxins or bacteria that could be dangerous for you or your baby. If you find yourself wanting to eat nonfood items, talk with your health care provider.

TAKING CARE OF YOUR MOUTH

It is particularly important that you take care of your teeth and gums while you are pregnant. Women with periodontal disease during pregnancy may be more likely to have babies who are born too early or too small, although the evidence for this claim is mixed.[7] Some pregnant women get a condition known as *gingivi-*

tis that involves swollen gums; it increases the risk of *periodontitis*. Periodontitis is a bacterial infection of the gums and surrounding structures that can spread to the bones that support the teeth.

Another reason to keep your mouth as healthy as possible during pregnancy and after birth is that the primary bacteria that cause tooth decay can be passed from you to your fetus or infant. The fewer bacteria you have in your mouth, the less likely it is that your child will develop dental cavities.

Seeing your dentist before and during your pregnancy is an excellent idea, as is daily care of your teeth and gums. Make an appointment to see your dental health provider as soon as possible after you become pregnant and discuss how frequently you should be seen. You may benefit from more frequent visits—such as once every three months—during this time.

Your daily routine for dental care should include:

- brushing morning and night with a soft-bristle brush and a toothpaste containing fluoride, which prevents tooth decay, and triclosan, an ingredient formulated to prevent periodontal disease[8]
- flossing once a day

As mentioned above, some women develop painful, swollen gums (gingivitis) during pregnancy. You may be able to prevent this with daily oral hygiene procedures, but if it does happen, talk with your dentist about an antiseptic mouth rinse you can use.

If you need to have some dental work done during pregnancy, be sure to tell your dentist you are pregnant. Keep the following in mind:

- Routine X-rays should be avoided during pregnancy. Have X-rays done only if you experience a dental problem that requires them.

Whether pregnant or not, you should always insist upon a lead apron to cover your belly, torso, and neck whenever you get dental X-rays. This protects you as well as your baby from stray radiation.
- Treatment of periodontal disease in pregnant women is considered safe.[9]
- The local anesthetic used by dentists for doing fillings or tooth extractions or other dental work is generally safe during pregnancy.
- For pain after dental work, acetaminophen with codeine is most commonly prescribed during pregnancy, and is considered safe. You should not take ibuprofen or aspirin.
- Some types of fillings have mercury in them. Questions have been raised about their safety, but there is no evidence that they cause problems. However, alternative fillings are available.

STAYING ACTIVE

BENEFITS OF EXERCISE

Being physically active during pregnancy can help you:

- have more energy
- sleep better
- feel happier
- maintain a healthy weight
- avoid or manage back and joint pain
- improve your posture and avoid pain in your arms and hands
- avoid constipation, bloating, and swelling
- reduce your risk of gestational diabetes and avoid the need for insulin if you develop gestational diabetes
- reduce your risk of some blood pressure problems
- improve your muscle tone, strength, and

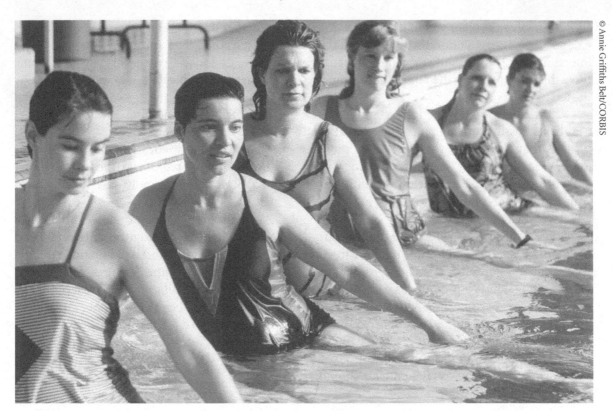

Group exercise sessions tailored specifically for pregnant women, like this water aerobics class, can help you stay active and meet other women who are pregnant.

endurance—which may help you through the hard work of labor![10]

BEING ACTIVE

If you have been physically active before, you can continue during pregnancy. If you weren't active before, now is a great time to start a daily walking or swimming program. Very few types of exercise are off-limits during pregnancy (see the list at the end of "Guidelines for Exercise," page 76). You may find that as your pregnancy progresses, you need to cut back on the intensity of your exercise routine. Let your body guide you.

You don't have to run a marathon every week to reap the health benefits of exercise. Getting 30 minutes of moderate physical activity most days is a good goal. The best exercise is exercise that you enjoy and that you can do regularly. Think about what will fit with your life.

For many women, walking is a great activity. It is free and it can be done in safe neighborhoods and malls. In order to get the most benefit, you have to walk pretty fast and swing your arms. Try to include walking in your regular routine.

Swimming is also excellent exercise during pregnancy. The water will support your pregnant belly, take strain off your back, keep you from overheating, and give you an overall massage. Water aerobics has many of the benefits of swimming. Many gyms and other community centers offer water aerobics classes especially for pregnant women.

Yoga is another great form of exercise. Yoga can promote muscle strength and flexibility, prevent and soothe back and joint pain, reduce stress, and help prepare the body for childbirth by opening the pelvis. Many yoga classes are designed specifically for pregnant women. If you take a yoga class that is not tailored for pregnant women, let the instructor know that you are pregnant so that she or he can modify activities that might be uncomfortable or unwise for you.

I've had back pain on and off since I was twelve. When I got pregnant, I was worried about what would happen when my belly got big—so many people had told me that was when their back pain started. Early in my pregnancy, a friend recommended the book Active Birth. *It has a mix of yoga and physical therapy exercises especially designed for pregnant women. I started doing the poses each morning, along with some specific exercises my physical therapist had given me. About halfway through my pregnancy, I found a prenatal yoga class, which was great. I really enjoyed the poses, and I loved getting to know other women who were also pregnant. I also tried to go for walks, do water aerobics, or swim a few times a week. To my surprise, my back pain actually got better, not worse, during my pregnancy! I did have my moments of aches and pains, but overall, I was pretty comfortable right up to the end. I think that the exercise—especially the yoga—really helped.*

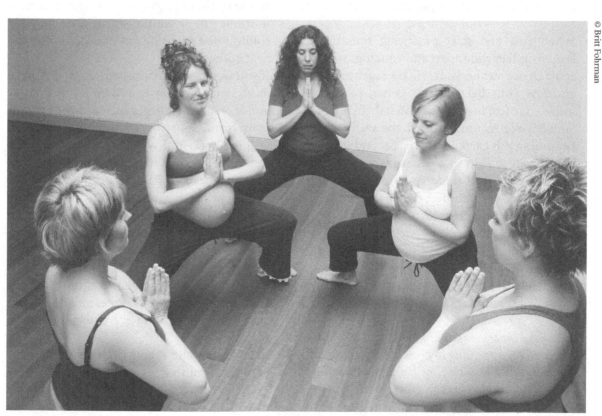

Squatting

One particular exercise that is helpful to pregnant women is squatting. Squatting is the natural position for giving birth. The pelvis is more open and gravity is on our side. But we don't do a lot of squatting in daily life in the United States or Canada (unlike people in some other parts of the world). As a consequence, we have a hard time squatting for labor even when we want to do so.

Squatting during pregnancy helps open the pelvis and strengthens the muscles needed for labor and delivery. If you are hoping to birth in the squatting position, discuss this with your health care provider and make sure the birth place you've chosen will allow it. Whether you plan to birth squatting or not, practicing squatting will help you during your labor and birth. A couple of tips to make squatting easier:

- When you first start practicing squatting, keep your feet wide apart and your toes wider apart than your heels. It will be easier to balance. As your balance gets better, you can move your feet in and straighten them.
- Squat while leaning against the wall when beginning this exercise. It is easier and safer.
- You may also find that squatting is easier if you put a support under your heels instead of trying to keep your feet flat on the floor. As you become more comfortable in the squat, you can lower the heel support gradually.
- If squatting is just too much, you can get many of the same benefits from sitting cross-legged on the floor. If it just doesn't work, don't worry about it.

There was a lot of complaining and most of it was from me. I gave up going to prenatal yoga class at seven months; I was tired of being reminded of how uncomfortable I was and how great some of the women felt. Sometimes the ligaments in my groin were so sore that it hurt to take a step or lift my foot on the stairs. And forget squatting—the position pregnant women are advised to practice every day—squatting made me cry.

Another set of exercises that may help you prepare for childbirth is pelvic floor (or Kegel) exercises. (For more information, see page 39.)

GUIDELINES FOR EXERCISE

General guidelines for exercise during pregnancy include the following:

- Wear comfortable clothing, including a well-fitting, supportive bra and comfortable shoes that are right for your activity.
- Drink lots of water to avoid dehydration and overheating.
- In the summer months, exercise in the early morning or evening or inside an air-conditioned building or mall to avoid the heat of the day.
- If you weren't exercising before you got pregnant, start start slowly and build up. For example, you might begin by walking out from your front door for 10 minutes and then walking back. You will have walked about a mile. If you do that five or six times this week, next week walk for 30 minutes at a time.
- Pay attention to your body. If you find yourself becoming exhausted, cut back on the intensity or duration of your activity.
- Be aware that your sense of balance shifts throughout your pregnancy. This is due not only to your growing belly but to hormonal changes that affect your bones and joints. Use care when performing exercises that involve balance.
- Keep an exercise log. It can be very encouraging and motivating to keep a log of your exercise—especially if exercising is new for you.

"Skiing was my salvation."

Edith Thys Morgan

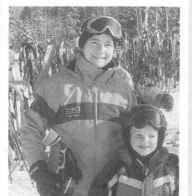

When I discovered I was pregnant in mid-August, my mind immediately raced forward to ski season. I had skied for thirty-one of my thirty-four years, and I didn't want my April 25 due date to force me off the slopes. I know, things as mundane as recreation should mean little when compared to creating a new life. But do women have to sideline the physical activities that keep us sane because we're pregnant?

First, I sought the counsel of my mother, expecting her to be on the conservative side. She had taken up skiing only a few years before my birth and surely would have exercised proper care. "Well, I don't remember exactly," she pondered, "but I know I didn't ski past your due date." So much for conservatism. I soon learned that pregnancy protocol has everything to do with where you live. Ask mountain dwellers, and they supply legends to accompany their business-as-usual philosophy. "My mother was skiing moguls the week I was born." "My wife skied the day before our daughter was born." "I went mountain biking when I was overdue."

Meanwhile, my urban friends were under the spell of the pregnancy police, the self-appointed experts who stalk you with advice and worries for nine months. "Don't do anything with your arms over your head or else the umbilical cord will wrap around the baby's neck." "Don't jog or you'll bounce the baby loose." And above all, "Don't ski because you might fall." Any form of recreation, it seemed, was tantamount to child abuse.

I decided to ignore all other advice and trust my doctor, whose casualness had immediately put me at ease. "No scuba diving or sky diving," she explained, "but other than that, you can do everything you did before. Just dial it back a notch or two."

This is not to advocate for skiing until your due date, or even skiing at all in pregnancy. Each woman's situation will be different. Fortunately, I had a very uncomplicated pregnancy through which I could stay active. Furthermore, as a former Olympic skier, I stress my body far less on skis than I do, say, walking or folding laundry.

Finally, I did dial it way back. I learned to ski early in the day, avoid crowds and daredevils, and mellow my own hard-driving technique to cruise control. With these modifications, skiing was my salvation. Working with gravity, my growing body still felt coordinated, agile, and liberated. Maybe skiing wasn't explicitly prescribed, but finding a way to stay healthy and happy while pregnant was exactly what the doctor ordered.

- Toward the end of your pregnancy, avoid exercises in which you lie flat on your back.
- Avoid extreme exertion, high-risk sports such as scuba diving and sky diving, and contact sports such as ice hockey and football. You also may want to avoid skiing, horseback riding, and other activities that could result in falls.

DEALING WITH DISCOMFORTS OF PREGNANCY

BACK PAIN AND BODY ACHES

During pregnancy, you will probably feel some discomfort in your back, arms, legs, or joints. Several factors may lead to this discomfort:

- Progesterone—one of the primary hormones of pregnancy—causes your joints and ligaments to loosen. This may cause aching in your hips and knees and even in your pubic bone.
- Your growing belly changes your center of gravity and may pull your neck, shoulders, and back out of alignment.
- The pressure of the growing uterus can constrict the veins and the nerves that go through the pelvis. This can lead to blood pooling in your legs, and to swelling, numbness, tingling, or cramping in your legs and feet.

Staying active may help avoid or manage the discomforts associated with these changes.

Most women have back pain at some point during pregnancy. The pain may be mild or severe, may be in your upper or lower back, or may be in your buttocks and radiate down your legs (a condition known as *sciatica*). Here are some strategies that may help prevent or reduce back pain:

- Exercise moderately. Moderate exercise—like walking each day—strengthens the back muscles, decreases muscle tightness and spasm, and keeps the joints in good position. Many women find swimming particularly helpful.
- Stretch regularly. This can include pelvic tilts (see illustration).
- If you are having back pain during the day, don't lie in bed for long periods of time.
- When you do lie down, avoid lying flat on your back.
- Try sleeping on your side in a "nest" of pillows or use a body pillow in your arms and between your knees.
- Avoid sitting for long periods of time. If you work at a desk, get up frequently and move around. You may also find that sitting on a birthing ball instead of a chair works better for your back.
- Take care to use good body mechanics when bending or lifting. Bend your knees, squat, get close to whatever you are trying to lift, and hold the object close to your body. When in doubt, get someone to help you.
- If you have back pain, alternate applying heat and cold packs on the part of your back that hurts. Twenty minutes of warmth followed by 20 minutes of cold often helps. A heating pad on a medium setting is a good heat source. Bags of frozen peas make handy ice packs.
- Treat yourself to a therapeutic massage, if possible.
- Wear comfortable, low-heeled shoes.
- Try an abdominal supporter.

POSTURE AND CARPAL TUNNEL SYNDROME

As our bellies grow, many of us compensate for the change in our center of gravity by arching our backs a bit. This change in posture, as well as the loosened joints caused by pregnancy

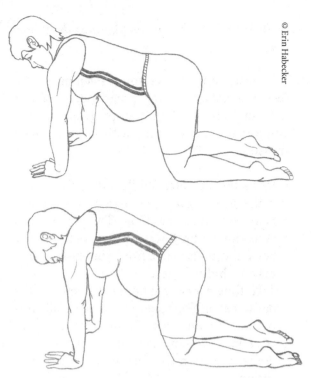

Pelvic tilt exercises can help strengthen your muscles and prevent back pain. Here's how to do them:

1. Get down on your hands and knees, keeping your back straight.
2. Slowly exhale, and tighten and pull in your stomach muscles so that your back rounds and arches upward. Hold for 5 seconds.
3. Slowly inhale as you relax and return to the first position.

Repeat as many times as you find comfortable. Over time, build up your number of repetitions to about 10 or 15.

hormones and the swelling caused by fluid shifts, may lead to backache and carpal tunnel syndrome—painful or numb wrists, hands, and fingers. For some women, carpal tunnel syndrome during pregnancy is very uncomfortable and interferes with everyday activities.

Sleeping during pregnancy always gets a little tricky toward the end, but the carpal tunnel syn-drome made it very hard. I found myself wishing I had detachable "Barbie" arms that I could take off at night, because if I turned onto my side at all that arm would be numb and throbbing within ten minutes. With my second pregnancy we got me a recliner to sleep in. This way I could stay off my sides, but not have to lie flat on my back.

To help with posture and prevent carpal tunnel syndrome during pregnancy, try the following:

• Wear a supportive, well-fitting bra, as changes in the size and shape of your breasts may be affecting your posture and comfort.
• Wear low-heeled, supportive shoes.
• Consider wearing an abdominal supporter (a wide elastic band that wraps beneath your belly), especially if you are carrying more than one baby.
• Pay attention to your posture and make it a point to consciously stretch and relax your shoulders every day. You can do this by "hunching" your shoulders up toward your ears and then relaxing them. Hold the "hunch" for a count of 10 and then relax. Rolling your shoulders in circles—10 times forward and then 10 times backward—may also help.
• Stretch and get moderate exercise.
• Drink plenty of clear water—at least eight large glasses every day.

If you do develop symptoms of carpal tunnel syndrome, you can try some home treatments:

• Continue all the strategies in the prevention section above.
• When you go to bed at night, make a "nest" for yourself with pillows that tip you slightly to one side and support your arms at your sides but slightly elevated.
• If you find that you curl your hands up dur-

ing the night, try using supportive wrist splints, which you can buy in most drugstores; they will hold your wrists in a neutral position while you sleep.

- Several times a day, exercise your wrists and hands by touching each of the fingers on the affected hand, one after another, to the thumb of that hand.

If carpal tunnel syndrome becomes severe, it may help to see a physical or occupational therapist and be fitted for custom wrist braces or have other medical treatment. Talk with your health care provider if you are having difficulty sleeping or doing your daily activities due to carpal tunnel symptoms.

SWOLLEN, CRAMPY LEGS

During pregnancy, the pressure of the growing uterus can slow down the return of blood from the legs. This may cause fluid to shift into the skin and muscles, producing swelling. It may also cause the blood to back up in the veins, producing varicose veins or making varicose veins you already have worse. In addition, the growing baby's need for fluid, vitamins, and minerals may cause the level of certain nutrients in the bloodstream to become too low, which leads to cramps. These changes can make for very uncomfortable legs, ankles, and feet.

The veins in my legs were increasingly swollen and sore. So every morning I'd have to pull on my therapeutic support hose. I was supposed to put them on before getting out of bed, but I'd usually be in a rush to pee and couldn't wait. Those hose were so tight, more than once I got a cramp in my hand trying to stretch one over my heel. Toward the end of the pregnancy, I'd get them all the way up over my belly and have to lie back down again, exhausted. Some days my two kids would watch, either laughing at the sight of their grunting and

oddly shaped mother or complaining about how long it was taking—or both.

Most women have some swelling in the feet and ankles during pregnancy. You can help minimize swelling, cramping, and the discomfort of varicose veins with some self-care measures:

- Drink lots of water. While it doesn't seem to make sense, getting enough water actually helps you avoid swelling. The water helps your kidneys flush waste products from your body and pulls water from your tissues that may be "hiding" there.
- Take time every few hours throughout the day to get off your feet. This is especially important if your work requires you to be on your feet for long periods. If possible, lie down. If you can't, lean to the side while sitting.
- Wear low-heeled, supportive shoes and avoid knee-high stockings that cut into your legs.
- A moderate-speed walk for 30 minutes each day will massage the muscles that support your veins and help prevent or ease varicose veins.
- Make sure you get at least 1,000 milligrams of calcium in your diet each day (see page 66). There is some evidence that getting enough calcium helps prevent leg cramps.

FATIGUE

Most women feel tired at some time in pregnancy. The first trimester, with its wildly changing hormone levels and huge physiologic changes, sends many women to the "nap couch" and most women to bed early at night. This fatigue often returns—but not usually so dramatically—in the third trimester, as your baby grows rapidly and your own body tries to keep up. The best thing you can do for yourself if you are feeling tired is to go with it. Ease up on yourself. Let go of some responsibilities for a while. Ask for some help from friends or family.

- If you work on your feet, try to build 10-minute breaks into your workday every couple of hours. When you do get a break, sit down and put your feet up, or lie down on your side.
- When you are at home during the day, take breaks. Set the alarm for an hour or so, and rest or nap. If it helps your comfort, lie on your side and maybe put a pillow between your legs when you sleep.
- Get some moderate exercise every day.

If you are so tired that you cannot walk or participate in your regular daily activities, talk with your health care provider. You may need to be tested for anemia or other medical conditions.

PROTECTING YOURSELF AND YOUR BABY

VIOLENCE AND ABUSE

Violent and abusive relationships can cause us to delay needed prenatal care or to deliver a premature or low-birth-weight baby. Physical violence and sexual abuse can also affect the fetus we are carrying. Freeing ourselves from violence may be the most important thing we can do to ensure our health and survival, and the health and survival of our children. (For more information, see page 104.)

WORKING DURING PREGNANCY

Most of us can continue working right up until we go into labor. All workplaces are required by law to be healthy and safe enough for women during pregnancy. If you work on your feet, take a break and sit down every couple of hours. If you work sitting down, take a break and walk around every couple of hours. In either case, keep some water close at hand so you can stay hydrated.

While you are pregnant, you have a right to job protection for up to twelve weeks. This means that even if you cannot do your job, your job must be held open for you during that time. Federal law does not require your employer to pay you for those twelve weeks, though, so even though your job will be there for you, the financial burden may be a consideration. You may be eligible for job transfer or paid or unpaid leave. Under an amendment to the federal Civil Rights Act, women "disabled by pregnancy" must be treated the same as other temporarily disabled workers, like those who have had heart attacks or accidents. (In this context, *disabled* is a legal term meaning "unable to work.") Some states also have pregnancy-disability acts.

If your employer has a policy that seems unclear or unfair on pregnancy, childbirth, or related issues, contact a committee on occupational safety and health (COSH) or other workplace health advocacy group for support.

TRAVEL DURING PREGNANCY

You can travel right up until you deliver your baby. Many health care providers advise against travel in the last four weeks of pregnancy, primarily because you might end up having your baby somewhere you didn't plan to. All types of travel are fine during pregnancy—unless you are an astronaut. Just keep the following guidelines in mind:

- Drink plenty of water while traveling. This can help you avoid swelling and headaches.
- Get up and go to the bathroom at least once every two hours. If you are traveling by car, stop hourly and get out and walk around. If you are traveling by air, walk up and down the aisle every hour or so.
- If you are traveling by air, leave your shoes on. The change in pressure during air travel can make your feet swell dramatically. If you take your shoes off at the beginning of the flight, you may end up having to depart from the plane barefoot.
- Most airlines do not permit women to fly during the last four weeks before their due date. Check this out when making your reservations.
- Consider packing your own food so that you have more control over your choices.
- If you are contemplating international travel, do some research to be sure that the place you are going has safe food and water.
- If you are traveling out of town, carry a copy of your medical records. Check with your insurance company about coverage far from home.

ALCOHOL

Alcohol use in pregnancy can be harmful to the growing baby. Heavy use of alcohol during pregnancy can result in a group of birth impairments known as *fetal alcohol spectrum disorders* (FASD). Children with FASD experience a range of physical disabilities, cognitive deficits, and behavior problems. It is estimated that about one in one hundred babies, including a disproportionately high number of American Indian and Native Alaskan babies, are affected by some form of FASD.[11] Prenatal alcohol exposure is one of the leading causes of birth impairments and developmental disorders in children.

There is no clear consensus on whether it is safe to drink small amounts of alcohol during pregnancy or how much alcohol it takes to put a fetus at risk. A recent meta-analysis found no evidence that low-to-moderate levels of alcohol use are harmful.[12] (The study defined low-to-moderate use as consuming less than 83 grams of alcohol in a week. Twelve ounces of beer contains 12.9 grams of alcohol; five ounces of wine contains 13.5 grams; and 1.5 ounces of distilled spirits [80 proof] contains 14 grams of alcohol.) However, because the threshold for harm is not known for sure, virtually all medical societies and expert groups recommend that women not drink alcohol at all during pregnancy. It is especially important to avoid drinking a large amount of alcohol at one time, particularly early in your pregnancy.

If you are drinking more than a small glass of wine or more than twelve ounces of beer a day, or any hard liquor regularly, and you can't stop, get help. (For more information, see "Getting Help with Alcohol, Drugs," page 85.)

TOBACCO

Smoke from tobacco is harmful to both you and your baby. This is especially true if you are the one smoking, but it is also true if you are exposed to secondhand smoke. Smoking and secondhand-smoke exposure damage your lungs, blood vessels, and heart, and make it much more likely that you will suffer from heart or lung disease at some time in your life. If you are smoking during pregnancy, your baby is exposed to harmful substances every time you inhale the smoke from a cigarette.

Women who smoke are more likely to have an ectopic pregnancy (a pregnancy where the fertilized egg implants outside the uterus) and to have abnormal bleeding during pregnancy. Babies whose mothers smoked while the babies were developing are smaller than babies whose mothers did not smoke. These small babies tend to have a more difficult time learning to breathe in the first moments of life and may struggle more to adjust to life outside the womb. After birth, babies exposed to secondhand smoke tend to grow more slowly and have more ear infections. They may have developmental delays and are at an increased risk for sudden infant death syndrome (SIDS).

Even when we know that smoking is bad for us and our babies, it is hard to quit. Most people who smoke make five to seven attempts to quit smoking before being successful. Pregnancy, and your concern for your baby, can be a great motivation to try to quit or cut back. The less you smoke, the less harm is done. If you can quit entirely, that will be even better for both of you.

If you are trying to quit, your odds of success will improve if you use some of the following methods: calling telephone "quit lines," using self-help materials and discussion boards on the Internet, attending classes or support groups, seeking counseling from your health care provider or a trained counselor, and avoiding secondhand smoke.[13] If you have been a heavy smoker, you may need nicotine replacement (patch, gum, or lozenge, all available over the counter, or nasal inhaler or spray, available by prescription) or a prescription medicine, bupropion (marketed under the name Zyban). Studies show that the risks associated with using nicotine replacement or Zyban are outweighed by the benefits of quitting smoking during pregnancy.[14]

If you smoke, let your health care provider know, so she or he can tailor your care to your needs.

CAFFEINE

Caffeine is a stimulant that tends to make us more alert and energetic. It is present in many commonly consumed foods, including coffee, tea, chocolate, and many soft drinks.

Caffeine affects the baby in the uterus: You drink a cup of coffee and get all buzzed up and so does your baby. But no lasting effects have been found after birth, as long as the daily consumption of caffeine is less than six 8-ounce cups of coffee each day (or about 150 milligrams of caffeine).[15]

More research is needed to clarify the effects of caffeine on pregnancy. Many women who consume significant amounts of caffeine during pregnancy also smoke cigarettes and/or drink alcohol, and the effects are hard to separate.

ILLEGAL DRUGS

The effects of illegal drugs on developing babies are not well understood. It is often difficult to separate the effects of the drugs from the effects of the home environment, alcohol and tobacco use, and poverty. Current evidence suggests the following:

- Women who use marijuana during pregnancy tend to have babies who are slightly smaller than the babies of women who do not use marijuana.
- Women who use cocaine (or any of its derivatives, such as crack) or methamphetamines are more likely to miscarry early in pregnancy or to experience *placental abruption* in the later stages of pregnancy than women who do not use cocaine. Placental abruption is when the placenta separates prematurely from the wall of the uterus, resulting in loss of oxygen to the baby. It is potentially deadly for the baby.
- Babies of women who use heroin or methamphetamine or one of many other street drugs are quite likely to be born addicted to the drug and to have to go through a withdrawal period that can be very difficult for them.
- Women who use opiates (e.g., heroin and morphine) during pregnancy are more likely to have miscarriages or stillbirths than women who don't use opiates.
- The use of cocaine and opiates during pregnancy may have a negative effect on the long-term development of babies, but the research is not definitive.[16]

Because illegal drugs can have serious health consequences for both you and your baby, it is best to avoid using them when you are pregnant. If you are unable to stop using drugs on your own, seek help. (For more information, see "Getting Help with Alcohol, Drugs," facing page.)

In a growing number of states, use of illegal drugs during pregnancy has been termed "child abuse" and has essentially been criminalized. The threat of arrest makes it difficult for drug-using pregnant women to seek prenatal care and help. Drug addiction needs to be addressed as a health issue, not a crime, and pregnant and parenting women need access to nonpunitive drug treatment services.

LEGAL DRUGS USED INAPPROPRIATELY

Drugs that are legal and prescribed by a health care provider can also become drugs of addiction if used inappropriately. Tranquilizers, sedatives, pain medications, and some kinds of amphetamines are often abused—sometimes unintentionally. Some women begin taking a medication for a specific problem and then become addicted. If this has happened to you, talk with your health care provider or seek help through a treatment program. Your provider can help you wean yourself from the drugs or can prescribe medications that will help you transition back to living drug free. (For information, see "Getting Help with Alcohol, Drugs," facing page.)

MEDICINES AND HERBAL TREATMENTS

With very few exceptions, everything you put in your mouth or inhale into your lungs when you are pregnant crosses the placenta and goes to your growing baby. This is true for almost all medicines and herbs, just as it is with food and drink. Keep the following thoughts in mind whenever you are making a decision about taking a medicine or herbal therapy during pregnancy:

- During the first trimester of pregnancy (the first 12 to 14 weeks), your baby is developing amazingly quickly. Babies are most vulnerable to toxins during this time.
- Talk with your health care provider before taking any medication or herbal therapy.
- If you are looking for more information about medications or herbal therapies, use reputable sources. Try to avoid getting your information on a drug or herbal treatment from the company that produces it. (For sources of good health information, see "Resources," page 325.)

Medicines

In the United States, all drugs go through an approval process at the Food and Drug Administration (FDA) before they are made available to the public. This testing is meant to protect the people taking the drugs from harm. Unfortunately, the testing that is done rarely includes specific testing on the effects of the drug on a developing baby. This is because the testing would have to be conducted on pregnant women, which would be dangerous and unethical. As a result, there is much we don't know about the effects on pregnancy of many drugs currently on the market.

In the United States, the FDA categorizes all medications for use in pregnancy. The categories are:

- **A.** Controlled studies in women taking these drugs have not demonstrated a risk to the developing baby in the first trimester, and there is no evidence of risk in later trimesters. The risk of harm to a developing baby appears remote.
- **B.** Animal studies have shown no risks for

these drugs, and the drugs have not been tested in pregnant women, *or* animal studies on these drugs may have shown a risk to the animal fetus, but controlled studies in women have not shown the same effect on human babies. These drugs are probably safe, but if there have been animal studies showing risk, those raise concerns.

- **C.** Animal studies have shown a risk of fetal harm from these drugs, but there are no controlled studies in women; *or* there are no studies in animals or women on reproductive effects of these drugs. Unfortunately, most drugs fall into category C. The safety of using them during pregnancy is unknown.
- **D.** There is evidence that these drugs may harm developing human babies, but the benefit of the drug may outweigh the risk of the harm. If you are taking a category D drug to preserve your own health or life, you will need to talk with your health care provider to weigh the risks and benefits.
- **X.** These drugs have been shown to cause problems for the developing baby, and the risks that come with using the drugs during pregnancy clearly outweigh any benefit. These drugs should not be used during pregnancy.[17]

Deciding which medicines to take during pregnancy, whether for a chronic condition or a new health problem, can be difficult. Some medicines that are taken without concern when you are not pregnant can cause disabling conditions for your baby if you take them during pregnancy, and a few can cause problems with the growth of your baby in your uterus. In most cases, there are alternative medicines or lower doses that can keep you healthy while protecting your baby.

Ideally, if you have a chronic health condition, you will have an opportunity to talk with your health care provider before you become pregnant so that you can make decisions about your medication before your baby is exposed. If you have just discovered you are pregnant and have been taking prescribed medicines, talk with your health care provider as soon as possible to make decisions about them. Stopping some prescription medicines quickly can cause problems, so it is wise to discuss changes with a knowledgeable provider.

No matter what your circumstances, doing your own research, talking with your health care provider, and seeking out support from knowledgeable organizations can help you make good decisions about medication during pregnancy. (For information about how a mother's exposure to certain medicines and other substances can affect the developing fetus, see www.motherisk.org/index.jsp.)

Sometimes it is better to take some medicine rather than take no medicine and end up in a worse situation. I had bad headaches with one of my pregnancies. It was my first experience with migraines. I didn't want to take any medicine at all, so I let one headache get so bad I started throwing up from the pain and had to be admitted to the hospital to have antinausea medicine and pain medicine so I could avoid dehydration. After that, my doctor advised that I take over-the-counter pain relief medicine at the onset of a headache, and I was able to avoid having such bad headaches.

Herbs

Many women think that because herbs are "natural," they are always safe. This is not true. Herbs can be potentially dangerous, just like other medicines. If you use an herbal treatment regularly or are considering using one during your pregnancy, do some research and talk it over with your health care provider.

In the United States, herbs are categorized

as supplements, not drugs. Because of this, the FDA does not have the same control over testing and labeling requirements for herbs as it does for conventional medicines. Manufacturers do not have to provide proof that the herbal therapy works or is safe, and they do not have to guarantee the consistent strength of their herbal products. As a result, accurate information about herbal therapies during pregnancy is even more difficult to find than accurate information about conventional medicines.[18]

OTHER TOXINS

It seems that hardly a day goes by without some warning of possible toxins in our food, our drinking water, the air we breathe, or our environment in general. You can easily make yourself crazy trying to keep up with all the recommendations and avoid everything that is potentially dangerous. The task is especially difficult because most research is done with nonpregnant volunteers first, and it may be years before a potentially dangerous substance is tested with pregnant women. There is a lot of conflicting information out there, and we often have to make decisions when much may be unknown.

If you can manage it, avoiding *solvents* during your pregnancy is a good idea. Solvents—like those used in working with artificial fingernails—have been connected with early miscarriage and long-term learning difficulties in children exposed in utero. Women who are exposed to solvents day after day are at most risk.[19] If you are a woman who works with solvents—applying and removing artificial fingernails, working with dry-cleaning chemicals, or house painting, for example—you can give yourself some protection by taking care to keep your work area well ventilated.

Concerns have been raised about *hair dye*, but research has not been conclusive. Some early studies showed a possible link to childhood brain tumors, but later studies contradicted those results.[20] If you dye your hair, you may want to wait until after the first trimester, to have someone else apply the dye, and to use supermarket brands rather than the stronger beauty parlor dyes.

Some *pesticides*, including some that may be used around homes and on farms, have been linked to miscarriage.[21] If your home needs to be sprayed during your pregnancy, stay out during the spraying and try to stay away for a day or two to allow the fumes to clear. Be sure to wash all your dishes and utensils after a home spraying.

As with drugs, food, and drink, if you are struggling to avoid something in the environment, put most of your energy into the first trimester (the first 12 to 14 weeks of pregnancy). This is the time period in which a developing baby is most vulnerable.[22]

KEEPING IT ALL IN PERSPECTIVE

Pregnant women are bombarded with advice and warnings all the time. Some of what we read and hear seems to imply that if we don't do everything perfectly, we are putting ourselves or our babies at great risk.

I mean, must they [pregnancy books] be so alarmist? 'You didn't paint your toenails before you knew you were pregnant, did you? Don't worry—if you're lucky, at least one hemisphere of your baby's brain should still develop normally.' It's as if you're already a bad mother—doomed from the get-go. And that whole 'best bite' pregnancy diet? Please. 'Is that the very best bite for the baby?' Michael likes to tease when I'm hunched like a criminal over a pack of gummy bears. 'Be sure to indulge yourself at least once a

CATS, STEAK TARTARE, AND GARDENING

Toxoplasmosis is an infection caused by a very tiny, common parasite. Most people who get toxoplasmosis feel like they have the flu. The illness comes and goes, and nothing really bad happens. During pregnancy, however, toxoplasmosis in the mother can cause an infection in the baby. A baby exposed to toxoplasmosis while in the womb—especially during the first trimester—may suffer blindness or brain damage. Toxoplasmosis infection in pregnant women is very rare, but potentially serious. By following some of the recommendations below, you can lower or even eliminate your risk for this illness.

For many years, pregnant women have been told to get rid of our cats or not touch them in order to avoid toxoplasmosis. It is true that cats—especially outdoor cats—may carry toxoplasmosis, but the parasite is also found in uncooked meat, garden soil, and untreated drinking water. You can't get toxoplasmosis from touching these things, but you can get it if you swallow or breathe in the parasites.

Here's how to protect yourself and your baby from toxoplasmosis infection:

- Avoid cat feces. If possible, have someone else clean out the litter box while you are pregnant. If you must clean out the box yourself, do it daily, as the toxoplasma eggs take a couple of days to become infectious. Wear gloves and a face mask and wash your hands thoroughly after cleaning the box. If your cat jumps up on the kitchen counters, be sure to wash the counters well before preparing food or eating.
- Keep your cat indoors. Outdoor cats eat birds and rodents and may pick up the parasite in that way. If your cat stays indoors and eats only canned or dry food, there is very little chance that its feces would have toxoplasma eggs.
- Wash your hands with soap and water after working in the garden.
- If you eat meat, cook it all the way through.
- Wash your hands and all food preparation surfaces and utensils before and after preparing food, including fruits and vegetables.

week,' the book advises. 'A fruit yogurt makes a nice treat.' A fruit yogurt! As if. A pound of cookie dough washed down with a quart of half and half—now that makes a nice treat.[23]

The conflicting and often rigid advice we hear can make us feel anxious, undermine our confidence in our bodies and ourselves, and contribute to the "climate of doubt" about birth so prevalent in today's culture. While making healthy individual choices and working together toward a safe environment are worthy goals, it's important to remember that women have an inherent capacity to grow and nurture our babies and that women in all sorts of circumstances around the world give birth to healthy babies. Remembering this can help us keep our perspective, celebrate our pregnancies, and reclaim the climate of confidence that we deserve during pregnancy.

NOTES

1. American Academy of Pediatrics, "Folic Acid for the Prevention of Neural Tube Defects," *Pediatrics* 104, no. 2 (August 1999): 325–327.

2. Food and Nutrition Board, Institute of Medicine, *Dietary Reference Intakes for Vitamin A, Vitamin K, Arsenic, Boron, Chromium, Copper, Iodine, Iron, Manganese, Molybdenum, Nickel, Silicon, Vanadium and Zinc* (Washington, DC: National Academy Press, 2001).

3. A. Rumbold, P. Middleton, and C. Crowther, "Vitamin Supplementation for Preventing Miscarriage," *Cochrane Database of Systematic Reviews* 2005, Issue 2. Art. No.: CD004073. DO1: 10.1002/14651858.CD 004073.pub2. See also Anjel Vahratian, Anna Maria Siega-Riz, David Savitz, and John Thorp, "Multivitamin Use and the Risk of Preterm Birth," *American Journal of Epidemiology* 160, no. 9 (November 2004): 886–892; Andrew Czeizel and Erica Medveczky, "Periconceptional Multivitamin Supplementation and Multimalformed Offspring," *Obstetrics & Gynecology* 102, no. 6 (December 2003): 1,255–1,261; L. C. Loffredo, J. Souza, J. Freitas, and P. Mossey, "Oral Clefts and Vitamin Supplementation," *The Cleft Palate—Craniofacial Journal* 38, no. 1 (January 2001): 76–83; and G. M. Shaw, L. Croen, K. Todoroff, and M. Tolarova, "Periconceptional Intake of Vitamin Supplements and Risk of Multiple Congenital Anomalies," *American Journal of Medical Genetics* 93, no. 3 (July 2000): 188–193.

4. Lisa M. Bodnar, Gong Tang, Roberta B. Ness, Gail Harger, and James M. Roberts, "Periconceptional Multivitamin Use Reduces the Risk of Preeclampsia," *American Journal of Epidemiology* 164 (2006): 470–477, accessed at http://aje.oxfordjournals.org/cgi/content/full/164/5/470 on September 12, 2006.

5. Lester Crawford, "Fish Is an Important Part of a Balanced Diet," U. S. Food and Drug Administration (March 2004), accessed at www.fda.gov/oc/opacom/hottopics/mercury/mercuryop-ed.html on June 3, 2006. See also U.S. Department of Health and Human Services and U.S. Environmental Protection Agency, "What You Need to Know About Mercury in Fish and Shellfish: 2004 EPA and FDA Advice for Women Who Might Become Pregnant, Women Who Are Pregnant, Nursing Mothers, Young Children" (March 2004), accessed at www.cfsan.fda.gov/~dsm/admehg3.html on June 3, 2006; Institute for Agriculture and Trade Policy, "Minnesota Smart Fish Guide: Safer, Sustainable Fish Consumption for Healthier Children and a Healthier Environment," (April 2004); and Katherine Mieszkowski, "Tuna Meltdown," salon.com (June 22, 2006), accessed at www.salon.com/news/feature/2006/06/22/tuna/print.html on June 22, 2006.

6. Rachel Westfall, "Use of Anti-emetic Herbs in Pregnancy: Women's Choices, and the Question of Safety and Efficacy," *Complementary Therapies in Nursing & Midwifery* 10, no. 1 (February 2004): 30–36. See also Galina Portnoi, Lu-An Chng, Lida Karimi-Tabesh, Gideon Koren, Michael Tan, and Adrienne Einarson, "Prospective Comparative Study of the Safety and Effectiveness of Ginger for the Treatment of Nausea and Vomiting in Pregnancy," *American Journal of Obstetrics and Gynecology* 189, no. 5 (November 2003): 1,374–1,377; and Mary Lou Moore, "Complementary and Alternative Therapies," *Journal of Perinatal Education* 11, no. 1 (2002): 39–42.

7. B. S. Michalowicz, J. S. Hodges, A. J. DiAngelis, et al., "Treatment of Periodontal Disease and the Risk of Preterm Birth," *New England Journal of Medicine* 355, no. 18 (2006): 1,885–1,894.

8. J. C. Gunsolley, "A Meta-analysis of Six-Month Studies of Antiplaque and Antigingivitis Agents," *Journal of the American Dental Association* 137 (2006): 1,649–1,657.

9. Michalowicz et al., "Treatment of Periodontal Disease."

10. Melanie Poudevigne and Patrick O'Connor, "Physical Activity and Mood During Pregnancy," *Medicine and Science in Sports and Exercise* 37, no. 8 (August 2005): 1,374–1,380. See also Jennifer Dempsey, Carole Butler, and Michelle Williams, "No Need for a Pregnant Pause: Physical Activity May Reduce the Occurrence of Gestational Diabetes and Preeclampsia," *Exercise and Sports Science Reviews* 33, no. 3 (July 2005): 141–149.

11. P. A. May and J. P. Gossage, "Estimating the Prevalence of Fetal Alcohol Syndrome: A Summary," *Alcohol Research & Health* 25, no. 3 (2001): 159–167. See also *Fetal Alcohol Syndrome: Diagnosis, Epidemiology, Prevention, and Treatment,* ed. K. Stratton, C. Howe, and F. Battaglia, Committee to Study Fetal Alcohol Syndrome, Division of Biobehavioral Sciences and Mental Disorders Institute of Medicine (Washington, DC: National Academy Press, 1996).

12. J. Henderson, R. Gray, and P. Brocklehurst, "Systematic Review of Effects of Low–Moderate Prenatal Alcohol Exposure on Pregnancy Outcome," *BJOG: An International Journal of Obstetrics & Gynaecology* 114 (2007): 243–252.

13. Centers for Disease Control and Prevention, Chapter 4, "Management of Nicotine Addiction," in *2000 Surgeon General's Report: Reducing Tobacco Use,* accessed at www.cdc.gov/tobacco/data_statistics/sgr/sgr_2000/00_pdfs/chapter4.pdf on May 17, 2007.

14. U.S. Department of Health and Human Services, "The Health Consequences of Involuntary Exposure to Tobacco Smoke: A Report of the Surgeon General" (2006), accessed at www.surgeongeneral.gov/library/secondhandsmoke/report.pdf on July 11, 2006.

15. Mark Klebanoff, Richard Levine, John Clemens, and Diana Wilkins, "Maternal Serum Caffeine Metabolites and Small-for-Gestational-Age Birth," *American Journal of Epidemiology* 155, no. 1 (January 2002): 32–37. See also G. Koren, "Caffeine During Pregnancy? In Moderation," *Canadian Family Physician* 46, no. 4 (April 2000): 801–803; and L. D. Devoe, C. Murray, A. Youssif, and M. Arnaud, "Maternal Caffeine Consumption and Fetal Behavior in Normal Third-Trimester Pregnancy," *American Journal of Obstetrics and Gynecology* 168, no. 4 (April 1993): 1,105–1,111.

16. Marylou Behnke, Fonda Eyler, Tamara Warner, Cynthia Garvan, Wei Hou, and Kathleen Wobie, "Outcome from a Prospective, Longitudinal Study of Prenatal Cocaine Use: Preschool Development at 3 Years of Age," *Journal of Pediatric Psychology* 31, no. 1 (January–February 2006): 41–49. See also Seetha Shankaran, Abhik Das, Charles Bauer, Henrietta Bada, Barry Lester, Linda Wright, and Vincent Smeriglio, "Association Between Patterns of Maternal Substance Use and Infant Birth Weight, Length, and Head Circumference," *Pediatrics* 114, no. 2 (August 2004): e226–e234; and Lynn Singer, Sonia Minnes, Elizabeth Short, Robert Arendt, Kathleen Farkas, Barbara Lewis, Nancy Klein, Sandra Russ, Meeyoung Min, and Lester Kirchner, "Cognitive Outcomes of Preschool Children with Prenatal Cocaine Exposure," *JAMA: The Journal of the American Medical Association* 291, no. 20 (May 2004): 2,448–2,456.

17. Springhouse, *Nursing 2005 Drug Handbook*, 25th ed. (Philadelphia: Lippincott Williams & Wilkins, 2005).

18. Diane Born and Mary Barron, "Herb Use in Pregnancy: What Nurses Should Know," *MCN: The American Journal of Maternal Child Nursing* 30, no. 3 (May–June 2005): 201–208.

19. Dionne Laslo-Baker, Maru Barrera, Dafna Knittel-Keren, Eran Kozer, Jacob Wolpin, Sohail Khattak, Richard Hackman, Joanne Rovet, and Gideon Koren, "Child Neurodevelopmental Outcome and Maternal Occupational Exposure to Solvents," *Archives of Pediatrics and Adolescent Medicine* 158, no. 10 (October 2004): 956–961. See also C. Till, Gideon Koren, and Joanne Rovet, "Prenatal Exposure to Organic Solvents and Child Neurobehavioral Performance," *Neurotoxicology and Teratology* 23, no. 3 (May–June 2001): 235–245.

20. Erin McCall, Andrew Olshan, and Julie Daniels, "Maternal Hair Dye Use and Risk of Neuroblastoma in Offspring," *Cancer Causes & Control* 16, no. 6 (August 2005): 743–748. See also Gerhard Nohynek, Rolf Fautz, Florence Benech-Kieffer, and Herve Toutain, "Toxicity and Human Health Risk of Hair Dyes," *Food and Chemical Toxicology: An International Journal Published for the British Industrial Biological Research Association* 42, no. 4 (April 2004): 517–543; and Elizabeth Holly, Paige Bracci, Mi-Kyung Hong, Beth Mueller, and Susan Preston-Martin, "West Coast Study of Childhood Brain Tumours and Maternal Use of Hair-Colouring Products," *Paediatric and Perinatal Epidemiology* 16, no. 3 (July 2002): 226–235.

21. Stephanie Brundage, "Preconception Health Care," *American Family Physician* 65, no. 12 (June 2002): 2,507–2,514.

22. Keith Moore and T.V.N. Persaud, *The Developing Human: Clinically Oriented Embryology* (Philadelphia: W. B. Saunders Company, 1998).

23. Catherine Newman, *Waiting for Birdy: A Year of Frantic Tedium, Neurotic Angst, and the Wild Magic of Growing a Family* (New York: Penguin Books, 2005).

CHAPTER 6

Relationships, Sex, and Emotional Support

During your pregnancy, your feelings may shift from joy and contentment to melancholy, with a whole range of possibilities in between. Many women report heightened perceptions, increased energy, and feelings of being in love during pregnancy. You may feel special, fertile, potent, and creative. You may also have surprisingly strong negative emotions and thoughts: "I'm losing my individuality." "I don't want to be a mother." "I'll never be sexy again." "I'm ambivalent about this baby growing in me." "I'm angry, scared, worried, tired, sick, in shock." "I feel so alone."

Negative or anxious feelings are natural. Most of us feel more positive as we get used to being pregnant, become attached to the growing baby, and prepare for labor and birth. Yet even during the most desired pregnancies, many of us have moments, hours, or days of anxiety, confusion, and feeling blue. Pregnancy may challenge and transform our relationships, whether intimate sexual partnerships or connections with friends and family. It also may shift our sense of self.

We can take active steps to find support and learn ways to cope better with the challenges of pregnancy. By taking care of ourselves and our emotional well-being, we foster the resiliency we will need as new mothers.

CHANGING IDENTITY

Whether you are single or in a committed partnership, over forty or in your teens, rich or poor or middle class, being pregnant will transform your identity and call on your emotional strengths and resources. You may gain confidence in your own abilities as your body accommodates to the new life growing within you. Learning to trust ourselves and our bodies during the changes of pregnancy, birth, and parenthood can help us as we face other challenges throughout life.

Yet if you have seen yourself as committed to your career, or as someone who does what she wants when she wants to, motherhood may not seem like a good fit. You may fear it will stifle your spontaneity, end your travel and hobbies, or curtail your career advancement. You may worry that others will see you as less strong and capable once you become a mother, or that you will lose your individuality, fall into economic dependence on a partner, or slip into your mother's identity. Thinking about ways in which you can maintain some continuity with your previous sense of self while celebrating and embracing the positive changes that will come with motherhood can help you navigate this transition.

I was always considered the "intellectual" one of the family, and I guess I became attached to this identity myself. So much so that I had moments of doubt that I could also be a good mother—that somehow being an intellectual would be incompatible with motherhood. I had to learn to trust in myself and believe that I was ready to grow into this new role just as my baby was growing inside of me. And that in becoming a mom, I was not leaving my "old self" behind, so much as expanding (physically and psychologically!) to incorporate both my old and new selves.

Depending on your relationship to your own mother and your experience of childhood, you may be fearful of being like your mother or fearful of not being as good a mother as she was. You may fear that you will not have time to spend with your friends, or that your friendships will be strained if your friends do not have children. Whatever concerns come up for you, it will take some time to resolve them as you get used to your new role.

For my husband and me, it was the first time in our marriage that we were moving away from being children ourselves and into [being] parents. At our birth class, there was a form that was titled "To the Parents." We looked at each other and said, "Why do we have to give this to our parents?" We both shrugged, and then slowly realized that it was not for our parents, that it was for us.

CHANGING RELATIONSHIPS

As a pregnant woman, you are moving into a new role. Your relationships with your partner, friends, and relatives—particularly your parents and siblings—may shift, too. Ideally, the people close to you can be a source of emotional support. But you may find that you need to seek out role models for mothering in people other than your own female relatives. Perhaps you will find role models in neighbors, friends, or coworkers. You may find it helpful to talk with other women about how they experienced the changes both in their sense of self and in their relationship to others in their lives. You are in the midst of an ongoing process of developmental change, and will learn as you go.

FRIENDS AND FAMILY

After finding out that I was pregnant . . . I was a bit freaked out. I was twenty years old, still in college, just moved back in with my mom temporarily, my boyfriend and I weren't exactly serious. I loved kids, but never thought about being a mom yet. . . . I [went] to work for the day and . . . a few hours [later], not being able to concentrate on a single thing, I called my mom and told her my news. I can't remember her exact reaction, but I do remember she wasn't angry. I think we both were trying to figure out how to be able to do this. . . . Up to that point we hadn't really had the

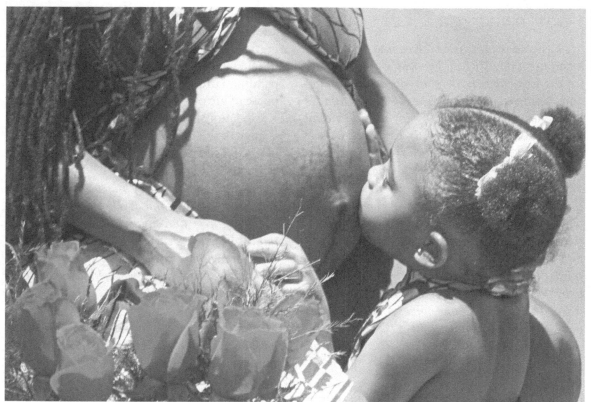

best relationship, but she stepped up and was really amazing.

Friends and relatives can offer you encouragement and information while you are pregnant. When women you know have had safe and satisfying birth experiences and their messages are supportive, you absorb their confidence, which makes it easier to approach birth joyfully and positively. If their experiences are more negative or they share "horror stories" with you, try to talk with others as well, and read stories by women whose births will offer you a more inspiring vision as you prepare for birth.

My mom had a lot of miscarriages, and one of my brothers passed away when he was three. During each of my pregnancies, I would think of my mom, and I would wonder: "Am I going to have this

baby? Am I going to go through this?" A lot of what my mom told me affected me and it was scary. Fortunately, I didn't have those experiences.

It is common to have fears and anxieties while standing on the threshold of the enormous and permanent change of becoming a mother. Not all fears and anxieties require "treatment." Rather, they require tolerance, patience, and compassion. Try acknowledging your anxieties as they arise, but not getting caught up in them. If you want to talk with other women about how they are navigating shifts in their relationships and sense of themselves, you may find support in childbirth classes and exercise classes designed for pregnant women, as well as on websites that offer information for pregnant women. (For more information, see "Getting Support," page 99.)

YOUR PARTNER'S FEELINGS

My husband made sure he talked into my belly at least once a day. "T.K. ('The Kid,' our nickname for the first baby) hears your voice all the time and I want to make sure he/she gets used to mine." It was fun for me to see how playful and sincere he was about this project of his. He sang, he read baby books, he read spy novels—just whatever struck his fancy. No matter what kind of stressful day I had had at work or how tired I was of the extra weight and bulk, I always loved the attention he gave my belly. When I was pregnant the second time, he nicknamed the baby A.K., for "Another Kid," and when I was pregnant the third time (in three years), he nicknamed the baby Y.A.K., for "Yet Another Kid." We never learned the gender of our babies until they were born, but it was important to our bonding with the babies and each other to give them a moniker.

If you have a partner, his or her feelings, questions, hopes, and fears are probably as complex as your own. Many partners will want to be actively involved in preparations for the arrival of your child.

My husband attended birthing classes with me, and the preparation brought us much closer together. He was very into having the bag for going to the hospital packed and would worry that we wouldn't be ready. The classes gave him checklists and made him feel included. Another way that he dealt with impending fatherhood was to completely strip the wallpaper in the nursery-to-be and paint and paper the whole room in a weekend. He needed to be a true provider and he was providing the space for the new baby.

Expecting a child can be a challenging period for couples. Both partners suddenly lose time for themselves and each other. Roles are being renegotiated, and concerns about the unknown surface. Your partner may be wondering: "How will my life change?" or "Can I juggle the financial and personal demands of an expanding family?" For some, entering this new phase of life may bring up fears of mortality.

Relationships between partners may change dramatically during pregnancy, particularly if other major shifts are taking place.

I was used to being very independent and felt very much on the same level as my husband in terms of career and finances. When I got pregnant, I began to depend on him to do more, in terms of my share of tasks, etc., and then when I decided not to go back to work, I had a hard time adjusting to my new role.

At times your partner may be feeling tired, left out, or neglected, or may find it hard to support you. Try to involve your partner in your pregnancy, so that the two of you can prepare, plan, and learn together. Childbirth classes offer guidance that can alleviate concerns about labor and delivery (see page 35). Preparing together often strengthens relationships and can create a buffer against resentment. Some couples choose to dedicate time together to non-baby-related activities, too, so that the baby is not always the center of the relationship.

You and your partner may find it helpful to talk about the fantasies you each hold of the other as a parent and what you expect of yourselves and each other. This way, you are sharing the experience of change and are able to begin to differentiate between your fantasies and the realities of early parenting.

I never felt so close to my partner as when I was pregnant. We had been trying to have a child for several years, so when I became pregnant the miracle of it all was present for us every day. We both read everything we could get our hands on to make the pregnancy the healthiest possible, and together we prepared wholesome foods, took . . . walks, and prepared the house for the new life that would turn us from a couple into a family. We took the journey together and it made us stronger.

In the best of circumstances, your partner can reflect back to you the ways in which you are changing, and help you care for yourself and receive care from others. If your partner cannot provide the support and reassurance you need, seek out a friend or family member who can. You may also want to seek counseling. (For more ideas, see "Getting Support," page 99.)

SEXUALITY

During my second trimester, sex was fabulous. I hadn't expected to feel sexy with a bulging belly, but I felt very sexy pregnant, and I was much more in awe of my body being able to make a life. All the anxiety surrounding cellulite and those few extra pounds was nothing compared to being pregnant, and I enjoyed those moments of not being so self-conscious of my body during sex. We were not worried about [preventing] pregnancy anymore and we were freer to enjoy the spontaneity of unprotected sex. I was also so hormonal that I'd be demanding sex daily. It was the only time in our relationship that he actually said, once, "I really can't, I'm absolutely exhausted."

Most of us discover that our sexuality changes in some way during the course of pregnancy. While some of us find that our sexual desire is stronger, others lose it completely. Often, we find that our orgasms feel different, or they make take longer to achieve than before or happen more quickly. Some women experience orgasm for the first time during pregnancy, while others become multiorgasmic. This is probably because increased blood flow and fluids in the genital area make the clitoris and vagina more sensitive.

CHANGES DURING PREGNANCY

For many women, sexual desire decreases during the first trimester of pregnancy due to fatigue, breast tenderness, and nausea. Other women find the freedom of not having to worry about birth control or conceiving makes sex more enjoyable. By the second trimester, many women feel less nausea and experience heightened sexual desire.

I felt sexy as soon as I started to show—but my husband was freaked out by the idea of making love to a pregnant woman.

Some of us enjoy our new curves and changing bodies without feeling hindered by them. Others may feel clumsy, awkward, or less sexually attractive. Your partner and others close to you can play a key role in helping you feel good about the changing contours of your body, but they may need to be told how much their acceptance and explicit comments make a positive difference.

As your body changes during pregnancy, you may need to try different sexual positions to find what is comfortable for you. Some women discover new or increased sexual pleasures during pregnancy because of such experimentation. "Spooning" while sitting up offers plenty of room for manual stimulation, side-lying allows for comfortable oral stimulation, and experimenting with pillows and support devices can help enhance and support a variety of positions and activities. Positions in which you face away from your partner can help with breast tenderness, as can wearing a sports bra.

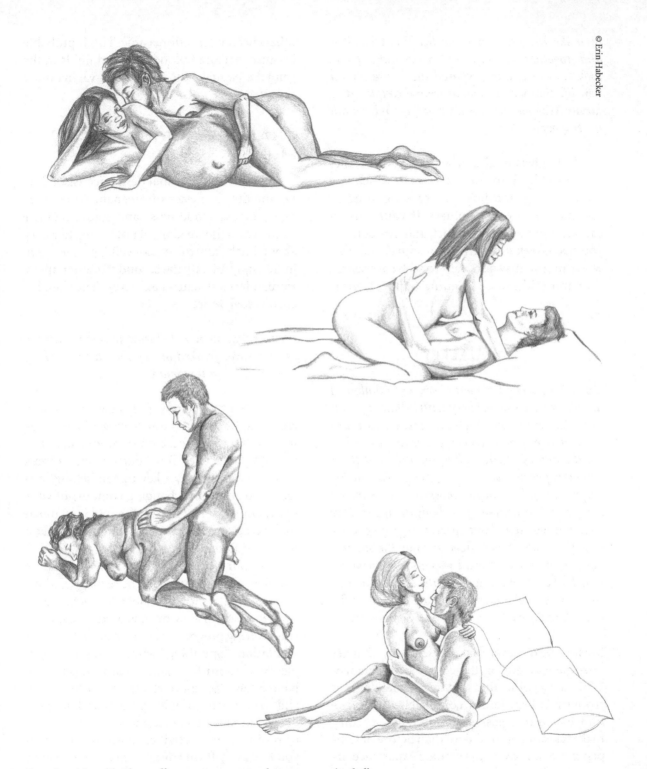

© Erin Habecker

Sexual positions like these offer ways to accommodate your growing belly.

By the time you are about halfway through pregnancy it may be uncomfortable to lie on your back during sex. If you feel sick or faint when on your back, it could be because the enlarged uterus is pressing on blood vessels in the lower part of your body. Be guided by how you feel and explore other positions to learn what makes you comfortable.

Due to a sense of fullness, some women find vaginal penetration uncomfortable at some points during pregnancy and opt for manual, oral, or self-pleasuring sex instead. This can be a period to explore various kinds of touch and find creative ways to enjoy our sensuality. If you want to continue having intercourse, the following positions may be helpful:

• pregnant partner on top (This puts no weight on your abdomen and allows you to control the depth of penetration and clitoral placement.)
• rear-entry or side-lying positions

• face to face: sitting on a sturdy chair, edge of the bed, etc.
• whatever is fun, is safe, and feels good

Some cramping after making love is normal throughout pregnancy. Your uterus contracts during orgasm and these contractions might be more noticeable during pregnancy as the uterus gets bigger. It can feel as if your uterus gets hard for a few minutes.

If you are past your due date and you want to induce labor, people may tell you that having sex will help. The evidence on this is mixed. (For more information, see page 148.)

PRECAUTIONS

Unless you are experiencing pregnancy complications, it is safe to continue having an active sex life until your water breaks or you are in labor. Sexual activity does not cause miscarriage and will not hurt your baby. The baby is

SAFER SEX

If you have unprotected sex with a partner whose sexual history is unknown to you or with someone who has a *sexually transmitted infection* (STI), you risk contracting an STI such as herpes, genital warts, chlamydia, or HIV. If you become infected, the disease may be transmitted to your baby, with potentially dangerous consequences. Safer sex practices can protect you from sexually transmitted infections. These practices include using a condom for intercourse and using a dental dam (a flat piece of latex that prevents transfer of bodily fluids) or condom during oral sex.

If you are sharing sex toys, either use a condom for each use or wash the toys well after each use. If you engage in anal intercourse, wash the penis or dildo with warm soap and water before inserting it into the vagina to avoid infection. Also be sure to use enough lubricant for comfort and to prevent injury.

(For more information on STIs and safer sex, see the chapters "Sexually Transmitted Infections" and "Safer Sex" in *Our Bodies, Ourselves*.)

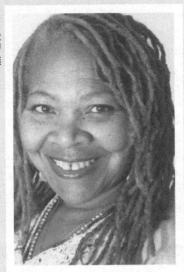

© Arnold Trujillo

MENTORS FOR MOTHERS-TO-BE

Kathryn Hall-Trujillo believes that supportive friendship and community can help women through pregnancy and improve health outcomes. That's why she created Birthing Project USA, a nonprofit organization dedicated to keeping babies alive by helping expectant mothers get the care, education, and support they need.

Birthing Project USA primarily serves women of color, but welcomes all women in need of support. Its unique approach involves the volunteer efforts of "Sister Friends." These are women in each community who are trained to navigate the health care system and provide one-on-one mentorship for a woman through pregnancy, birth, and her baby's first year of life. One participant in the program recalls:

My pregnancy was not planned. My baby's father was not thrilled about it, and neither was my family. I was living with my sister at the time and our relationship was not close. But having a "sister friend" made being pregnant a wonderful experience. I was able to understand the changes in my body and how to deal with the emotional part of pregnancy. I still remember that day my "sister friend" went with me to the hospital. She picked me up at 6:30 A.M. She stayed with me at the hospital until I delivered. She was the only one with me when my baby arrived into this world.

In keeping with an extended-family model, the project celebrates milestones in children's lives as they grow. It also offers a program for fathers.

Hall-Trujillo, who is a former public health program adviser for the state of California, says that Birthing Project babies tend to be of better birth weight than expected for African-American babies because the mothers more often carry them to 40 weeks rather than the 36 weeks average for African-American women. She credits social support for this difference.

Birthing Project USA has helped ensure the health of more than ten thousand babies since 1988. The group has expanded into eighty-six communities in the United States, Canada, and Honduras. (For more information, contact Birthing Project USA at 1-888-657-9790 or www.birthingprojectusa.com.)

kept safe by the amniotic sac, cervix, and uterine muscle. There is also a thick mucous plug that seals the cervix and protects the baby from infection.

You may need to abstain from some or all sexual activity if you have symptoms of preterm labor; vaginal bleeding; leakage of amniotic fluid; *placenta previa* (when the placenta is covering the cervix); or what is called "incompetent cervix," a condition in which the cervix is weakened and dilates (opens) prematurely, raising the risk for miscarriage or premature delivery. (For more information on these conditions, see Chapter 8, "Special Concerns During Pregnancy.")

If you are experiencing these pregnancy complications, your health care provider will advise you to stop having sex. Be sure to talk openly with your provider about why, and what specifically she or he recommends that you stop doing. If you have preterm labor, you will want to avoid uterine contractions; therefore, nipple stimulation and orgasms are not a good idea. With other conditions, these sexual activities are fine, but you should avoid vaginal penetration.

SUSTAINING YOUR EMOTIONAL WELL-BEING

Many of us feel overwhelmed and exhausted at times during pregnancy. Finding support and other ways to take care of ourselves at these times can help foster the resiliency we need to cope with the challenges of pregnancy.

You can take care of your emotional well-being in many ways: You may call a friend, go for a walk, cry, join a water aerobics class for pregnant women, make love, make art, garden, seek spiritual guidance, watch a funny movie, protest an injustice, cook, write in a journal, or find your own creative, individual response.

One key to staying "sane" was a weekly prenatal yoga class I began taking [during] my tenth week of pregnancy. . . . Yoga kept me focused on all the positive, miraculous things happening within my body. The strengthening and limbering work we did in class gave me more energy and [helped me feel] fit and pain-free for the duration of my pregnancy. I also listened to a relaxation CD that helped a lot with visualization and breathing techniques. I rested as much as I could and napped when I felt like it. I had to remind myself that I wasn't lazy if I let some tasks and activities slide: I was pregnant, after all, and there are few things more important than maintaining perspective and avoiding stress at such a precious time in your life.

GETTING SUPPORT

As during other times in our lives when we experience great changes or challenges, having good support is key. Women who are supported by a partner, friends, and/or family cope better with stress during pregnancy and are less likely to feel anxious or depressed.[1] Yet finding support can be difficult. One hurdle for many of us is asking for the help we need.

There were certainly people I could have relied on for support during my pregnancy with the twins, like my mother, mother-in-law, and friends. But I felt I didn't want to burden anyone with my worries. My mother was busy with a demanding full-time job, and besides, she was able to do it all with four kids without help. My mother-in-law was there and not working but I had the fear of appearing weak in her eyes so I rarely asked her for help.

Local support groups for pregnant women can be great sources of support and practical information. Special swimming and yoga sessions for pregnant women may provide you

WAYS TO TAKE CARE OF YOUR EMOTIONAL WELL-BEING

- Pay attention to what you think and feel. Identifying and understanding the sources of distress in your life are the first steps toward coping.
- Eat well, get enough rest, and be physically active. These wellness strategies can help you feel calm and more resilient. Exercise and regular movement in particular can help you release the pain of anger, grief, fear, or depression.
- Stay connected to people you care about; develop and nurture your relationships. Consider joining a support or common-interest group; reach out to neighbors.
- Cultivate peace of mind and relaxation. Some of us find meaning and comfort in meditation, prayer, or being part of a religious community. Others relax through activities such as singing, painting, reading, or gardening. Engage in activities that foster your gratitude, appreciation, and compassion.
- Work for social/political change. When the stressors in our lives are too big and powerful to tackle on our own, working with friends, neighbors, or colleagues to change the conditions that make our lives difficult can give us a sense of purpose and help us see our individual concerns within a larger societal context.

with such a group. Many groups offer emotional support for women with specific concerns (for example, depression) or identities (over forty, lesbian, etc.). Birth Networks are a specific type of support group dedicated to providing women with information about research regarding best birth practices, informed consent, informed refusal, and providers who will help you work toward the goal of a safe and satisfying birth. Most Birth Networks use the Internet to distribute information. (Although Birth Networks operate independently, the Lamaze Institute maintains information about them; to find one near you, go to www.lamaze .org/institute.) If there is no support group in your community, you may want to start one. (For more information about childbirth classes and support during labor and birth, see Chapter 3, "Preparing for Childbirth.")

While you're pregnant, you may also want to think about what type of support you will need after you give birth and line it up in ad-

vance. (For more information about postpartum support, see page 282.)

I was lucky in that I knew about five other women who were pregnant at the same time as me. It was so helpful to compare "war" stories. And certainly women who were not pregnant got really tired of our obsession! I think that hearing all kinds of stories helped me keep things in perspective and realize that we all have our own experience of pregnancy and labor and not to think it's going to be or has to be any certain way.

PROBLEM SOLVING

Knowing when to take action is an important part of effective coping. Although we can't control all of the external circumstances of our lives, if we can focus on solutions to specific problems, we are more apt to take the actions that will ultimately benefit us. Problem solving during pregnancy may involve reassessing a relationship, seeking out advice or support, changing a schedule, or fighting for a cause. When our relationships are a source of stress, working together to learn effective communication styles can be extremely helpful. You may also need to set boundaries, say no, take time for yourself, or seek outside help if you continue to feel a lot of stress or anxiety.

STRESS MANAGEMENT

Some women use specific techniques to help manage the stress of our everyday lives. Meditation, prayer, deep breathing, yoga, t'ai chi, and a variety of other techniques, such as mindfulness, imagery, and progressive muscle relaxation, may help us relax. Some of us also use them as part of our spiritual practice. Many of these techniques have two components in common: the *focusing of attention* through repetition of a word, prayer, phrase, or physical activity; and the *disregard of everyday thoughts* when they occur. Specific techniques can be learned through classes, books, and videos.

Many of us find that small relaxation breaks throughout the day—taking a few deep breaths, or creating a soothing image to focus on (like swimming in a cool pool), or doing gentle stretches—help us relieve tension.

DEPRESSION DURING PREGNANCY

People sometimes assume that pregnant women are always joyous and enthusiastic, but this isn't true. We also experience ambivalence, fear, sadness, and sometimes anxiety or depression that may require special help. According to some estimates, about one in every ten pregnant women experiences some depression, which is about the same rate as for women who are not pregnant. Yet pregnancy can make de-

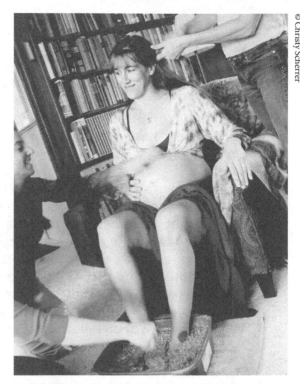

Community rituals have long been used to help pregnant women through the transition of becoming a mother. A baby shower or other creative ritual may offer you both practical and emotional support. Blessingway ceremonies like this one focus on celebrating and pampering the mother-to-be.

pression more difficult to diagnose. For example, sleep disturbances and lack of energy could be related solely to pregnancy, but they could also be related to depression. You may be depressed if you experience significant changes, including total loss of pleasure in activities that you used to enjoy; persistent feelings of worthlessness, sadness, or hopelessness; stark changes in appetite; prolonged periods of fatigue; uncharacteristic tearfulness; and suicidal thoughts. About half of all episodes of postpartum depression begin during pregnancy and may also be accompanied by persistent, intense anxiety that does not respond to reassurance or the

HOW TO MEDITATE

To try a simple form of meditation, follow these steps:

1. Assume a comfortable position and close your eyes.
2. Take a few deep breaths to calm your mind and body. Inhale deeply, allowing your abdomen to expand. As you exhale, imagine that you are blowing out a candle.
3. Then concentrate on a mental focus, such as a sound or word or phrase or prayer that you repeat silently to yourself in rhythm with your breath.
4. If a thought or something from the outside world distracts you, take a deep breath and return to your mental focus. Instead of getting caught up in an internal dialogue, gently redirect your attention to your out-breath, focus word, or phrase. You will find that with time and practice, this redirection becomes easier.
5. Continue for 10 to 20 minutes. (Place a clock nearby, so that when you feel your time is up, you can take a quick look and then choose to continue or stop.)
6. Take a few slow, deep breaths, stretch, and slowly open your eyes.

usual support needed by women during this period.

Women may feel depressed during pregnancy because of hormonal changes; the circumstances of the pregnancy (for example, an unplanned pregnancy or a hostile or unsupportive partner and/or family); severe and extended nausea; earlier experiences with infertility and/or pregnancy loss that may give rise to anxiety about the current pregnancy; obstetric complications; or a long period of bed rest.

I became depressed during my second pregnancy. . . . I had very little emotional support during that pregnancy and my daughter became very sick for a few months, the stress of which triggered an intense emotional roller coaster in me. It turned out that I had an ovarian cyst that was too big to be removed until my son was two months old, so I had to have major surgery when my son was an infant. Also, my son had terrible

colic until he was six months old. But we did get through it, and the process taught me a lot about myself, ultimately making me a better parent. . . . My advice would be to go to therapy if you can or feel you need to, and surround yourself with other mothers . . . [and] deepen the connections you already have.[2]

Ever since my eighteenth week of this pregnancy, I have been feeling depressed. I feel flat/unhappy all the time, I cry a lot, I can't sleep, I can't concentrate, I'm impatient with everyone, and not even playing with my toddler makes me happy anymore. This is a much-wanted pregnancy and there is nothing going on in my life that should be making me so unhappy. My only explanation is the high hormone levels in my body right now (I was at my all-time best while nursing, when hormone levels are quite low!).[3]

Depression can affect your ability to care for yourself during pregnancy and to care for yourself and your baby after giving birth. Depression in pregnant women is associated with low weight gain, alcohol and substance abuse, and sexually transmitted infections, all of which can harm mothers and babies.[4] In addition, depression may make bonding with your baby difficult, thus possibly affecting your baby's overall development.

Whether you have experienced depression before or you experience new symptoms during pregnancy, it is important to seek help. You can begin with making sure you have enough sleep, exercise, good food, and practical help with coping with any stressful situations. Seek emotional support by reaching out to friends and family, talking with your health care provider or religious counselor, or joining a specialized support group. If such support is not enough to help you through a difficult period, ask for assistance from a mental health professional—such as a counselor, social worker, or psychologist—who is knowledgeable about depression in pregnancy. A skilled therapist can provide support and guidance, assess whether medications may be helpful for you, and, if necessary, refer you to a provider who can prescribe them.

If you cannot find an appropriate therapist or if your insurance won't cover therapy, ask your prenatal care provider to recommend a psychiatrist, clinical nurse specialist, or other medical provider who is experienced with prescribing medication. The potential benefits and harms of antidepressant medicines during pregnancy should be considered on an individual basis, taking into account the severity of your depression.

Many medicines for depression belong to a class of drugs known as *selective serotonin reuptake inhibitors* (SSRIs).* SSRI medications include Prozac, Zoloft, Paxil, Luvox, Celexa, and Lexapro. Wellbutrin, Remeron, and Effexor are also widely prescribed; while these drugs are not SSRIs, they act on the brain in similar ways. All of these drugs are considered "second-generation" antidepressants because they have largely replaced the older tricyclic antidepressants. These psychotropic medicines affect the central nervous system and may restore emotions or moods to normal.

While antidepressant medications are widely believed to be effective and are clearly helpful for some people, there is some controversy over how effective and how safe they are. One large review of research studies found that these drugs are only slightly more effective than placebos. The 2006 FDA review looked at 372 placebo-controlled antidepressant trials that included nearly a hundred thousand people. It found that four out of ten people who received a placebo improved, while five out of ten people who received an antidepressant improved. This means that only one additional person out of ten responded to treatment with antidepressants.[5]

Like many drugs submitted for FDA approval, the second-generation antidepressants have often been studied only for relatively short periods of time before being approved, and their negative effects, such as sexual problems, tend to be downplayed or even concealed by the companies that sell them. One rarer effect, *akathisia* (a severe state of agitation and restlessness that can lead to suicide), can be confused with other, similar states of agitation and distress.[6] You should use drugs such as these only under the care and guidance of an experienced psychiatrist or other professional who will monitor you regularly for certain behavioral and psychiatric changes, including increases in suicidal thinking, that may warrant a change in medication.

The potential problems with SSRIs must

* It is misleading to refer to these medications as "selective," because they are not necessarily selective. The more appropriate term is *SRIs*, but it is not commonly used.

be weighed against observational evidence that pregnant women who stop taking antidepressant medication are more likely to experience symptoms of depression than women who continue with the medication.[7] Although it is wise to avoid medication during pregnancy unless it is absolutely necessary, severe depression can be harmful to both a woman and her baby, so medication may be the best treatment for some women.

Some health providers may recommend reducing an SSRI gradually before the birth of a baby to reduce the effects on a breast-feeding infant, but this approach must take into account your level of depression and your ability to tolerate reduced medication. (For more information about breast-feeding and medications, see page 263.)

Sometimes depression is confused with *post-traumatic stress disorder* (PTSD), a condition in which a woman experiences flashbacks, panic attacks, and nightmares. If this distress is treated with antidepressants, the woman may be even less able to cope. However, one of the complications of PTSD is that it can also lead to depression. Some women who have had traumatic birth experiences develop PTSD in another pregnancy. It is also possible for women who have experienced traumatic events in childhood (in particular, sexual abuse) to have a resurgence of anxiety and PTSD-type symptoms during pregnancy.[8] (For more information about the effects of sexual abuse on pregnancy, see following section.)

Pregnant women who are struggling with other problems, such as *bipolar disorder* (commonly called "manic depression") and anxiety, may be offered other medicines in addition to or instead of the second-generation antidepressants. If a doctor suggests any medicine, make sure that you are fully informed about all the possible benefits and adverse effects of the medicine. You can consult the package insert, which is available from your pharmacy or on the Internet at www.fda.gov/cder. You and your health care providers can also get free information on the possible pregnancy effects of medications from a teratology* information service. (For detailed information, go to www.otispregnancy.org/otis_fact_sheets.asp or call 1-866-626-6847 if you don't have Internet access.)

SEXUAL ABUSE AND DOMESTIC VIOLENCE

THE EFFECTS OF SEXUAL ABUSE

Some of us have experienced sexual abuse in childhood or as adults. The aftereffects of abuse vary in severity, but they can last a long time. Abuse issues are sometimes triggered unexpectedly during pregnancy, labor, and birth, in the form of conscious memories or flashbacks to the abuse, or unconscious body memories (tension, anger, sick feelings, or other discomfort) when a woman is reminded of the abuse in some way.

Common triggers for those of us who are survivors include vaginal exams or other invasive procedures, and pain during or after childbirth, especially in the vagina, but also in the abdomen, back, breasts, and perineum. Our interactions with our care providers—authority figures who may expect compliance and trust—may remind us of our perpetrator or perpetrators, with whom we may have felt helpless, unequal, submissive, or overpowered. Control—over our bodies, our contractions, or the emergence of the baby—and being controlled by the baby, whose needs come before our own, can be major issues for us. We may associate a

---

* Teratology is the study of the causes and biological processes leading to abnormal development and birth defects.

lack of control with being abused. We may have learned that remaining in control is essential to safety and being out of control is threatening.

Reminders during pregnancy or labor to "relax and it won't hurt," to "yield" or "surrender" to the contractions, to "trust your body" or "do what your body tells you to do" may have an effect opposite to the one intended, if we have learned to guard against giving up control in abusive situations. Abuse experiences may also leave us feeling that our bodies are damaged and untrustworthy.

HOW TO RESPOND TO THESE CONCERNS DURING CHILDBEARING

1. Recognize and accept that some fears and concerns make sense. Sexual abuse (or any other abuse) rarely leaves the victim free from aftereffects. Give yourself permission to be afraid or concerned.
2. Try to separate your present pregnancy and upcoming birth and parenthood from your past abuse. Now you are older and more able to bring your wisdom and self-knowledge to these new challenges. Consider working with a trauma therapist or counselor who is knowledgeable about childbearing, or reading books for survivors that contain suggestions for dealing with triggers and reducing your concerns. (For help in locating resources, see "Hotlines" page 330.)
3. Decide whether or not to disclose your abuse history, along with issues it has brought up for you, to your care provider. Some caregivers are interested in emotional issues and are both willing and able to respond to your needs, while others may not have the skills needed to help you. If you are comfortable disclosing your history to your midwife or doctor, you can work together to plan your care so that it will be sensitive to your history. If you are uncomfortable with your provider, you may want to change to another person with whom you can establish a trusting relationship.
4. If possible, have a doula (birth assistant) at your birth, one whom you trust. Share your fears or concerns with her, so that she can help you deal with them. She does not need to know about your abuse history in order to provide emotional support and help. (To learn more about doulas, see page 33.)
5. Write a birth plan that is friendly and flexible yet clearly explains your preferences and fears. (To learn more about birth plans, see page 37.)
6. If you have a partner or other support person, enlist his or her support in dealing with this. You may want to tell your support person about specific settings or examinations that make you uncomfortable and work with her or him ahead of time on some ways to help you in these situations.

With good communication, self-help tools, and caring support from your loved ones, doula, and health care providers, your chances of having a rewarding pregnancy, birth, and postpartum experience are greatly increased.

VIOLENCE

Physical assault, rape, sexual abuse, and psychological and emotional abuse can result in health problems for pregnant and birthing women and for infants. The vast majority of this violence is inflicted by husbands, boy-

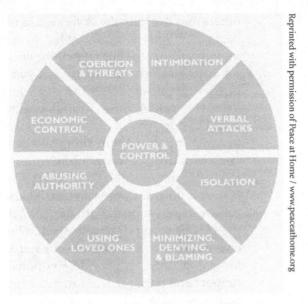

The Power and Control Wheel, developed by the Domestic Abuse Intervention Project of Duluth, Minnesota, is one model for understanding the dynamics of violence and abuse.

friends, partners, and other family members. Violence in intimate relationships can prevent women from getting necessary health care, choosing when we become pregnant, and protecting ourselves against sexually transmitted infections.

My partner said he hated condoms and wouldn't use them. He got very angry and threatening and [had intercourse with me] anyway. It wasn't until *I found out I was pregnant that they told me I had the virus, too.*

Domestic violence can cause us to delay our prenatal care or deliver a premature or low-birth-weight baby. It can also cause trauma to the fetus.[9] Exposure to violence and trauma also makes us more likely to use cigarettes, drugs, and alcohol, putting us and our babies at risk.

I tried to stop drinking when I found out I was pregnant, but then my husband began to resent the pregnancy. So I continued to drink with him to prevent a blowup, even though I knew it could hurt the baby.

Pregnancy and childbirth offer a chance for women who are being abused to receive help. In private prenatal visits with our health care providers, separate from our partners, we can talk about violence in our relationships. Health care providers should tell us about the warning signs and the dynamics of domestic violence and refer us to appropriate services within our community. There is no need to suffer alone when confronted by an abusive partner.

Leaving a violent relationship can be very difficult. The emotional ties that bind relationships are frequently most powerful when we are pregnant or have just given birth. We are

GETTING HELP

Toll-free, twenty-four-hour national hotlines such as the National Domestic Violence Hotline (1-800-799-SAFE, or 1-800-799-7233) can connect you with help in your area.

also vulnerable, and we depend on our partners for help and support. Although we may hope that a violent partner will change and become a loving parent, we also may fear that if we try to stop the violence, worse things may happen. During the process of leaving an abusive relationship, we need to create a good safety plan and use the resources of battered-women's programs, the police, the courts, and health care providers.

Freeing ourselves from violence in our relationships may be the most important thing we can do to ensure our health and survival, and the health and survival of our children. Becoming a mother may propel us to take action.

He abused me for a long time, punching me, kicking me, and burning me with his cigarettes. But when I came home from the hospital and my baby was crying and he threw him into his crib, I knew I had to leave. I couldn't let him do it to my kid.

FINDING SUPPORT

Each of us has different sources of support for celebrating or coping with the emotions that our pregnancy brings up. Good prenatal care, safety in our work lives and homes, and financial security are all vital to sustaining emotional well-being during pregnancy. In addition, our emotional well-being is supported when we have loving, caring people in our lives; nourishing food to eat; time to rest and to exercise; guaranteed paid maternity leave; and encouragement from confident, skillful health care providers. Yet many women do not have access to these essential supports. Some of these factors are beyond our personal control and will be improved only with broader social and political advocacy. (For more information, see Chapter 18, "Advocating for Mothers and Families.")

Other factors may respond to changes we can make ourselves. We can develop coping strategies—from laughing with friends to going swimming, writing in a journal, or joining a support group—to boost our resiliency. As your pregnancy progresses, try to engage in activities that will promote your health: taking time for socializing, for relaxation, and for building relationships that are meaningful to you.

NOTES

1. R. H. Glazier, et al., "Stress, Social Support, and Emotional Distress in a Community Sample of Pregnant Women," *Journal of Psychosomatic Obstetric Gynaecology* 25, nos. 3–4 (September–December 2004): 247–255, accessed at www.ncbi.nlm.nih.gov/entrez/query.fcgi?db=pubmed&cmd=Retrieve&dopt=AbstractPlus&list_uids=15715023&queryhl=7&itool=pubmed_DocSum on October 10, 2006.
2. Excerpted from "Depression During & After Pregnancy," a series of personal stories and advice on the Berkeley Parents Network website, accessed at http://parents.berkeley.edu/advice/pregnancy/depression.html on February 26, 2007.
3. Excerpted from "Depression During & After Pregnancy," accessed at http://parents.berkeley.edu/advice/pregnancy/depression.html on February 26, 2007.
4. American College of Obstetricians and Gynecologists, "Committee Opinion No. 354: Treatment with Selective Serotonin Reuptake Inhibitors During Pregnancy," *Obstetrics & Gynecology* 108 (2006): 1601–1604.
5. L. Jones and M. Stone, "Clinical Review: Relationship Between Antidepressant Drugs and Adult Suicidality," Food and Drug Administration, Center for Drug Evaluation and Research, accessed at www.fda.gov/ohrms/dockets/ac/06/briefing/2006-4272b1-index.htm, on November 16, 2006, p. 41.
6. This treatment-induced form of severe agitation occurred in most clinical trials of SSRIs, where research participants receiving the drug dropped out at a rate

of 5 percent for agitation compared with a rate of 0.5 percent for those who had a placebo. Up to 20 percent of people in clinical trials show short-term increases in agitation/anxiety, but the severity is not enough to cause a person to drop out of the study.

7. L. S. Cohen et al., "Relapse of Major Depression During Pregnancy in Women Who Maintain or Discontinue Antidepressant Treatment," *JAMA* 295, no. 5 (February 1, 2006): 499–507, available online at www.womensmentalhealth.org/topics/PDF/cohen_relapse_JAMA.pdf.

8. Sheila Kitzinger, *Birth Crisis* (New York: Routledge, 2006.)

9. Jana L. Jasinski, "Pregnancy and Domestic Violence: A Review of the Literature," *Trauma, Violence, and Abuse* 5, no. 1 (January 2004): 47–64.

CHAPTER 7

Prenatal Testing

For many of us, the months of pregnancy are filled with anticipation, mental preparation, and fantasy about life with our child-to-be. We dream about the child's and the family's future. As prospective parents, we might imagine our child smiling, walking, talking, playing, going to school, making friends, playing sports, falling in love, leaving home, taking a job, and someday also becoming a parent.

Often we have many expectations about what our lives will be like with a new child. We imagine a child who will give us joy and possibly make us proud someday. Perhaps we are counting on sharing our favorite interests with our child. We might wish for a girl because we think we will be closer to her than we would be to a boy. Or we might prefer a boy this time because we already have a girl.

Ever since the 1970s, it has been possible to get information during pregnancy about characteristics of the developing baby. In recent years, the number of tests available to pregnant women has multiplied, allowing increased scrutiny of the fetus. Usually, women choose prenatal testing to learn about health problems, diseases, or disabilities that might occur, but sometimes women want to know the baby's sex or to learn for sure who the father of the child is. As technology changes, more and more information about the baby will likely be available through testing—future height or predisposition to health problems that may occur in later life.

Some prenatal tests provide information about characteristics of the developing baby, while other tests give information about the mother's health. Prenatal tests that provide information about your health, such as blood testing to find out if you are anemic, have gestational diabetes, or are HIV-positive, are important because they detect conditions that often can be treated. (For more information about them, see Chapter 4, "Your Developing Pregnancy and Prenatal Care.")

This chapter focuses on tests that detect information about the developing baby. Because learning about the health of the fetus is the most common reason that doctors or midwives offer testing and is usually why women want it, this chapter concentrates on testing for conditions that can affect the health of your baby. The chapter also raises questions about other information that tests can provide.

Tests are available for a variety of conditions—some considered "mild," some considered "severe," and some that affect life expectancy. If you learn through prenatal testing that your baby will likely be born with a correctable, treatable, or lifelong impairment, you may want to make special plans before the child's birth. Or you may decide to end the pregnancy if you know that your future child would have a disabling condition.

While prenatal tests may offer useful information, they also raise concerns. Rarely, some tests lead to miscarriage or have other adverse effects on women and babies. Even when they do not cause medical problems, tests can create anxiety and expense and add to the medicalization of pregnancy and birth.

I was really nervous when my husband and I were about to have the ultrasound to determine the sex of our baby. Part of me wanted to change my mind and not go through with the ultrasound. I was thinking, "Can this test cause any harm to the baby, even though the doctor said no? Do I really want to know the sex after all? How will I know how to decorate the nursery? Is this really the halfway point? We can finally choose a name and start identifying the baby by name." I had so much on my mind I couldn't relax.

I had a CVS [chorionic villus sampling; see page 121] done, which was both physically and emotionally painful. We found out there were some irregularities, so I ended up needing an amnio as well. It turned out the irregularity was some

fluke in the test, and we finally got a clean bill of health [for the fetus]—six months into the pregnancy. The waiting was excruciating. To be pregnant but not be able to let yourself feel the joy and hope of it was truly horrible.

Tests for fetal traits give us the opportunity and the responsibility to decide whether we want to become parents of a child with a particular set of characteristics. Some of us may decide that we don't want this information. Others of us will be extremely eager to know all we can about our developing baby. Your doctor or midwife may strongly recommend testing, but it should not be automatic; decisions about testing are up to you.

As you consider testing, think about what you want to know about the fetus during your pregnancy and how knowing might influence your actions and decisions. Decisions about whether to have prenatal testing and what to do about the results are very personal. Many factors, including your feelings about parenting, disability, and abortion; your upbringing; and the community you live in, will influence your decisions. The way that your health care provider presents your options can also influence you.

In addition to raising difficult personal decisions, prenatal testing raises ethical questions for society. As more tests are available, will there be increased pressure on women to abort any fetus with an impairment? Will fewer resources be available for those of us who choose to continue such a pregnancy? Does the ability to test for disabilities and for sex foster a tendency to try and create children to order?

Our choices, whatever they are, will shape our society and the way it understands parenthood, children, family, health, disability, and choice. In this way, our decisions about testing are both private and public, personal and political.

QUESTIONS TO CONSIDER ABOUT TESTING

As you are deciding whether or not to have tests that will give you information about your developing baby, consider the following questions:

- Do I want to know whether or not my baby might have a condition such as Down syndrome, sickle-cell anemia, cystic fibrosis, or deafness?
- What do I know about life with these conditions?
- Would knowing that my baby will have a particular condition make a difference in my decision to continue my pregnancy? If so, why?
- Would knowing any other characteristics detectable by prenatal testing, such as the sex of my baby, the identity of the father, or whether I'm carrying twins or triplets, affect my decision about continuing my pregnancy? If so, why?

As you consider testing, think about your own dreams of parenthood. What are the central values of your family, and how do future children fit into your values and your life goals? How may a child's possible disease, disability, or health problem influence your parenting experience? How may a child's Down syndrome, cystic fibrosis, or other condition affect your life, your hopes for your child, your partner, your time with your other children?

Before choosing to have any test, it is important to know what the test is capable of telling you and what the advantages and disadvantages are. Ask your health care provider, and do your own research, to find out the following:

- What information is this test intended to provide?

- Does the test pose any risk to you and/or your developing baby?
- Why is this test recommended for you? Are you in a group that makes your baby more likely to have this condition?
- When can you expect the results to come back?
- How reliable is this test? If you get a result described as abnormal or unusual, what kind of follow-up testing or counseling will be offered?
- Who can help you understand what your result means?
- What are your options after receiving the result? Are there any treatments available for you or for the fetus if the result is abnormal, or will the choice be between continuing or ending the pregnancy?
- How much will this test cost? Will your health insurance cover part or all of the cost of this test? If not, can you get any financial assistance?

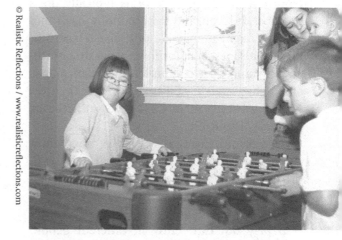

© Realistic Reflections / www.realisticreflections.com

A child with Down syndrome shows off her foosball skills. Although prenatal tests can identify conditions like Down syndrome, they cannot tell you exactly what the physical, cognitive, and life-span effects would be.

LIFE WITH DISABILITY

About one in thirty-three babies is born with what is called a "birth defect" or disabling condition.[1] Some factors, such as environmental toxins and maternal use of alcohol, are known to increase the likelihood of impairment for a baby. But the causes of most impairments are not known.

Many women today don't have much first-hand experience of living, studying, or working with people who have some of the conditions for which tests are now available. As you consider testing for certain conditions, learn about the conditions, as well as about what life with them is like on a daily basis for the individual with the disability and her or his family.

WHAT TESTS CAN'T TELL YOU

No prenatal test can guarantee that your child will be born without any health problems or will not develop them later in life. The most common disabling conditions typically don't occur in children, and many conditions cannot be detected by prenatal tests. Prenatal tests cannot at present detect cardiovascular disease, diabetes, cancer, or certain learning, emotional, and behavioral disabilities; nor can they tell you about traits such as eye color, athleticism, or musical aptitude.

No test can accurately predict exactly how a condition such as Down syndrome, cystic fibrosis, sickle-cell disease, or spina bifida will affect your child. This is true for two very different reasons. First, the biological effects of a condition play out differently in different people. Prenatal tests are not able to tell you exactly what the physical, cognitive, and life-span effects will be for your child.

For example, some children with cystic fibrosis experience significant medical problems and have short lives. However, most people living with cystic fibrosis who follow current treatment guidelines will live at least into their thirties.[2] Although they will likely have some periods of intensive medical therapy, most will also be able to go to school, play with friends, and get jobs. Many people with cystic fibrosis find partners, and some become biological or adoptive parents. Similarly, Down syndrome, the condition for which prenatal testing is most often recommended, can cause a range of impairments. It typically causes intellectual disability and medical problems. Available treatments or surgeries lessen or correct most of the heart, intestinal, and other medical conditions. The possible cognitive impairments range from mild to severe, with only a small percent of affected children having severe mental disabilities.[3] Almost all children with Down syndrome can be expected to participate in school, and many adults will go on to get jobs, form relationships, and live in the community. No prenatal test can tell you whether your developing baby will be seriously or mildly affected with cognitive or medical impairments.

But beyond the varying biology of the conditions, the main reason that a test won't give you as much information as you might like is that knowing your child has Down syndrome, cystic fibrosis, or spina bifida tells you little or nothing about your child's future interests, talents, appearance, or personality. The test provides only one piece of information. You will need to consider how a child's spina bifida, for example, will be part of the child's life and yours. Imagine that one of your family activities is camping. Can you learn what you would need to know to help a child with mobility impairments to camp with you? If your family loves reading and intellectual conversation, can you imagine raising a child who has cognitive impairments from Down syndrome and won't always understand what others are talking about? You may want to consider that a child without a disability might not want to go camping, or might not like books and intellectual conversation, either. How easily can you accept a child's own unique strengths and limitations, and make the child a part of your family life? What positive changes could this child bring to your family despite the impact of impairments?

DISCRIMINATION, ADVOCACY, AND COMMUNITY

Social acceptance of disability is another factor in how a child's disability may affect the child's life or yours. Even if you can love and accept a child who has muscular dystrophy or Down syndrome, how will your extended family react? Will your child make friends? Will teachers, your religious group, or employers give your child a chance to show her or his whole self? Do you have the resources to help this child interact with the world?

In the past, living with a disability has included living with a certain amount of prejudice and societal discrimination, and this will probably be true in the future. Like people of color and women, people with disabilities have formed support groups and political action groups. The work of these groups has improved laws, services, and opportunities. Antidiscrimination laws make it illegal for schools, restaurants, theaters, or employers to prevent people with disabilities from learning, working, or enjoying ordinary life. Many parks, campgrounds, museums, and tourist attractions are now more open to people with mobility, hearing, or visual impairments than they once were. Unfortunately, there is resistance to implementing laws and services fully. Parents of children with disabilities will likely have to advocate more than parents of typical children to find good schools, medical and social services, friends, and activities for our children.

FAMILY LIFE

Many of us imagine that raising a child with a disability is much harder, more costly in dollars and emotion, and much less rewarding personally than raising a child who doesn't have a disability. We fear that our marriage will break up under the strain, or that we won't have the money for medical care or special equipment, and that our other children will be neglected because of the particular needs of the child with the disability.

These are understandable concerns. You will need to get information from knowledgeable people—such as genetic counselors and parent/advocacy groups—to help you think about these realities. The community of people with disabilities and their families is generally better than health care professionals at telling you what life is really like.

Families of children with disabilities have periods of stress and hardship, especially when the diagnosis or prognosis is uncertain. Yet recent research has found that families raising children with disabilities are much more like other families than they are different.[4] Studies conclude that families also have more periods of going about ordinary life and figuring out ways to adapt to their child's disability than they do periods of stress and hardship.[5] All families everywhere must adapt to features of each person in the household, with or without disabilities.

All parents face the challenges of getting enough emotional and practical support from family and friends, taking enough breaks from child raising to pursue other parts of their lives, and having the money, the time, and the social situation to make parenting more joyful than it is exhausting. If a parent cannot find funding or services to help accommodate a child's disability, the stresses and struggles of child raising will be compounded.

In some ways, raising my son and my daughter feels similar. My daughter with Down syndrome is [like] her older brother—active, feisty. She struggles to keep up with him, to do whatever he is doing. . . . She needs more help than he did at every stage—you have to be hypervigilant to see that she is getting what she needs, learning to put on her clothes herself, to climb, to read. [But] the hardest part isn't my daughter, it's the social responses. . . . You have to explain to people that you are fine with your life and with your child. People take it for granted that my life is more stressful and not as good as theirs, that my child is not as good as theirs. It is not that we have to work harder to catch her words or to go slower when we walk so that she can keep up with us; it is that people devalue her. That's the hardest thing.

TYPES OF TESTS

Three types of tests screen for or diagnose potential impairments in the fetus. The first type is **genetic-carrier screening.** It consists of blood tests that can be performed before you get pregnant or in early pregnancy. The tests determine if you or your partner is a carrier of diseases such as cystic fibrosis that can be inherited by your children. (For more information, see facing page.)

The second type of prenatal test is a **screening test.** Such tests measure the likelihood that your fetus has a particular condition, but cannot tell you for certain whether the fetus has the condition.

Finally there is the **diagnostic test,** which gives a yes-or-no answer and tells you that the fetus does or does not have a particular condition. The availability of such tests raises many complicated questions for prospective parents, because treatments for the conditions they di-

HOW FETUS SELECTION AFFECTS SOCIETY

In some parts of the world, babies of one sex or the other are very much preferred. Sometimes women experience great pressure from their families and society to have children of the preferred sex. This pressure can lead to situations like those in China and India, where more boys than girls are now being born because of prenatal testing and selective abortion.[6] The practice of aborting female fetuses is a threat to the gender balance that will have long-term consequences.

What is true for sex selection can be said of disability-based selection as well. Fewer people are born today with the disabilities that we can test for than were born with the same disabilities before we could test for them. This reduction in the diversity of the population may affect people's attitudes toward individuals with disabilities, including those who develop disabilities later in life. Some advocates wonder if such changes will decrease tolerance for people with disabilities and reduce support for necessary social services.

agnose are limited. Treatment can essentially "cure" only a few conditions, such as clubfoot or cleft palate. For other conditions, such as cystic fibrosis, sickle-cell disease, or spina bifida, a range of medications and therapies can improve the child's health and functioning, but cannot end the disability. And for some conditions, no treatment currently exists.

GENETIC-CARRIER SCREENING

Genetic-carrier screening involves testing the blood or saliva of prospective parents to see if they are carriers of certain genes. (Genes are basic biological units that determine hereditary characteristics and transmit them from parent to child.) This type of screening is used to check for diseases that can be passed on through genes from either parent or both parents. The screening can be performed before conception or early in pregnancy to determine the chance that a child might be affected with certain diseases that either run in her or his family or are more common among people of the family's ethnic background than they are among the general population.

We have a son who has a very rare metabolic disease of which I am a carrier. We found this out after I gave birth to him. It only affects boys. Girls can be carriers but be perfectly healthy. Luckily my son has a very mild case—most kids don't make it past three years. At six years he is doing great. He is extremely handicapped—cannot sit unassisted, walk, or talk—but he is an inquisitive, happy child. [After he was born, we decided to try to get pregnant again naturally, but abort if genetic testing showed the baby would have the disease.] We found out it was a girl (sigh of relief!) Three years later I am grateful. Grateful that we have two children that have brought so much joy to our lives. Grateful that our son is

thriving despite his limitations. Grateful to see my daughter develop and grow normally, which has helped heal a sadness in my husband and me. Grateful that genetic testing was available to us, for I don't know if I would have taken the risk of having a second child without it.

Some conditions are more common in certain populations. For example, Caucasians whose families came from Northern Europe are more likely to have cystic fibrosis; African-Americans are more likely to have sickle-cell disease; people of Southeast Asian or Mediterranean background are more likely to have anemias known as *thalassemias;* and people of Ashkenazi Jewish, French-Canadian, or Cajun background are more likely than others to experience Tay-Sachs disease and several other conditions. Genetic-carrier screening can test for these conditions and others that occur at higher rates in certain groups. If you and your partner are both found to be carriers for such a genetic condition, a fetus would have a one-in-four chance of being affected; diagnostic prenatal testing can be done to determine whether or not the fetus has the condition.

Some rarer genetic conditions, such as hemophilia, fragile X syndrome, and Duchenne muscular dystrophy, are passed to children in a slightly different way, known as *X-linked inheritance.* These conditions are more likely to affect boys than girls.* Genetic-carrier screening can test for these conditions as well.

If you have a family member who has a genetic condition, tell your doctor, midwife, or

---

* For example, X-linked inheritance in muscular dystrophy usually means that the mother carries the mutation for the disease on one of her two X chromosomes. In this situation, she has a 50 percent chance of passing the affected gene to her sons and daughters. Since her daughters receive another X chromosome from the unaffected father, they will be carriers like their mother. Her sons who inherit the affected X chromosome will inherit a Y chromosome from the father and will have Duchenne muscular dystrophy.

genetic counselor if you are interested in getting testing for that condition. In some cases, there may be prenatal genetic testing available that can help you determine if your fetus is affected. This genetic testing is offered only if you have a family member with a specific condition. Genetic-carrier screening is routinely offered for cystic fibrosis, sickle-cell disease, and Tay-Sachs disease at an early prenatal visit, depending on your racial and ethnic background.

If you choose to undergo genetic-carrier screening, it is important to talk with a genetic counselor and to think through what you might do if the screening shows that you are a carrier for a certain condition. Genetic-carrier screening tests you and your partner, and describes only your likelihood of passing along certain conditions. If both you and your partner are carriers and you want information about your fetus, you may decide to have a diagnostic test such as amniocentesis to determine if your developing baby has the condition. (For more information on genetic counseling, see page 122. For more information on considering your options, see "Responding to Test Results," page 123.)

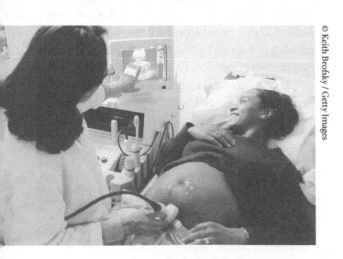

© Keith Brofsky / Getty Images

SCREENING TESTS

The most common screening test performed during pregnancy is *ultrasound*, which produces an image known as a *sonogram*. This procedure has many uses, including screening the fetus for physical malformations. In addition to ultrasound, a number of screening tests for Down syndrome and other characteristics of your developing baby are available.

Most screening tests give an estimate of the likelihood that a certain condition is present in the fetus. For example, the likelihood of a fetus having Down syndrome may be stated as 1:150, meaning that there is one chance in one hundred fifty that the fetus is affected. (This is based on the rate at which the condition occurred among babies of women who had similar test results and who shared the same age, ethnic background, smoking status, and other characteristics.) Because screening tests are designed to identify as many potential cases as possible, they sometimes suggest that a condition is likely to be present when in fact it is not present. This outcome is called a "false-positive" result. Screening tests allow many false positives because that ensures that almost all true positives will also be caught. For this reason, if a screening test is positive and you want to determine whether the condition is really present or not, you will need diagnostic testing.

The American College of Obstetricians and Gynecologists recommends that all women, regardless of age, be offered either screening or diagnostic tests for Down syndrome and related chromosomal conditions. (For more information on commonly offered tests, see the "Screening Tests" table.)

The screening tests offered to pregnant women are numerous, and they change often. For up-to-date information, see the March of Dimes website, www.marchofdimes.com.

SCREENING TESTS*

TEST	WHEN OFFERED	WHAT IT TELLS YOU AND HOW	SAFETY AND ACCURACY†	FOLLOW-UP
First-trimester serum screen (Nuchal translucency sonogram or combined test)	11 to 14 weeks; most reliable results at 11 to 13 weeks	• Estimates the chance that the fetus has Down syndrome • Ultrasound is used to measure the amount of fluid at the back of the fetus's neck • Combined test adds a blood test to provide a more accurate assessment	• Generally considered safe (See box on page 119 for some concerns about ultrasound.) • The combined test will detect about 8 out of 10 fetuses who have Down syndrome • One in 20 of the test's positive results are false positives (the test will be positive even though the fetus does not have Down syndrome)	• If chance of Down syndrome is higher than a 35-year-old's chance, a diagnostic test (CVS or amniocentesis; see page 121) will be offered as follow-up to confirm results
Multiple-marker screen (Maternal serum screening test, triple test, triple screen, quad screen)	15 to 20 weeks; most reliable results at 15 to 18 weeks	• Estimates the chance that the fetus has: • Down syndrome and a few other chromosomal conditions • Neural tube defects (spina bifida, anencephaly) • Abdominal wall defect (gastroschisis) • Tests your blood for levels of three (triple screen) or four (quad screen) different substances	• The blood test is safe • The triple screen detects about 6 to 7 out of 10 fetuses that have the condition; the quad identifies about 8 of 10 • Some positive results are false positives. False positives are more common when the test uses one to three markers instead of four and in older women.	• If the chance of any of these conditions is higher than a set standard, a diagnostic test (ultrasound or amniocentesis, as appropriate) will be offered as a follow-up *(continued)*

* These tests may be offered as standard care for certain groups of women, but that does not mean that they are medically necessary. Rather, each pregnant woman may decide whether she wants to have her fetus tested for potentially disabling health conditions. For a longer discussion of this issue, see the main text of the chapter.

† Accuracy of prenatal tests depends on the age, race, and smoking status of the woman on whom the test is performed. It also depends on the accuracy of the estimated gestational age of the fetus.

TEST	WHEN OFFERED	WHAT IT TELLS YOU AND HOW	SAFETY AND ACCURACY†	FOLLOW-UP

Ultrasound (Sonogram)	18 to 20 weeks	• Screening to check fetus's
		  • Growth and well-being
		  • Placental location
		  • Sex (on request)
		• Can detect some types of physical impairment, including neural tube defects (spina bifida, anencephaly); some heart conditions; and major problems in the limbs, nervous system, abdomen, or other organ systems
		• Uses sound waves to create an image of the developing fetus. Sometimes it is difficult for untrained people to see this image as a picture.
			• Ultrasound is thought to be safe, but there are some concerns about the intensity and repeated exposure (See box on facing page.)
			• Accuracy depends on the position of the fetus during the ultrasound and the skill of the person performing the test
			• Cannot detect every form of physical impairment; able to detect the most serious forms
				• If a screening ultrasound raises concerns, diagnostic testing will be offered

* These tests may be offered as standard care for certain groups of women, but that does not mean that they are medically necessary. Rather, each pregnant woman may decide whether she wants to have her fetus tested for potentially disabling health conditions. For a longer discussion of this issue, see the main text of the chapter.

† Accuracy of prenatal tests depends on the age, race, and smoking status of the woman on whom the test is performed. It also depends on the accuracy of the estimated gestational age of the fetus.

ULTRASOUND: MEDICAL TEST, BONDING OPPORTUNITY, OR CONSUMER ENTERTAINMENT?

Though it is used in many branches of medicine, ultrasound is perhaps most familiar as the source of grainy-gray images of fetuses. Practitioners use ultrasound to confirm fetal life; to check fetal age, size, and number; and to determine the location of the placenta. They also use it to screen the fetus for physical malformations or developmental problems.

Unlike other tests, however, the ultrasound examination has come to be valued by many expectant mothers in the United States as an opportunity to see and "bond with" an awaited child. Women often bring along family and friends eager to "see the baby" and are given an image to keep.

Capitalizing on public enthusiasm for "seeing" the baby, and taking advantage of the more realistic images afforded by new 3-D devices, a number of businesses now offer "keepsake" ultrasounds directly to the public for a fee, bypassing the medical system. The FDA regards this practice as an unapproved use of a medical device, and has issued public warnings against it. The research that determined that ultrasounds are reasonably safe was done in the 1970s and 1980s. Today's equipment produces sound waves that are eight times higher in intensity. In addition to concerns about the unapproved use of a medical device, the FDA is concerned about repeated and prolonged exposure, unskilled technicians, poorly maintained equipment, and the lack of trained counselors in case of suspected fetal impairments.[7]

Even within a medical setting, women may ask for or be offered multiple ultrasounds without true medical justification. Given that some questions about long-term safety still exist, this practice is questionable.

Safety is not the only troubling issue. Some people are concerned about the psychological and ethical implications of subjecting our fetuses to ever-closer scrutiny. Ultrasound may serve to foster the belief that a "perfect" baby is the only desirable (or acceptable) baby. We may find it difficult to fully accept and celebrate a pregnancy before testing suggests that the baby is healthy and has no disabling condition that might lead to ending the pregnancy. In this way, prenatal testing puts women in the position of experiencing pregnancy as "tentative," in the words of feminist critic Barbara Katz Rothman.

At the same time, however, ultrasound encourages women to embrace weeks-old fetuses as babies and persons. This view is invoked when we describe fetal ultrasound as "baby pictures" and expect that the sight of them will cause a woman to "bond" emotionally with her fetus.

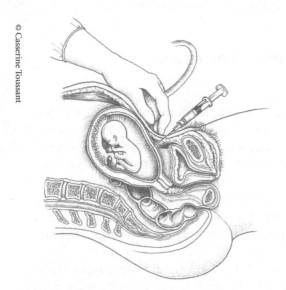

© Casserine Toussant

During an amniocentesis procedure, a needle is inserted through your abdomen to draw out a few teaspoons of amniotic fluid for testing.

DIAGNOSTIC TESTS

Diagnostic tests confirm the presence or absence of a particular condition in your developing baby. They are offered to women whose screening-test results detected a higher likelihood of a genetic or chromosomal condition, to women over age thirty-five, and to women with a family history of certain conditions. Diagnostic tests involve a small risk of miscarriage or infection. They give highly accurate information.

The two most common diagnostic tests are chorionic villus testing and amniocentesis, which can be used to detect several different conditions. Both these tests involve having a needle passed through your abdomen or vagina to obtain a very small sample of tissue or fluid. The tissue or fluid is tested for chromosomal impairments. (For more information on commonly offered tests, see the "Diagnostic Tests" chart.)

The diagnostic tests offered to pregnant women are numerous, and they change often.

For up-to-date information, see the March of Dimes website, www.marchofdimes.com.

CHOOSING TESTING

Since my husband had Down syndrome in the family and I would be thirty-five when the baby was born, I knew I wanted as much information as possible. It wasn't that we even knew what our decision would be if there were genetic problems, but my husband and I wanted [to know the results].

As you get information from other people who know about some of the diagnosable disabilities, you may conclude that it won't be so different to raise a child who has sickle-cell disease than it is to raise one who doesn't. Or even if you believe that raising a child with a known disease or disability will be substantially different, your beliefs and values may still lead you to accept such a child. You may choose to get tested simply to have more information and be prepared if results suggest that the baby may have a disability. Or, you may decide that, if possible, you want your child to begin life only with the physical, sensory, and mental abilities typical of children without disabilities. You may feel that if your child developed an illness or disability later in life, you would do everything you could to help, but you want to do everything you can—including ending the pregnancy—to prevent this situation.

My husband and I really wanted more children. We had a 75 percent chance of having a healthy baby on our own. We crossed our fingers and got pregnant naturally with the agreement that we would get genetic testing done and if necessary abort. We love our son [who has a disability] but did not emotionally, spiritually, or financially want to bring another handicapped child into the world.

DIAGNOSTIC TESTS*

TEST	WHEN OFFERED	WHAT IT TELLS YOU AND HOW	SAFETY AND ACCURACY	FOLLOW-UP

Chorionic villus sampling (CVS)	10 to 13 weeks	• Tests for:
		  • Down syndrome and some other chromosomal conditions
		  • Some genetic conditions can be diagnosed if both parents are known carriers (these include Tay-Sachs disease, cystic fibrosis, and sickle-cell disease)
		• A needle is inserted through your abdomen or cervix to collect a tissue sample from the placenta
			• About 1 in 100 chance of miscarriage for most women
			• More than 99 percent accurate, depending on the condition in question
			• Cannot tell the severity of the condition
				• No treatments available before birth
				• Pregnancy can be terminated
				• Preparations can be made for care after your child's birth

Amniocentesis (Amnio)	15 to 20 weeks	• Tests for:
		  • Same genetic and chromosomal conditions as CVS (see above)
		  • Neural tube defect conditions (spina bifida, anencephaly)
		• A needle is inserted through your abdomen to draw out a few teaspoons of amniotic fluid
			• About 1 in 200 to 1 in 400 chance of miscarriage
			• In rare cases, procedure can cause infection or injury to the fetus
			• More than 99 percent accurate
			• Cannot determine the severity of the condition
				• Almost no treatments before birth for most conditions
				• New surgery techniques being developed to correct neural tube defects (spina bifida) before birth
				• Pregnancy can be terminated
				• Preparations can be made for care after your child's birth

* The American College of Obstetricians and Gynecologists recommends that all women, regardless of age, be offered either screening or diagnostic tests for Down syndrome and related chromosomal conditions.

COUNSELING

Pre-testing Counseling

Your health care provider should give you some information about the prenatal tests you are being offered. However, there is no standard information that providers are required to supply during prenatal counseling. As more and more tests are offered, busy providers may opt to give you a bunch of booklets about tests rather than discuss the tests with you. These booklets are important to read, but some of them use terms that make the discussion too technical for the layperson to follow. Sometimes it can be very difficult to read or hear descriptions of conditions that might affect your developing baby. You may tune out or let your imagination and fear take over. Language barriers and differences in communication styles may sometimes make it difficult to get good information from your health care providers.

In addition, your doctor or midwife may not know much about the lives of people with Down syndrome or spina bifida or muscular dystrophy. She or he may believe that impairments have only negative effects on the lives of children and their families. If this is so, your health care provider's fears and stereotypes may bias the advice you are given.

As you gather information to help you make decisions about prenatal testing, your options should be presented to you clearly and your questions answered thoroughly. Health care providers should not present optional tests as if they are essential or required and should not pressure you or direct your decision. Ask questions if something is confusing. Your health care provider should want to help you understand. It is okay to ask for more information and to talk about your concerns so that you can make the best decisions for yourself and your growing family.

The doctor really didn't give me a choice per se. She just said that it is the only test they offer and I really should have it done. She made me feel like I should, and since she is the doctor, I did. Really, I felt kind of like I would be doing something bad by not having it done. I don't know if she even looked at me when she was talking to me—I have memories of her talking to me while writing in my chart.

Genetic Counselors

Sometimes your health care provider may refer you to a genetic counselor. Genetic counselors are health professionals who have special skills in presenting information and providing support to pregnant women and families who are thinking about prenatal testing.[8] They are trained to provide information about testing and about the conditions that a fetus may be affected by or might develop, and to provide resources and connections to families and support groups so that you can obtain more information and make a decision that fits with your values. Many genetic counselors belong to a professional society, whose code of ethics describes how genetic counselors should allow their clients to come to their own decisions, without pressure.

It is common for a session with a genetic counselor to be scheduled right before an amniocentesis. The counseling session is meant to provide information and allow for time in which to make a decision. Therefore, you may want to try to have the genetic counseling session apart from—and in advance of—the amniocentesis session. You are free to turn down the amniocentesis in any case.

PAYING FOR PRENATAL TESTING

Most health insurance plans, including Medicaid, will pay for prenatal visits, care, and medically necessary tests. If you are concerned that you cannot afford a prenatal test that you have decided is best for your pregnancy, your health care provider or a genetic counselor may be able to help you find some financial assistance to cover the cost of the test.

RESPONDING TO TEST RESULTS

When you hear test results, you may feel exhausted, relieved, exhilarated, despairing, joyful, or terrified, depending on the results and your hopes and expectations. If a screening test suggests an increased chance of a condition being present, you can decide whether you want follow-up testing or not.

If you find out through diagnostic testing that your baby has a disability, deciding whether or not to terminate your pregnancy can be very difficult. Some women and families may believe that it is wrong to end a pregnancy, regardless of the potential problems a child may bring. Other women and families believe that the decision depends on the particular condition involved and the family's circumstances. If you believe the decision depends on your situation, you will need to consider whether you think you and your child will have a life that you will both enjoy, despite the obstacles and limitations that a disability can impose. If you have enough time, energy, support, and possibly money in your own life to give your child what she or he will need, and you expect to have many of the same joys and rewards you would have received in raising any other child, you may be comfortable continuing your pregnancy.

If your test results show that the baby has an impairment, no one should pressure you into having an abortion, just as no one should pressure you to have an abortion for any other reason. But if your test results tell you something you think will be too difficult for you and your child, you don't have to continue the pregnancy, even if other people think you should.

NEXT STEPS

If you have received a test result that indicates a disability, ask your health care provider to give you as much information as she or he has about what the results mean. You may be referred to a genetic counselor or social worker. These professionals can clarify and further explain any information you have received. They should provide additional information on abortion, adoption, and raising a child with the diagnosed condition. They should offer you information about what life with the condition is like, and they should make it possible for you to meet children and families living with the condition that has just been diagnosed, as well as families who decided not to continue pregnancies after learning about the condition in the pregnancy. If they don't offer such opportunities, ask them to help you learn where you can find them. If you are thinking about terminating the pregnancy, you may have only a few weeks to make your decision in some cases. Even so, try to make time to consider your decision.

Continuing the Pregnancy

If test results indicate that the baby you are carrying is almost certainly going to be affected by a specific condition, you can use this information to prepare for the birth of your child. You can learn more about any immediate or long-

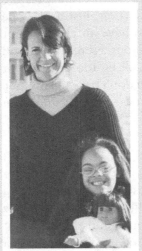

"The miracle you ask for may not be the miracle you receive."
Tierney Temple Fairchild

I was having a wonderful pregnancy, filled with all the joy that expecting a firstborn can bring. Then the technician said during a routine ultrasound at 21 weeks that she was having difficulty seeing the heart and its chambers.

My husband Greg and I soon learned that the baby had only three heart chambers, and that this condition was highly correlated with Down syndrome. Our doctor encouraged us to have an amnio in order to have enough information to make a decision. We were immediately connected with a genetic counselor, who would be our lifeline for the next two weeks.

The days and weeks that followed tested our fortitude, challenged our faith, and required honesty and constant communication. We collected all the information we could about the heart defect, Down syndrome, and the two in combination. We talked frequently with our genetic counselor about the options, the statistics, and our emotions.

Three days in, the FISH [fluorescence in situ hybridization] test confirmed the diagnosis with 97 percent accuracy. It was another seven days before the amnio results created the certainty and urgency to decide. We saw every specialist we could and spoke with families about their experiences. At one point Greg even contacted an adoption agency specializing in Down syndrome. We tried to ask every question that could be answered.

The unanswerable questions nagged. What if the baby is among the 10 percent who are severely mentally disabled? How will the heart surgery at five months affect her development? Will we experience the social stigma we know exists?

We changed our minds a few times each, finally converging on a critical question: What is it about us with all our resources that make us unwilling to take on this challenge when many stand waiting to adopt? With no good answer, we overcame our fears and decided to continue the pregnancy. We mourned the baby we might have had and turned our attention to preparing for the special needs our child would bring with her.

Naia Grace Fairchild is now eight years old, fully included in her second-grade class, reading nearly on grade level. She is a happy, healthy child with two younger brothers and many friends. Greg and I often reflect on how big our concerns were during the decision. Our fears never materialized and we continue to watch Naia excel.

During our decision process and into her first year, there were many dark days. One sermon I heard during the process stuck with me. "The miracle you ask for may not be the miracle you receive." Indeed.*

* For more information about Tierney Temple Fairchild's experience, see Mitchell Zuckoff, *Choosing Naia: A Family's Journey* (Boston: Beacon Press, 2003).

term needs that may be different for your child because of the condition and start gathering whatever information and support you need.

We somehow came to believe that we could handle whatever came our way. We knew that some of the dreams we had for our baby were in doubt and that our definition of normal was about to change. The scariness of it all set in as the weeks went by. We found ourselves questioning our decision. Yet, we always seemed to return to the same conclusion. That Kevin had the right to show us what was meant for his life.[9]

Abortion

If you decide that abortion is the best option for you, your health care provider should be able to provide you with information about abortion options, which will be affected by how far along your pregnancy is and the availability of abortion services in your area. You can also contact Planned Parenthood or a genetic counseling center to find out where you can get an abortion. (For more information on abortion, see *Our Bodies, Ourselves.*)

You will likely have significant feelings of loss and sadness if you decide to end the pregnancy that you had previously wanted and had been planning to carry to term. You may have many of the same feelings as women who have miscarried, yet your experience is different also. (For information on grieving childbearing losses, see Chapter 9.) Those of us who have experienced this kind of loss often do not speak openly about it because we fear being judged. If you can, seek the support of others who have suffered similar losses, through local or online support groups.

Getting amniocentesis seemed a foregone conclusion at age forty. Then we got a diagnosis of Down syndrome. My husband and I cried to-gether and then we talked. Having an abortion was NOT a foregone conclusion, but neither was carrying the baby to term. I prayed intensely to make a decision that was correct according to my own moral and religious standards, and was best for our marriage and the family we hoped to create. I have always been pro-choice.

Because we were older, we knew too much. My husband, a lawyer, at one point in his career was suing on behalf of institutionalized mentally retarded adults, to force placement of those for whom [such placement] was appropriate in community residences. I had written about the horrible conditions in these large warehouse institutions. We knew what a strain having a severely mentally disabled child can have on a marriage, and ours was still in its infancy. We were concerned about whether we would have emotional and physical energy left to give to any other children.

The issue that in the end determined my decision was what kind of life we could offer this child over the long term. I began visiting institutions for retarded adults and found that they were still appalling.

I had a saline abortion, with hard back labor. . . . In my own mind, I named that baby, and I mourned him.

THE DECISION IS YOURS

For some of us, the possibility of learning more about our developing baby during pregnancy makes us anxious and unhappy, because we feel required to decide, rather than leave things to occur as they will, as our grandmothers and great-grandmothers did. Others feel just the opposite, welcoming testing because we want to go ahead with a pregnancy only if we can know about the health of the baby before it is born. There is no one "right" way to feel about tests or about continuing or ending a preg-

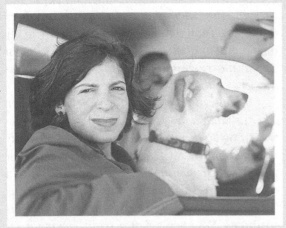
© Thayer Allyson Gowdy

"Part of what was so awful was the uncertainty."

Elizabeth Weil

The five-month sonogram raised some concerns, so I was asked to go back for a follow-up. This time there appeared to be all sorts of small anomalies—the fetus's liver seemed too big, there seemed to be some spots on the baby's brain, and the bowels did not look right.

After several weeks, I was diagnosed as having CMV, or cytomegalovirus, infection. It's a common virus that's dangerous only if a woman gets it for the first time when she's pregnant. I had apparently passed the virus along to the fetus. We were told that the baby I was carrying would almost certainly be deaf, would almost certainly be blind, and would probably have very severe mental retardation.

Deciding what to do was an awful process, and part of what was so awful was the uncertainty. We were told that these things were very, very likely—though it was possible we would have a healthy baby. That was maddening. My husband and I, being who we are, dove into doing tons and tons of research, assuming that if we researched enough, we would get to really firm ground with it. But we never did. We just kept hearing the same thing: It's very, very likely your baby will be born in this extremely impaired condition.

There wasn't one moment when it became clear that we were going to terminate the pregnancy. It was just something that slowly, and very painfully, came to feel like the right thing to both of us. I had lots of fears of feeling endless sadness about the decision, but I didn't feel it was unethical. I very much believe that these are decisions to be made by families, and that the fetus I was carrying was not yet a person with the same rights and privileges that I had or my husband had.

I was deeply upset by the loss of that baby and felt like the only way to get back on my feet was to get pregnant again. I got pregnant again about four months later and gave birth to my second daughter. Sometimes when I see my children, I have this vision of the boy we didn't have being with them. He is really present in our lives in these unexpected ways, and I imagine he will stay there for a long time.

nancy after you learn particular test results. Don't let people pressure you into testing or not testing. Try to help the people supporting you understand what you want, whatever it is. The more you learn, the more you may decide that testing and then abortion if the results identify a particular impairment are best for you, even if you otherwise would never have wanted an abortion. But if you conclude that you want this pregnancy and child regardless of what you learn about a possible disability, that decision should also be yours to make. True reproductive choice means the choice to get the information and support you need in order to make the right decision for your life and the lives of the people you love.

NOTES

1. Centers for Disease Control and Prevention, National Center on Birth Defects and Developmental Disabilities, "Basic Facts About Birth Defects: Frequently Asked Questions" (2005), accessed at www.cdc.gov/ncbddd/bd/facts.htm on May 13, 2006.
2. Cystic Fibrosis Foundation, *Patient Registry 2004 Annual Report* (Bethesda, MD: Cystic Fibrosis Foundation, 2005).
3. March of Dimes website, accessed March 2, 2007, at www.marchofdimes.com/professionals/14332_1214.asp. See also National Down Syndrome Society brochure "About Down Syndrome," accessed on March 2, 2007, at www.ndss.org/index.php?option=com_docman&task=doc_view&gid=110.
4. Philip M. Ferguson, "Mapping the Family: Disability Studies and the Exploration of Parental Response to Disability," in *Handbook of Disability Studies,* ed. Gary L. Albrecht, Katherine D. Seelman, and Michael Bury (Thousand Oaks, CA: Sage, 2001): 373–395. See also Stanley D. Klein and Kim Schive, eds., *You Will Dream New Dreams: Inspiring Personal Stories by Parents of Children with Disabilities* (New York: Kensington Books, 2001); and Janet Read, *Disability, the Family, and Society: Listening to Mothers* (Buckingham, UK: Open University Press, 2000).
5. Ferguson, "Mapping the Family." See also Klein and Schive, *You Will Dream New Dreams*; and Read, *Disability, the Family, and Society.*
6. World Health Organisation, "Sex Selection and Discrimination," Genomic Resource Centre (2006), accessed at www.who.int/genomics/gender/en/index4.html on May 13, 2006.
7. Carol Rados, "FDA Cautions Against Ultrasound 'Keepsake' Images," *FDA Consumer Magazine* 38, no. 1 (January–February 2004), accessed at www.fda.gov/FDAC/features/2004/104_images.html on July 15, 2006.
8. National Society of Genetic Counselors, "About Us," "FAQs About Genetic Counselors and the NSGC," and "Code of Ethics" (2006), accessed at www.nsgc.org/about/faq.cfm on May 13, 2006.
9. Molly A. Minnick, Kathleen J. Delp, and Mary C. Ciotti, *A Time to Decide, a Time to Heal,* 4th ed. (St. Johns, MI: Pineapple Press, 2000), 19.

CHAPTER 8

Special Concerns During Pregnancy

Every pregnancy is a unique experience. But some pregnancies involve particular differences or challenges. This chapter is about pregnancies that are more challenging for the health of the mother or baby because of the age of the mother, the number of babies she is carrying, difficulties staying pregnant, or other health concerns that require extra attention during pregnancy.

If you experience any of these complications during your pregnancy, or have experienced them in the past, you may need additional or specialized prenatal care. You may also feel more anxious and need extra emotional support. Having a comprehensive plan for care, coordinated with your health care providers, and talking with friends and family about your concerns can help reduce anxiety. It also can be helpful to join a support group, reach out to other women in similar circumstances, or seek counseling from therapists who specialize in high-risk pregnancies. The nonprofit Sidelines National High Risk Pregnancy Support Network (www.sidelines.org) offers one-on-one support and online services through a network of volunteers. The group is also working on legislation to promote better care and more research dedicated to complicated pregnancies.

PREGNANCY WHEN YOU ARE YOUNGER OR OLDER

PREGNANCY IN YOUR TEENS

Becoming pregnant as a teenager can present many challenges, but you can have a healthy pregnancy and birth. Younger teens (thirteen to fifteen years old) have a higher rate of complicated births, but you can help prevent problems by taking good care of yourself and getting support.

The suggestions for nutrition and exercise in Chapter 5, "Taking Care of

Yourself," will help you have the healthiest pregnancy possible. It will be especially important that you gain enough weight, so don't diet while you are pregnant. If getting enough food is difficult for you, contact the WIC program (Special Supplemental Program for Women, Infants, and Children) in your community or call your local food bank. (For more information, see page 65.)

You may have many changes to negotiate and plans to make as you prepare to give birth. You will need to know where you and the baby will live, and you may need to figure out how to stay in school or at your job, arrange for health insurance, and ensure that you will have enough money. It can seem overwhelming. Take advantage of any support systems available to you; the more helpful people (family; friends; the baby's father; a school counselor, public health nurse, social worker, midwife, or nurse-practitioner) you can surround yourself with, the better. They can encourage you to be and to stay healthy, to feel positive about pregnancy and birth, and to plan for and make decisions about your and your baby's future.

I'm fifteen and when I got pregnant it was really hard for me in school to do gym. You know, the running and all. The gym teacher was kind of mean, so I talked to my counselor and she got me into this school that is just for girls who are pregnant. It is better for me, 'cause we just walk for exercise and everybody helps you.

Just because you are having a baby does not mean you have to leave school. Ask your school guidance counselor or health care provider if there are schools in your community especially for pregnant or parenting students. Many communities have such schools. They may offer classes in parenting as well as day care for your baby so that you can attend classes. Your continuing with school is very important for both you and your baby. Getting an education that opens the door to a job you enjoy will help you be happier and you will be able to parent your baby more successfully, too.

I'm sixteen and this is my first baby. My mom had me when she was sixteen, too. When I went into labor, I told my mom I wanted my little sister to be with me. She's twelve. After my baby was born, I told my sister, "You are smart and pretty. Don't do this. Don't do what me and mom did. You can be anything you want." I love my baby, but I want my sister to have a better life. Later, my midwife told me I was smart and pretty, too, and that I could do anything I want. She said I could still go to college. I hope I can. I know it will be a lot of work, but I would like to be a lawyer.

PREGNANCY IN YOUR LATE THIRTIES OR EARLY FORTIES

Many of us are becoming pregnant for the first time in our late thirties and early, middle, and sometimes even late forties. If you are over thirty-five years old, medical providers may label you as an "elderly primigravida" or a woman of "advanced maternal age," consider you high-risk, and view your baby as a "premium baby." However, elevated risks associated with becoming a mother after the age of thirty-five are limited. There is an increased chance that you will have a baby with Down syndrome, and you have a higher chance of developing age-related conditions such as diabetes and high blood pressure.[1] Women who are pregnant and over the age of thirty-five are offered more interventions during pregnancy and birth. But if you are in good health and you do not have any medical or pregnancy complications, you should not need a lot of special care. The vast majority of "older" women have healthy pregnancies and births.

Because you are over age thirty-five, your health care provider will offer you blood testing, ultrasounds, and/or an amniocentesis to help determine if there are any chromosome problems in your baby. Deciding to have a test or which tests you think will be best for you can be difficult. Some of the tests offered (such as ultrasound) don't tell you for certain that your baby does or does not have a chromosome problem, and the tests (such as amniocentesis or chorionic villus sampling) that do give you a certain answer about your baby's chromosomes are more invasive and involve a small chance of causing miscarriage. (For more information, see Chapter 7, "Prenatal Testing.")

Some of us find our age and our experience a benefit as we progress through our pregnancies and motherhood.

For much of my life I had been convinced that I didn't want kids. Then I settled into my career and found myself in a really great relationship. We talked about kids and realized that we really wanted them. We got married when I was thirty-eight, and I got pregnant three days later. . . .

As an older mom I think—no, I know—I'm a better mom than I would have been at a younger age. I'm healthy, so I'm still able to do all the active things with the kids—biking, snowboarding. And I am much more patient than I used to be. We do struggle a bit with balancing preparing for retirement with trying to save for the kids' college, but in the grand scheme of things, that's a pretty good challenge to have.

TWINS AND BEYOND

The number of pregnant women carrying more than one fetus at a time has been increasing over the past few decades. Assisted reproduction is responsible for most of this increase.

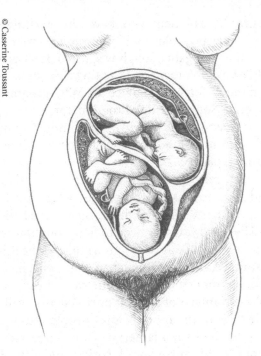

© Casserine Toussant

Nonidentical (fraternal) twins occur when two eggs are fertilized and both implant in the uterus. The twins have separate placentas and sacs.

Drugs that stimulate the ovaries to produce multiple eggs or in vitro fertilization may result in a woman's carrying more than one baby at once.

Women who are pregnant with *multiples*—twins, triplets, and more—require some specialized care. You will be offered frequent visits and a few extra ultrasounds to monitor the growth of your developing babies. The type of multiple pregnancy you have will determine what other care you will need.

Identical multiples occur when a fertilized egg splits into two or more embryos. Depending on how early or late in the pregnancy the split occurs, the babies may have a single placenta and amniotic sac or they may be in separate placentas and sacs. It is rare for twins to share a single sac and single placenta. When this occurs, the babies are at greater risk for having complications and you may need to give birth by cesarean section as soon as they are believed to have a good chance of surviving outside the womb.

Nonidentical (fraternal) multiples occur when more than one of a woman's eggs are fertilized and each of the fertilized eggs grows. Nonidentical multiples are especially likely to occur in women whose mothers or other female relatives had multiple births and in women who use assisted-reproduction techniques. Nonidentical multiples have separate placentas and sacs and are less likely to have growth problems during gestation than identical twins.

Whenever our bodies are carrying more than one baby at a time, it is more work. Two or more babies in a uterus take up a lot more space and stretch the uterus, which becomes larger and heavier and pulls more on the back. The babies need more nutrients and send more waste to the mother's kidneys than a single baby would. Still, our bodies are wonderfully able to handle the additional burden—especially if we take a little extra care of ourselves.

If you are carrying more than one baby, you will probably find the following suggestions helpful:

• Get plenty of rest.
• Add an extra 200 calories per day for each additional baby you are carrying. (For nutrition guidelines, see Chapter 5, "Taking Care of Yourself.")
• Do stretching exercises each day to ease the strain on your back. Prenatal yoga classes may be especially helpful for you.
• Get gentle exercise every day to keep your energy up and your muscles strong. Swimming is great for you if you are carrying multiples because, for a glorious hour or so, your weight is suspended in water.

The urine pregnancy test was immediately positive, and I knew I was pregnant with my second set of twins. . . . The older twin girls were five. Questions raced through my mind. How would my body adapt, especially when it was so difficult the first time? . . .

During my first pregnancy, I tried to eat over 100 grams of protein per day. Everything that entered my mouth contained peanut butter or tofu, and I ate a lot of our homegrown meat and fresh eggs. But now, with three kids, I barely had time to care for myself. . . . I was quite fearful that my body was not capable of carrying these babies; I had so many doubts.

I reread Birth Reborn, *by Michel Odent, a book that years earlier had instilled confidence in my ability to nourish my babies and achieve a very healthy pregnancy and birth. I began to get excited about the challenge and knew that my body could grow and gracefully accommodate twins again. Although I was considered higher risk because of my age (thirty-six), I considered my age a benefit—I had a greater understanding of my resources and what my body was capable of. . . . I gained fifty pounds again, and I learned about receiving versus giving; I gracefully accepted my own limitations and wisely asked for help when I needed it! I gave birth [vaginally] to full-term fraternal twins weighing seven pounds, two ounces and seven pounds, eight.*

Women with multiple gestations are more likely to have complications during pregnancy. Generally, the more fetuses you have, the greater the chances of complications. The most common complication for women carrying multiples is preterm birth. This may be due to the stretching of the uterus and the pressure of the weight of the babies on the cervix, but the reason is not known for sure. Your health care provider will teach you the signs of preterm labor, and you will both watch carefully for these signs, such as cramping in your back or lower abdomen or pain in your groin. This may mean occasional vaginal exams or ultrasounds to check whether your cervix is becoming shorter (effacing) or opening (dilating).

If your cervix begins to shorten or open or you begin to have preterm labor contractions, your health care provider may recommend that you limit your activity or even go on bed rest. While good research has not proven the benefits of bed rest for women in preterm labor, some women find that our preterm labor symptoms get worse when we are more active. Talk with your health care provider to decide what self-care is best for you in this situation. (For more information about preterm labor, see page 134. For more information about premature birth, see page 219.)

I was twenty-one weeks into the pregnancy and expecting twins when I found out that my cervix was dangerously short. My doctor sent me home on bed rest. . . .

The weeks that followed brought ups and downs. . . . Physically my energy levels were being sucked away and my muscles and joints were aching from lying down. In addition to the expected changes of pregnancy, my body was adjusting to new medications that left me feeling nauseated, bloated, weak, and shaky. I longed to be outside in the sunshine or meeting with friends. Emotionally I felt unproductive and isolated.

*The hardest part was the uncertainty. No one could be sure that bed rest would make a difference. The babies might be born severely premature in spite of bed rest. Would they survive? If they survived, would they be disabled because of complications related to being premature? I knew bed rest would end when the babies were born. But how long would that be? For their sakes, we were hoping for several months. How could I possibly cope that long? I found comfort in my spiri-*tuality. *I put my trust in God and found strength and peace.*

REDUCTION OF MULTIPLES

In rare cases, and almost always as a result of infertility treatments, a woman may find herself pregnant with three or more fetuses. *Selective reduction* is a medical procedure that causes a woman to lose some but not all of the fetuses. Selective reduction is done to decrease the chance of preterm birth or problems with fetal growth as well as to avoid complications that may threaten the health or life of the mother.

The procedure is usually performed early in pregnancy, between 9 and 12 weeks of gestation. Some women who have a family history of a specific genetic problem may choose to use genetic testing to determine if the condition is present in any of the fetuses, and if it is, abort that fetus or those fetuses. (For more information on prenatal testing, see Chapter 7.) Though selective reduction is done to decrease the risks of complications from multiple births, the procedure itself has risks, including the possible death of a remaining fetus or fetuses.

The decision to have selective reduction can be very difficult. Find out as much as you can from your health care providers about their experience with the procedure and ask if you can be put in contact with women who have had the procedure to learn more about their experiences.

BLEEDING

Any amount of vaginal bleeding during pregnancy can be scary, as it can mean a miscarriage is beginning. However, many women have some spotting or bleeding during healthy pregnancies.

BLEEDING IN THE FIRST TRIMESTER

You may have a bit of spotting—a small amount of blood on your underwear or on the toilet paper after you wipe—at about the time you would have expected your period. Some women will even have what seems like a very light period. At the time that the fertilized egg implants in the wall of your uterus—usually about one week after conception or three weeks after your last menstrual period—you may have some slight spotting as well. This spotting rarely lasts more than a day or two.

Spotting may also occur at other times throughout your pregnancy. Sometimes, sexual intercourse or other vaginal penetration will cause the cervix to bleed a little. Most of the time, the cause of spotting is not known, but it may be a sign that you have a cervical polyp or an infection such as a yeast infection or bacterial vaginosis, or a sexually transmitted infection that is irritating to the cervix. If you have spotting that continues for more than a day, check with your health care provider.

Bleeding without any cramping may be the beginning of a miscarriage or it may be from some other source that does not harm the baby. Heavy bleeding that requires wearing a sanitary pad or tampon and that is accompanied by painful cramping is usually a sign of a miscarriage. (For more information about miscarriage, see page 153.)

BLEEDING IN THE SECOND AND THIRD TRIMESTERS

Spotting may also occur during the second and third trimesters. As in the first trimester, contact your provider if it lasts more than a day.

Bleeding that is like your period or is a bright red gush of blood may be a sign that you are having preterm labor or that there is a problem with your placenta. If you experience such bleeding in your second or third trimester, see your health care provider immediately. Two serious concerns that may be present if you have heavy bleeding are placental abruption and placenta previa.

When the placenta separates from the wall of the uterus before the birth of the baby, it is called a *placental abruption*. This sometimes occurs if the mother is injured in some way. Smoking, pre-eclampsia, using cocaine or crack cocaine, chronic high blood pressure, and a previous history of placental abruption also increase the chances of abruption. When a placenta "abrupts," all or part of the oxygen and nutrition supply to the baby is cut off. This type of bleeding is usually accompanied by pain. If the placenta separates from the uterine wall quickly and completely, the mother and her fetus may bleed heavily. If a woman is experiencing an abruption she needs medical help immediately.

When the placenta grows across the opening of the cervix, it is described as a *placenta previa*. A placenta previa can be complete, covering the entire opening, or partial, with just an edge of the placenta covering part of the opening.

The location of the placenta is noted when you have an ultrasound. If you do not have a placenta previa during the first ultrasound you get during pregnancy, this complication will not occur and you don't have to worry about it. If you do have a placenta previa that is seen on ultrasound before 28 weeks, it is likely that the placenta will move away from the cervix as the uterus continues to enlarge. In this case, you will be offered one or two more ultrasounds later in pregnancy to check where the placenta is. If the placenta is still over the cervix late in the second trimester, your health care provider will help you plan the care you need during the last part of pregnancy and birth.

When labor begins, a placenta previa will be loosened from where it touches the cervix as the cervix opens. The loosened portion of the placenta will not be able to provide oxygen and nutrients to your baby. As the placenta separates from the cervix and uterine wall, the blood vessels that attach it to the uterus will break and cause the mother to bleed. The bleeding from a placenta previa is usually not painful and often occurs for the first time in the third trimester. The first bleeding event usually does not cause a problem for the mother or baby, but the condition will be dangerous for both during labor. If labor begins before you can schedule a cesarean section, call your health care provider immediately. An unscheduled cesarean will be done.

If you are having bleeding that is like a heavy period in your second or third trimester, call your health care provider and go to the hospital right away, so that you can get medical assistance rapidly.

WHEN LABOR COMES TOO SOON

PRETERM LABOR

Preterm labor—labor that begins more than three weeks before your due date—is a relatively common complication of pregnancy. About one in every twenty women has a preterm delivery. The most common symptom of preterm labor is a regular, painful tightening of the uterus that may feel like light or strong menstrual cramps or like the back pain you may feel before your period starts. Other signs are increased discharge of mucus from the vagina, sometimes blood-tinged, and cramplike pressure low in the abdomen. Just like full-term labor, preterm labor feels different for each woman. If you have signs of preterm labor or you feel something new in your body that you are not sure about, contact your provider.

Preterm labor contractions don't always continue. Most women who have preterm contractions go on to give birth to a full-term baby.

Contractions that feel like a tight nonpainful band around your abdomen are normal during pregnancy. They are known as *Braxton-Hicks contractions*. These contractions can occur with increasing frequency as you get closer to your due date, and occur more often if you have previously given birth. Braxton-Hicks contractions do not open the cervix and do not mean you are likely to have a premature baby. They often occur when you have intercourse, lift heavy items, or urinate. You can have one a day or several, but they do not come at regular intervals.

If it is difficult for you, your midwife, or your doctor to tell the difference between normal Braxton-Hicks contractions and true preterm labor that will cause the cervix to dilate, your provider can check the length of your cervix via a vaginal exam.

Some new tests can help determine which women with symptoms of preterm labor are at low risk for giving birth early. The *fetal fibronectin* (FFN) test is a simple test done on fluid collected in the vagina with a cotton swab. If your FFN test is negative, chances are very low that you will give birth in the next two weeks. Another test is ultrasound to measure the length of the cervix. A longer cervix means you are unlikely to deliver preterm. These tests are not available in every hospital, and they are new. Ongoing studies will help figure out how useful these tests are in predicting preterm labor.

If you are diagnosed with preterm labor, you will likely be given medication, put on bed rest, admitted to the hospital, or otherwise monitored frequently. The goal will be to keep you pregnant and allow your baby to keep growing inside of you for as long as it is safe.

If the preterm labor begins after 34 weeks' gestation (about six weeks before your due date), labor may be allowed to proceed. Babies born after 34 weeks' gestation may need a longer stay in the hospital than full-term babies and may have some minor short-term health problems. They are more likely to take longer to learn to breast-feed well and may need to feed more frequently than a full-term baby, so a certified lactation consultant or a nurse who specializes in helping mothers breast-feed near-term infants can be especially helpful. Babies born after 34 weeks usually do just fine, however, and often can go home within a week or two after birth.

A woman in preterm labor *before* 34 weeks is usually given a steroid injection to help develop the baby's lungs and medication to stop labor for a few days. The steroids reduce several complications of prematurity and improve the survival chances of premature babies. The steroids work best if they are given at least forty-eight hours before the premature baby is born. This is the most important treatment that can be given if you are at risk of delivering your baby at 34 weeks or less of gestation (six weeks or more before the due date).

Other medications, known as *tocolytics*, help delay delivery for at least forty-eight hours, the amount of time needed for steroids to work. Tocolytic drugs may be given by mouth, intravenously, or by injection. If your doctor suggests that you take a tocolytic drug for several weeks, discuss the plan in detail. Ask about the anticipated benefits in your situation and the expected negative effects.

Bed rest is another common treatment for women with symptoms of preterm labor. Research on the treatment of preterm labor has not shown that bed rest prolongs pregnancy or improves the outcome for the baby. For some women, however, limiting activity does seem to calm down contractions.

Once real labor begins, there is no clearly effective treatment to stop the baby from being born early. If it looks likely that you will have a preterm delivery before 34 weeks, talk with your provider about the possibility of transferring to a hospital that has a specialized intensive care nursery. Babies born in these facilities have better outcomes than babies who do not have access to such care.

A woman's chances of having a preterm birth due to preterm labor are increased if she smokes or uses cocaine or methamphetamine during pregnancy or if she is severely underweight prior to pregnancy. There is no evidence that moderate exercise or normal physical activity during pregnancy increases the risks of preterm birth. Recent randomized trials have shown that women who have already had one preterm birth may reduce their risk of another preterm birth by getting progesterone injections during pregnancy.[2] It's a good idea to consult an obstetrician with expertise in high-risk pregnancy (a perinatologist or maternal-fetal medicine specialist) if you have already had one baby born preterm. (For information about premature birth, see page 219.)

I was 32 weeks pregnant when I went into preterm labor. When I was first diagnosed, I kept thinking about all the things I had planned for the next month. I had to finish my childbirth classes, get things at work finished before my maternity leave, and get the house ready for a baby. It was hard to let go of all the things I had planned to do before the baby came.

After a weekend in the hospital, I was sent home on bed rest for five weeks. In retrospect, those were actually the best five weeks of the pregnancy. Once I was on bed rest, I had the time to take all the naps my body wanted and it was easier to eat several small snacks (instead of larger meals) and drink enough water. Also, I didn't feel guilty anymore for not being productive. I had permission to just do what I needed to do for myself and the baby.

. . . I had been pretty physically active before the pregnancy and had hoped to be active enough during the pregnancy to stay in pretty good shape. Bed rest put an end to those hopes. . . . By the time I got off bed rest . . . I was much weaker and was low on energy. I'd lose my breath just walking around the block. After my son was born, it took a long time and a lot of exercise before I felt like I was in shape again.

PRETERM PREMATURE RUPTURE OF MEMBRANES (PPROM)

If your bag of waters breaks more than three weeks before your due date, this is known as *preterm premature rupture of membranes* (PPROM). The condition is similar to premature labor and birth (see page 219). In fact, most women will develop preterm labor and will give birth preterm within a week after PPROM. One reason PPROM may occur is that the woman has *chorioamnionitis* (an infection; see page 218), which can weaken the membranes of the amniotic sac (bag of waters) and cause them to break. Also, PPROM is more common in women who smoke. But most women with PPROM and preterm labor have no identifiable reasons for developing the condition.

If you have PPROM before week 34 of your pregnancy, you will probably receive steroid injections to help mature your baby's lungs (see page 135). You may also receive intravenous antibiotics, which have been shown to delay birth somewhat in women with PPROM. If you have signs of infection or other health problems or your baby begins to show signs of health problems, your health care provider may recommend that labor be induced. In these situations, delivering preterm reduces the risk of worsening infection or other health problems for you and your baby. Still, it is always a difficult decision to induce labor before the due date, as early delivery also carries risks to the baby.

My daughter was born at 34 weeks, five days after I broke my bag of waters. I stayed in the hospital getting some medication to stop labor and the shot of steroids to help her lungs mature. Then we decided to induce labor because we didn't want the baby to get an infection. She weighed five pounds, six ounces at birth. She looked so small in the incubator, but she was breathing without any problem. Over the next few days she got jaundiced, and lost some weight. She was very sleepy and didn't nurse well, so we gave her some water in a bottle to keep her hydrated. She stayed in the intensive care nursery for ten days and then we took her home. Nursing was an all-day and all-night chore. She just got tired easily and nursed often but never for very long. She and I slept and nursed and slept and nursed and slept and nursed all day and all night for about three weeks. At ten weeks she finally woke up and started smiling and nursing better with longer intervals between. . . . I was exhausted but so happy to see her smile. . . . I felt like she really joined us when she was ten weeks old.

"INCOMPETENT CERVIX" / "CERVICAL INSUFFICIENCY"

Very rarely, a woman will have a condition called "incompetent cervix" or "cervical insufficiency," which means that her cervix doesn't stay firm and closed. When this happens, the baby may be born quickly in the second or early third trimester, following minimal or no labor pains. Typically this occurs when the baby is too premature to survive outside the womb. It is not known why this happens, but in some women it may be related to having prior surgery on the cervix.

If you have been diagnosed with this condition in one pregnancy and get pregnant again, you may have your cervix sewed closed with a procedure known as a *cerclage*. This is usually done at the end of the first trimester. As with all medical procedures, there are risks to cerclage. The risks include breaking the bag of waters, infection, and triggering labor. Cerclage should not be done if you have painful preterm contractions or signs of infection. With most cerclages, the stitches are removed if you have contractions or signs of infection, or when you reach about 36 weeks' gestation (four weeks before the due date).

Evidence is mixed on whether cerclage is effective at preventing the cervix from opening. Many health care providers think it helps, and some women with prior experience of an "over-eager" cervix get through a second pregnancy more easily when a cerclage is in place.

Bed rest is usually recommended in addition to cerclage, but research does not suggest it is effective. There is no evidence that bed rest alone improves the outcome for the baby, and studies have not compared cerclage *with* bed rest to cerclage *without* bed rest.

THE RH-NEGATIVE MOTHER

At your first prenatal visit, a blood test will be done to find out what your blood type is and whether you have a factor in your blood called Rh. Rh is one of the antigens—markers—found on the surface of blood cells. Most people—about 85 percent—are Rh positive. However, some of us discover during pregnancy that we are Rh negative. If you are Rh negative and the baby's father is Rh positive, you may be carrying a baby who is Rh positive. When this happens, the baby's Rh positive cells may get into your bloodstream, and your body will make antibodies against them. This can cause health problems for any future babies you may have.

If you are Rh negative and this is your first pregnancy, it's highly unlikely that you've been exposed or will be exposed to the Rh marker.* The most likely time to be exposed to the Rh marker in your baby's blood is at the time of birth.

To prevent antibodies from being made, women who are Rh-negative are tested for antibodies to Rh and are given RhoGAM shots during pregnancy and after delivery. The RhoGAM shot blocks your body's immune system from making antibodies to the Rh marker. The shot is safe for you and your baby.

If you are Rh-negative, expect to be tested for antibodies two times during your pregnancy. You will be offered a RhoGAM shot at about 28 weeks and another right after birth if your baby is Rh positive. If you had an earlier pregnancy and did not receive RhoGAM, your health care provider will monitor your pregnancy closely. If Rh antibodies are found in your blood, a specialist will be consulted and your baby may receive special treatment while still growing in your uterus. Due to the availability of RhoGAM, the risk of developing the Rh antibodies is very low, almost to the point of being nonexistent.

---

* Although it is rare, it is possible to have been exposed to the Rh marker even if you have never been pregnant. The most common way this happens is from a blood transfusion with inappropriately cross-matched blood. It is also possible to have been exposed if you had a miscarriage that was undetected, or if you had an invasive prenatal procedure and didn't receive RhoGAM.

DIABETES IN PREGNANCY

About one in every twenty-five pregnancies is complicated by diabetes. Some women develop diabetes during pregnancy; this is known as *gestational diabetes mellitus,* or GDM. Some of us have diabetes before becoming pregnant; this is known as *pre-existing diabetes.*

GESTATIONAL DIABETES

Gestational diabetes is caused by hormonally induced resistance to insulin, the substance that helps the body use and store glucose (a type of sugar). This leads to *high blood sugar,* (hyperglycemia). Women are usually tested for gestational diabetes in weeks 24 to 28 of pregnancy. (For information on the test, see page 56.) You are more likely to develop this condition if you are overweight, have had gestational diabetes before, have close relatives with diabetes, are over twenty-five years old, or are Latina, African-American, or Native American.

Managing Gestational Diabetes

The main goal of managing gestational diabetes is to keep your blood glucose at a normal level, so that excess sugar does not cross the placenta and cause high blood sugar in the developing baby. High blood sugar in the developing baby can lead to excess fetal weight gain (a condition known as *macrosomia*). If this happens, you may experience problems with birth, and your baby may be at risk for injury during birth. Babies with macrosomia can also experience breathing problems and have an increased risk of developing obesity and type 2 diabetes as they grow older.

Most of us can keep our blood sugar at normal levels by adjusting our eating habits, although some of us will need insulin therapy as well. When you have gestational diabetes, your blood sugar rises in response to the amount and type of carbohydrates you eat. This is called "carbohydrate intolerance." "Simple" carbohydrates—such as those in soft drinks, candy, and even milk—are generally not recommended. On the other hand, "complex," or unrefined, carbohydrates—such as those in beans and whole grains—can be eaten in controlled amounts.

Your provider will probably ask you to monitor and record your blood sugar levels; this involves pricking your finger to obtain and test a drop of blood. Moderate exercise is recommended for women with gestational diabetes since exercise can temporarily lower blood sugar levels.

Because managing gestational diabetes is complex, it is very important to receive one-on-one counseling after diagnosis. Your provider will probably advise you or refer you to a nutritionist or diabetes educator. If not, ask for a referral or seek another, experienced health care provider with whom you feel comfortable.

The Emotional Impact of Gestational Diabetes

I was a mess, unable to eat anything without the fear of my blood sugar skyrocketing, making [my baby] even bigger. I gained no weight. She kept on gaining. I felt trapped by my strict diet and four-times-a-day blood testing. My fingers were bruised, yet the life within me kept on going.

Managing gestational diabetes can cause stress, as well as a sense of alienation from other pregnant women and even our partners and families. Fortunately, we are rarely alone. Many university hospital programs offer support groups for women with gestational diabetes, and there are also many online resources available.

Even though gestational diabetes is challenging, some of us have found that, as we become more used to its day-to-day management, we feel pride in being able to take steps so early on to safeguard our own and our child's future health.

Since women with gestational diabetes are at a higher risk for developing type 2 diabetes later, it is important to continue to check in with your health care provider after you give birth. Although postpartum weight loss should never be rushed, implementing a gradual, long-term weight loss plan is a good way to protect yourself from future diabetes if you are above the recommended weight for your height and build.

PRE-EXISTING DIABETES

Pregnant women with pre-existing diabetes share many of the concerns of women with gestational diabetes, but they have unique issues, too. Although those of us with pre-existing diabetes are used to managing our condition, the stricter blood glucose goals imposed during pregnancy require extra attention.

Research shows that if we start our pregnancies with our blood sugar controlled, and maintain this throughout pregnancy, we have as good a likelihood of delivering a healthy baby as any woman.[3] However, since many health care providers are inexperienced in treating pregnant women with pre-existing diabetes, and since some believe incorrectly that it is always more dangerous for women with pre-existing diabetes to have a child, working with a skillful health care provider who is knowledgeable about diabetes is critical.

If you become pregnant and already have type 1 or type 2 diabetes, your provider will ask you to have blood tests done during an early prenatal visit to measure your long-term blood sugar levels (also known as *glycated hemoglobin*, or Hb_{A1c}, testing) and kidney function. The results will provide information to help you manage your pregnancy. In addition, you can expect that your health care provider will arrange for the following special exams and tests for you:

- periodic visits with a nutritionist or diabetes educator to help you plan your diet and insulin doses
- a check-up with an ophthalmologist or optometrist before conception or during the first trimester to monitor the health of your eyes during the stress of pregnancy
- possible follow-up eye exams later in the pregnancy
- more frequent ultrasounds to make sure your baby is growing at a normal rate
- non-stress tests (monitoring the baby's heart rate and pattern as well as any contractions you may be having) later in pregnancy

It is imperative to educate and empower ourselves. Read, talk to others, ask questions, speak up, and become active in ongoing conversations about your treatment. Sometimes we need to uproot and replant ourselves with doctors who are more knowledgeable and more open to our input.

In some cases, your insurance plan may not cover treatment by a specialist. If you are in this situation, you may need to appeal to your insurance company or pay for some of your care yourself.

PRE-ECLAMPSIA/HYPERTENSION

High blood pressure (hypertension) during your pregnancy can cause complications for you and your baby. If you have high blood pressure, the placenta may be smaller and less able to transfer nutrients to your baby. Some women with high blood pressure do very well and have big, healthy babies, and some develop problems that result in a smaller baby who may need to be delivered early.

If you develop high blood pressure for the first time toward the end of your pregnancy, you may have a condition known as *pre-eclampsia*. Between five and eight out of every one hundred pregnant women in the United States will have pre-eclampsia.

Checking for pre-eclampsia is one of the main reasons prenatal visits are every week or every other week toward the end of pregnancy. Your clinician will check for it by measuring the amount of protein in your urine and taking your blood pressure at each visit. Symptoms of pre-eclampsia include headaches; swelling in your face, hands, or legs; visual disturbances; bleeding problems; upper abdominal pain; and, in severe cases, convulsions (eclampsia). Eclampsia can be life-threatening to both mother and fetus.

The cause of pre-eclampsia is not clear, but current research points to a combination of genetic, hormonal, and nutritional factors. A woman is more likely to develop pre-eclampsia if she is pregnant for the first time, if she has high blood pressure before pregnancy, if she is overweight, if she is carrying more than one baby, or if she has another medical condition such as pre-existing diabetes, sickle-cell disease, lupus, or kidney disease. If you have any of these problems or you've had pre-eclampsia in a previous pregnancy, it's a good idea to consult an obstetrician or a specialist in maternal-fetal medicine before you get pregnant again.

Taking a multivitamin supplement regularly three months before you conceive and during the first three months of pregnancy may reduce your risk of developing pre-eclampsia.[4] If you are at risk for developing pre-eclampsia, your health care provider may suggest taking antioxidants or increasing your calcium intake.[5]

The only real "cure" for pre-eclampsia is to give birth to the baby, usually by inducing labor. (For more information about induction, see page 146.) If you develop pre-eclampsia before the baby is mature enough to breathe spontaneously after delivery, you may be advised to stop work and refrain from other strenuous activities, and to rest as much as possible. Your health care provider may want you to go to the hospital, where you can be treated with medication to lower your blood pressure and to prevent seizures. You may also get medication to help the baby's lungs develop faster, so you can give birth. Pre-eclampsia is not in itself a reason for a cesarean birth. The baby can usually be born vaginally.

INFECTIONS DURING PREGNANCY

HIV/AIDS

HIV (human immunodeficiency virus, the virus that causes AIDS) can pass from mother to fetus (this is known as *vertical transmission, mother-to-child transmission,* or *MTCT*) during pregnancy and childbirth. It can also pass from mother to infant during breast-feeding.

It's a good idea to get an HIV test as early as possible in your pregnancy, so that you will know your HIV status and can take steps to pre-

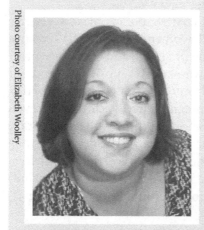

Photo courtesy of Elizabeth Woolley

"It was like playing pin-the-tail-on-the-donkey with a donkey that was constantly moving away."

Elizabeth "Bjay" Woolley

When I was 7 weeks pregnant, I had uncontrolled type 2 diabetes and I feared for my baby. Eight years earlier I was diagnosed with diabetes, and didn't take the disease seriously. Treatment had progressed from diet and exercise to a combination of oral medications. My lax attitude and pregnancy hormones were causing out-of-control blood sugar levels. I asked my general practitioner for insulin and to see a dietician. Insulted, he angrily said he knew what he was doing, and walked out. I ducked into a bathroom and cried for almost an hour.

Up to this point, I had always mindlessly followed my doctor's instructions. But no longer. I found a diabetes educator who listened to me and helped me assemble a health care team. She encouraged me to learn more and be more involved in my care. I was started on insulin and a diet, and given blood sugar goals and supplies.

It was not easy, but I did it all—testing eight times a day, insulin shots five times a day, and the diet. I didn't have a baby yet, but I lugged a large insulated diaper bag everywhere I went. It was filled with my needles, insulin, log, meter, snacks, ice, and other supplies. Tight blood sugar control was an ongoing battle, as my insulin needs increased through pregnancy. It was like playing pin-the-tail-on-the-donkey with a donkey that was constantly moving away.

Fortunately, I was motivated and took self-education seriously. I became an active member of the team who had a good idea of what was going on and even offered suggestions. I am thankful my body responded favorably to my efforts and I was able to keep hitting my goals without complications.

My beautiful son was born in April 2001. After his birth, it was scary to no longer have such intense support, but the knowledge I gained will allow me to continue to care for myself in order to care for him. Because of my experience, I have started a website, DiabeticMommy.com, to help other mothers get information and support.

vent transmission if you are HIV-positive. The Centers for Disease Control and Prevention recommends that women who have specific risks for HIV or live in states where HIV is more common get a second test in the third trimester.[6]

If you are HIV-negative, it is important to take steps to stay that way. Some research has shown that it is easier for women who are pregnant to become infected with HIV if exposed to it.[7] Therefore, it's important not to engage in behaviors during your pregnancy that could put you at risk for HIV, such as injection-drug use or unprotected sex with someone who is HIV-positive or whose HIV status is unknown to you.[8]

If you are HIV-positive, treatment can improve your health and dramatically reduce the chance that your baby will be born infected with the virus. Transmission of HIV is strongly correlated with your *viral load* (how much of the virus is in your blood).[9] Antiretroviral drugs lower viral load. In some clinical studies, antiretroviral drugs taken during pregnancy and at the time of birth have reduced the rate of vertical transmission to less than one in fifty births.[10] If you are HIV-positive and not taking antiretroviral drugs, there is about a one-in-three to one-in-six chance that your baby will be infected.[11]

In the past, it was recommended that all pregnant women who were HIV-positive give birth by cesarean section. Now the recommendations depend upon your viral load. If your HIV infection is untreated, or if you are taking antiretrovirals but your viral load is more than 1,000 copies per milliliter, having a planned cesarean will reduce the chances of your baby becoming infected.[12] If your viral load is less than 1,000 copies per milliliter, the current recommendations support giving birth vaginally, as cesarean sections have known risks and the benefits of a cesarean in these circumstances are uncertain.[13]

As new research is done, the guidelines for treating HIV continue to change rapidly. If you are pregnant and HIV-positive, it is important that you receive care from a specialist who treats women with HIV or that your health care provider consults with such a specialist.

Since HIV can pass to an infant through breast milk, it is safest for mothers in the United States who are HIV-positive not to breast-feed. Researchers are investigating whether certain types of antiretroviral therapy may help prevent transmission from mother to baby during breast-feeding.[14]

Some HIV/AIDS policy makers actively discourage all women who are HIV-positive from becoming pregnant, and encourage pregnant women who are HIV-positive to end our pregnancies. Ironically, though, if you are HIV-positive and pregnant and wish to abort, you may find that abortion clinics will refuse to take you or will charge extra. Advocates are fighting to preserve the reproductive rights and freedom of women who are HIV-positive, including access to nondiscriminatory health care.

In my fourth month I started my prenatal visits. I invited my baby's father to join me. We both got to hear the baby's heartbeat for the first time. I fell in love with my baby. My boyfriend looked nervous and uneasy. The doctor sent me to the lab to get numerous blood tests done. She asked me if I was interested in getting an HIV test. I went ahead and consented to getting the test done. I didn't think I had any problems because I was tested about a month after I started seeing my boyfriend, and I tested negative. To my surprise, I received a phone call at my job from my physician. He wanted to see me the next day in regard to one of my blood tests. My heart sank. . . .

The next day I went to see my doctor. . . . When he told me I had tested positive for HIV I couldn't stop crying. I was so worried for my baby. I did not want him to have it. For a few minutes I though of going home and cutting my wrists. I was so afraid of what people would think of me. I thought about how young I was. I thought of my two boys at home and how I failed them. Of course, the idea of cutting my wrists didn't last very long. I have too much to live for.

. . . I gave birth to a beautiful boy. I named him Malachi. Malachi is Hebrew for "God's Messenger." I believe if it weren't for my Malachi I probably would have found out when it was too late. I am eternally grateful for being able to give

birth to all three of my boys and I will do my best to see them grow up to be young men!

HEPATITIS

Hepatitis is a viral infection of the liver. There are many different types of hepatitis. The most common are hepatitis A, B, and C. *Hepatitis A* is a virus spread by eating food or drinking water that has been contaminated with feces—usually because of poor hand-washing by restaurant workers. Hepatitis A may make you very sick, but it will not usually cause lasting problems for you or your baby.

Hepatitis B and *hepatitis C* are viral infections spread by sexual contact and contact with infected blood. They are most commonly spread through sexual contact or sharing needles in IV drug use. Both hepatitis B and hepatitis C may be transmitted to a baby during birth. Today, most young people in the United States have been immunized against hepatitis B. There is no vaccine for hepatitis C.

All pregnant women should be screened for hepatitis. If you have had hepatitis B or C, you may be a carrier and can transmit the infection to others. If you know that you are a carrier for hepatitis B or C, be sure to let your health care provider know as early as possible in your pregnancy. Your health care provider will monitor your health and possibly consult with a specialist in infectious diseases to prepare for protecting your baby. There is no evidence to suggest that a cesarean section is safer than a vaginal birth and there is no evidence that a cesarean section will protect the baby from becoming infected. Since it is safer in general, vaginal birth is recommended unless another problem arises that indicates you need a cesarean section.

If you are a carrier of hepatitis B or C, your baby will be given a full bath soon after birth (to avoid prolonged exposure to your blood)

and will receive both hepatitis B immune globulin (HBIG) and the first dose of the hepatitis vaccine. Your baby will be monitored closely during the first year of life to see if she or he has contracted the virus.[15] Women who are carriers of hepatitis B or C can breast-feed.

HERPES

Herpes simplex virus (HSV) is a virus in the chicken pox family. It is spread from person to person by skin contact. Herpes comes in two types—type 1 and type 2. Type 1 is more often found on the mouth, but it can also be transmitted to the genitals. When on the mouth, it gives people what we call "cold sores." Type 2 is more often found on the genitals, but it can also be transmitted to the mouth. Ordinarily, herpes of either type is just an annoying inconvenience. But during pregnancy it may be cause for special concern.

One in every four pregnant women in the United States has herpes of some type. Most of us who have the virus have no idea that we do.[16] If you have genital herpes, and you have the virus in your birth canal during delivery, your baby may contract *neonatal herpes*. If you have oral herpes, your baby may contract neonatal herpes if you kiss her or him when you have an active cold sore. Neonatal herpes can cause serious problems for your baby.

If you had herpes before becoming pregnant or you contract it early in your pregnancy, the likelihood of passing the virus to your baby is very, very low—less than one in one hundred.[17] Your immune system has learned to handle the virus and you probably have few outbreaks. Even if you have an outbreak, your immune system will make antibodies against the herpes virus that cross the placenta, and the antibodies will protect your baby.

Your baby will be most at risk if you have your very first outbreak of herpes (*primary her-*

pes) near the time you give birth. This is because, with a new infection, your body has not had a chance to make antibodies against the virus. You will likely be having more frequent and more severe outbreaks. If you have primary herpes near the end of your pregnancy, your health care provider may consult with a specialist in infectious diseases to determine the best way to protect your baby from infection.

If you know you have herpes, tell your health care provider at your first pregnancy visit. Discuss the plan of care and the best ways to protect your baby. The following suggestions will help prevent spreading the infection to your baby:

• Some health care providers routinely recommend that women with a history of getting herpes sores take antiviral medicines near the end of pregnancy to suppress outbreaks. The most common medicine for this is acyclovir. Antivirals have not been approved for use in pregnancy, but they have been used a lot without any apparent harm to the baby. Studies have not shown that routine antiviral therapy is a good idea for all women with herpes.[18] However, if you have frequent outbreaks of herpes, you may want to consider antiviral therapy near the end of your pregnancy to avoid an outbreak at the time of birth.
• As much as possible, avoid interventions during labor that may break your baby's skin and make her or him more vulnerable to infection. These include artificial rupture of membranes, fetal scalp electrode, and vacuum or forceps delivery.
• If you have a genital herpes outbreak at the time of delivery, you and your provider will discuss the pros and cons of having a vaginal birth or cesarean section. The best choice will depend on where the sore is and what you and your provider think is safest.
• After your baby is born, if you have a cold sore on your mouth, do not kiss your baby until the cold sore has completely disappeared. Wash your hands carefully before touching your baby.

If you do not have the virus, and your partner is unsure whether he or she has the virus, your partner may want to be tested. If your partner has the virus, abstain from sex during active outbreaks. Between outbreaks, use a condom or dental dam every time you have sexual contact.[19]

OTHER INFECTIONS

Other infections that can cause problems for your developing baby include *cytomegalovirus (CMV), listeriosis, toxoplasmosis, rubella* (German measles), *chicken pox, parvovirus,* and *coxsackie virus.* Most women of childbearing age in the United States have either had rubella or been vaccinated against it. Toxoplasmosis is transmitted from cat feces or spores that are found in dirt. (For more information about preventing toxoplasmosis infection, see "Cats, Steak Tartare, and Gardening]" page 88.) Chicken pox is highly infectious, but most adults have had it as children and therefore cannot get it again. (A vaccine is available for those who have not.)

While most of these infections are generally mild and cause few problems for a woman who is not pregnant, they can cause serious problems for the baby inside the uterus. Complications tend to be worse if you get the infection early in your pregnancy (up to 12 to 15 weeks). If you have any symptoms of an infection during your pregnancy, call your health care provider right away. Signs of infections include fever, rash on your upper torso, or swollen glands behind your ears or on your neck. Most of these infections have a low rate of transfer to the developing baby inside you.

If you have an infection that could cause serious harm to your baby, talk with your health care provider about the following:

- **Options for determining if the baby is infected or not.** For some diseases, tests can help you know how the baby is affected.
- **Options for treatment.** For some infections, medications may lessen the effects on your baby.
- **Potential impact of the infection on your baby.** If the impact is likely to be very severe and your baby is infected, you can talk to your provider about terminating or continuing the pregnancy.

BREECH BABY

Sometimes a baby will settle in the mother's pelvis in a sort of seated position, with the baby's head up instead of down. This is known as the *breech position*. Breech babies can be feet-first (a "footling breech"), buttocks-first with the feet up by the arms and head (a "frank breech," the most common breech position), or legs crossed (a "complete breech").

It is fairly common for a baby to be breech early in pregnancy, but most babies turn so that they are head-down by 34 weeks. If an abdominal exam or ultrasound after the eighth month of pregnancy shows that your baby is in the breech position, a provider can try to turn the baby to head-down before labor starts, by pressing on your uterus from the outside. This is called *external cephalic version*. The fetal heart rate is monitored with ultrasound at the same time the baby is being turned. You will feel a lot of pressure as the baby is moved. The main risks of external version are placental abruption and inducing labor, both of which are rare. Turning the baby in this way works in

about three out of five cases, although some providers have more success than others.[20]

Two other techniques for turning the baby, used by practitioners of Chinese and alternative medicine, are *moxibustion* and *acupuncture*. Moxibustion involves burning a stick of moxa, made from a ground herb, near a particular body part. It's hard to know, from existing research, how well moxibustion works.[21] One study was stopped early because too many women found the moxibustion unpleasant and didn't complete the treatment.[22] Acupuncture has been shown to have a modest effect.[23]

If turning the baby does not work and he or she is in a breech position as you near your due date, you will face a decision about how the baby will be born. Both vaginal breech deliveries and cesareans pose some risks to mothers and babies. In some circumstances, the safest way for your breech baby to be born is for you to have a cesarean section. If the baby is positioned so that the feet are first (footling breech), there is a chance that the umbilical cord will fall through the cervix into the vagina before the baby is born or that the cervix will not open wide enough for the baby's head to come out. Because of these risks, a cesarean section is recommended when a baby is a footling breech. Alternatively, you are a good candidate for a vaginal birth if the baby is in frank breech or complete breech position, you have had a previous vaginal birth of a full-term baby, the baby is judged to be full-term and not too big, and your health care provider has experience with vaginal breech deliveries.

The main risk in vaginal birth of a breech baby is that difficulty may be encountered in the delivery of the head, usually the largest part of the baby, with resulting compression of the umbilical cord and loss of oxygen to the baby. The American College of Obstetricians and Gynecologists used to recommend routine cesareans for all breech babies, but it no longer does so.[24] Research suggests that routine cesarean section for breech babies does not lead to better outcomes than vaginal birth.[25]

If your baby is in the breech position as you approach your due date, learn all you can about the benefits and harms of the different modes of giving birth and talk with your provider about the various options. Most obstetricians will recommend that a breech baby be delivered via cesarean section, but some are willing to attend you throughout a vaginal birth. If you plan to give birth vaginally, be sure that your provider and any other providers who might be attending you have experience with breech births. (As cesarean sections for breech babies have become more common, fewer providers have learned the hands-on skills necessary to safely attend a woman giving birth to a breech baby.)

Occasionally, babies who are in the breech position will turn to head-down when labor contractions begin. If your baby is breech and you are planning a cesarean, you can request that the cesarean not be done until the natural onset of labor. Discuss this plan with your provider, so that you know how soon to come in after labor starts. In early labor, an ultrasound can be done. If the baby is head-first, you won't need a cesarean. By waiting until labor starts on its own, you also allow for the fetal lungs to develop more. On the other hand, if you wait for the onset of labor, the operation may not be with your doctor of choice as the surgeon. (For more information about breech birth, see "Breech Presentation," page 221.)

THE LONG PREGNANCY

The average length of pregnancy is 40 weeks, but some women naturally have pregnancies that are a bit shorter or longer. In addition, many of us don't know for sure exactly when we got pregnant. Therefore, the "due date" we get at our first prenatal visit may be off by days or even weeks.

Even knowing how uncertain the due date is, most of us become utterly focused on our due date as the end of pregnancy draws near. The last weeks of pregnancy are often filled with little (or big) aches and pains. We are eager to meet the little person growing inside of us. If our due date comes and goes with no sign of labor, the days really begin to drag. It doesn't help that family and friends keep calling to ask if we are in labor yet!

If we go more than a week past our due date, our health care provider may begin to be concerned as well. In pregnancies that go longer than 42 weeks, the placenta may "run out of steam" and not provide oxygen and nutrients to the baby as effectively. When this happens, babies may develop something called "post-maturity syndrome." Post-maturity babies actually lose weight, and their skin becomes wrinkled. They may have difficulty breathing and eating after they are born. When a pregnancy continues more than a week to ten days after the due date, your health care provider may order weekly or twice-weekly non-stress testing or biophysical profiles to assess your baby's health (see "Tests for Your Baby's Well-Being," facing page). Your provider may also ask you to do daily kick counts and give you instructions on how to do so.

INDUCTION OF LABOR

If you and your health care provider are becoming concerned that the pregnancy is continuing too long, you may consider inducing your labor. Here are some things to think about in such a situation:

• Babies generally do best if they get to grow to their full size inside the uterus. This usually

TESTS FOR YOUR BABY'S WELL-BEING

The non-stress test and the biophysical profile are tests that are done in the health care provider's office or the hospital to check on the well-being of your baby. Either or both may be offered to a woman who has a health concern in pregnancy, whose baby is moving less than usual, or whose pregnancy has gone past the due date.

For the **non-stress test,** you will lie in a reclining chair or bed with belts around your belly holding two monitors in place. One monitor will pick up your baby's heart rate. The other will monitor your uterus for contractions and your baby's movement. The non-stress test is considered "reactive," or good, if your baby's heart rate goes up and down and really speeds up for about 20 seconds (an "acceleration") at least two times in a 20-minute period. A reactive result is a sign that your baby has enough oxygen and nutrients and is doing well.

The **biophysical profile** combines the non-stress test with some measurements that are done with ultrasound. During the ultrasound, the technician or nurse will measure the amount of fluid surrounding your baby and will look for movements of the baby's arms, legs, and chest. The biophysical profile is scored with points for the non-stress test, the fluid, and the different types of movement. The best possible score is 10. A score of 6 or less may mean that your baby is not getting enough oxygen and may need closer evaluation. Because the biophysical profile includes several different measures, it is a more accurate predictor of how well your baby will do over the next couple of days than the non-stress test alone.

takes about 40 weeks, or anywhere from 38 weeks to 41½ weeks. If the due date is not accurately calculated so as to be in the middle of this normal time frame, inducing labor could force a baby out into the world a few days to a few weeks early.

- When it is time to go into labor, the cervix (the mouth of the uterus) becomes soft and stretchy and "points" toward the vaginal opening. Trying to induce labor before the body is ready may result in a long, hard labor or a cervix that cannot open. This can lead to a cesarean section. (Women who have labor induced have a higher chance of giving birth by cesarean.)

- There are a number of ways of inducing labor in the hospital. These include *cervical ripening* (putting medicine into the vagina or putting a small, soft latex balloon into the cervix), *breaking the bag of waters* (artificial rupture of membranes, or AROM), or encouraging contractions with *Pitocin* (synthetis oxytocin). Cervical ripening or AROM may give you a "jump-start" to get your labor going on its own. Many women report this is easier than a Pitocin induction. In a Pitocin induction, the medicine is making labor for you, which may be more uncomfortable.

There are also things you can try at home to encourage labor:

- Some women report success with drinking a "cocktail" of prune juice, orange juice, and castor oil. There is no research to say this works, but some women believe it helps get contractions started. It will certainly give you diarrhea!
- Many people believe that sex and orgasms will get labor going. If you have a male partner, his semen is rich in substances called prostaglandins. Prostaglandins make the cervix soft and make the uterus ready to contract when labor begins. Whether or not semen is present, when you have an orgasm, your own body will secrete a bit of oxytocin, and this may cause the uterus to contract. Some recent research has shown that sex doesn't consistently induce labor,[26] but it does seem to work for some women.
- Nipple stimulation usually makes contractions happen, but does not always start true labor. Since this stimulation sometimes happens during sex, it may be a part of why sex sometimes starts contractions or labor. Nipple stimulation can cause contractions that are longer than usual and therefore it is not recommended unless you are in a hospital and your baby is being monitored with continuous electronic fetal monitoring.
- Acupuncture has been used to induce labor in some cultures. However, very little research has been done, so it is difficult to know whether it is effective.

If you are considering induction of labor, talk with your health care provider about the risks and benefits and about the options—which method of induction is likely to be most successful and easiest on you and your baby.

CONCLUSION

Women who have health problems during pregnancy can become very anxious and worried about all the extra care and tests that are offered. If you have a chronic health problem or develop a problem during pregnancy, the extra prenatal visits, tests, and time to talk to a specialist will offer you an early opportunity to gather information. You can use the resources and knowledge to help take care of yourself and your baby. When your baby is born, you may be more prepared than most to move into the next stage of being a mother.

NOTES

1. M. Prysak, R. P. Lorenz, and A. Kisly, "Pregnancy Outcome in Nulliparous Women 35 Years and Older," *Obstetrics & Gynecology* 85, no. 1 (January 1995): 65–70. See also B. Jacobsson, L. Ladfors, and I. Milsom, "Advanced Maternal Age and Adverse Perinatal Outcome," *Obstetrics & Gynecology* 104, no. 4 (October 2004): 727–733.
2. Paul J. Meis, Mark Klebanoff, Elizabeth Thom, Mitchell P. Dobrowski, and Baha Sibai, "Prevention of Recurrent Preterm Delivery by 17 Alpha-Hydroxyprogesterone Caprote," *New England Journal of Medicine* 348, no. 24 (2003): 2,379–2,385.
3. John L. Kitzmiller, Thomas A. Buchanan, Siri L. Kjos, Christian A. Combs, and Robert E. Ratner, "Preconception Care of Diabetes, Medical Malformations, and Spontaneous Abortions," *Diabetes Care* 19 (1996): 514–541.
4. Lisa M. Bodnar, Gong Tang, Roberta B. Ness, Gail Harger, and James M. Roberts, "Periconceptional Multivitamin Use Reduces the Risk of Preeclampsia," *American Journal of Epidemiology* 164 (2006): 470–477, accessed at http://aje.oxfordjournals.org/cgi/content/full/164/5/470 on September 12, 2006.
5. G. J. Hofmeyer, A. N. Atallah, and L. Duley, "Calcium Supplementation During Pregnancy for Preventing

Hypertensive Disorders and Related Problems" *Co-chrane Database of Systematic Reviews* 2006, Issue 3. Art. No.: CD001059. DOI: 10.1002/14651858.cd00105 .pub2.

6. Centers for Disease Control and Prevention, "Revised Recommendations for HIV Testing of Adults, Adolescents, and Pregnant Women in Health-Care Settings," *Morbidity and Mortality Weekly Report* 55, no. RR14 (September 2006): 1–17.

7. R. H. Gray, Li X, G. Kigozi, et al., "Increased Risk of Incident HIV During Pregnancy in Rakai, Uganda: A Prospective Study," *Lancet* 366 (2005): 1182–1188.

8. B. Warren, R. Glaros, S. Hackel et al., "Residual Perinatal HIV Transmissions in 25 Births Occurring in New York State," in *Proceedings of National HIV Prevention Conference*, Atlanta, GA, June 12–15, 2005.

9. D. M. Thea, R. W. Steketee, V. Pliner, et al. for the New York City Perinatal HIV Transmission Collaborative Study Group, "The Effect of Maternal Viral Load on the Risk of Perinatal Transmission of HIV-1," *AIDS* 11, no. 4 (March 15, 1997): 437–444.

10. A. P. Kourtis and A. Duerr, "Prevention of Perinatal HIV Transmission: A Review of Novel Strategies," *Expert Opinion on Investigational Drugs* 12, no. 9 (September 2003): 1,535–1,544.

11. L. M. Mofenson, "Mother-Child HIV-1 Transmission: Timing and Determinants," *Obstetrics and Gynecology Clinics of North America* 24, no. 4 (December 1997): 759–784.

12. Perinatal HIV Guidelines Working Group, "Public Health Service Task Force Recommendations for Use of Antiretroviral Drugs in Pregnant HIV-1 Infected Women for Maternal Health and Interventions to Reduce Perinatal HIV-1 Transmission in the United States" (July 6, 2006), U.S. Public Health Service, Rockville, MD.

13. Ibid.

14. C. Thorne and M. L. Newell, "Prevention of Mother-to-Child Transmission of HIV Infection," *Current Opinion in Infectious Diseases* 17, no. 3 (June 2004): 247–252.

15. Centers for Disease Control and Prevention, "STD Treatment Guidelines," *Morbidity and Mortality Weekly Report*, August 2006; accessed at www.cdc.gov/std/treatment/2006/rr511.pdf on October 16, 2006.

16. American Social Health Association, "Herpes and Pregnancy," 2006; accessed at www.ashastd.org/herpes/herpes_learn_pregnancy.cfm on October 15, 2006.

17. Centers for Disease Control and Prevention, "STD Treatment Guidelines," accessed at www.cdc.gov/std/treatment/2006/rr5511.pdf on October 16, 2006.

18. Ibid.

19. American Social Health Association, "Herpes and Pregnancy" (2006), accessed at www.ashastd.org/herpes/herpes_learn_pregnancy.cfm on October 15, 2006.

20. J. Zhang, W. A. Bowes Jr., and J. A. Fortney, "Efficacy of External Cephalic Version: A Review," *Obstetrics & Gynecology* 82 (1993): 306–312. One very small study found 59 percent success with epidural versus 24 percent without: S. J. Carlan et al., "The Effect of Epidural Anesthesia on Safety and Success of External Cephalic Version at Term," *Anesthesia & Analgesia* 79, no. 3 (September 1994): 525–528. Other studies, however, show (a) no difference between spinal and no anesthesia: L. Dugoff, C. A. Stamm, O. W. Jones III, S. I. Mohling, and J. L. Hawkins, "The Effect of Spinal Anesthesia on the Success Rate of External Cephalic Version: a Randomized Trial," *Obstetrics & Gynecology* 93, no. 3 (March 1999): 345–349; or (b) a 60 percent success rate without epidural and 71 percent success with epidural: R. Neiger, M. D. Hennessy, and M. Patel, "Reattempting Failed External Cephalic Version Under Epidural Anesthesia," *American Journal of Obstetrics & Gynecology* 179, no. 5 (November 1998): 1,136–1,139

21. I. Neri, G. Airola, G. Contu, G. Allais, F. Facchinetti, et al., "Acupuncture plus Moxibustion to Resolve Breech Presentation: A Randomized Controlled Study," *Journal of Maternal-Fetal and Neonatal Medicine* 15, no. 4 (2004): 247–252. See also M. E. Coyle, C. A. Smith, and B. Peat, "Cephalic Version by Moxibustion for Breech Presentation," *Cochrane Database of Systematic Reviews* 2005, Issue 2. Art. No.: CD003928. DOI:10.1002/14651858.CD003928.pub2.

22. F. Cardini, P. Lombardo, A. L. Regalia, G. Regaldo, A. Zanini, et al., "A Randomised Controlled Trial of Moxibustion for Breech Presentation," *BJOG* 112 (2005): 743–747.

23. Neri et al., "Acupuncture Plus Moxibustion."

24. American College of Obstetricians and Gynecologists, ACOG Commitee Opinion no. 340, "Mode of Term Singleton Breech Delivery," *Obstetrics & Gynecology* 108, no. 1 (July 2006): 235–237.

25. H. Whyte, M. E. Hannah, S. Saigal, W. J. Hannah,

S. Hewson, K. Amankwah, et al., "Outcomes of Children at 2 Years After Planned Cesarean Birth Versus Planned Vaginal Birth for Breech Presentation at Term: The International Randomized Term Breech Trial," *American Journal of Obstetrics & Gynecology* 191, no. 3 (2004): 864–871.

26. Jonathan Schaffir, "Sexual Intercourse at Term and Onset of Labor," *Obstetrics & Gynecology* 107, no. 6 (June 2006): 1,310–1,314.

CHAPTER 9

Childbearing Loss

The loss of a pregnancy or the death of a baby during late pregnancy or in child-birth or infancy is often an immense and shocking blow. The grief that follows can be intense, and because it is not widely recognized in our culture, it may not be well understood.

I was hysterical with grief and jealous of all those pregnant moms, and moms push-ing strollers. I didn't know anyone who had had a miscarriage. That was a terrible thing. Even though intellectually you know miscarriage is quite common, there is still a great deal of secrecy and shame surrounding the experience.

The vast majority of women who experience childbearing loss go on to have successful pregnancies and deliver healthy babies. But such a loss affects future childbearing decisions and experiences, as well as relationships with family and friends. Understanding the most common causes of childbearing loss in the United States, as well as ways to get support in grieving a loss, can help prepare you to cope with the loss of a pregnancy or infant in the event that it happens to you or someone you know.

Childbearing loss occurs in many different ways, from miscarriage and still-birth to the decision not to carry to term a baby with impairments. Whatever our experience, loss of a pregnancy or an infant can be devastating. It challenges us physically, psychologically, and spiritually and can affect the core of our identity as a woman.

Women experiencing childbearing loss need emotional support and sensi-tive care and attention from health care providers, families, and friends. Many hospitals now have bereavement teams and organize pregnancy-and-infant-loss support groups. Sensitive providers and support groups (whether face-to-face or online) can help women and our partners with the isolation that often follows a

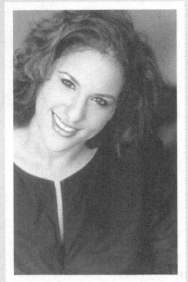

© Fadil Berisha

"I expected to hear the baby's heartbeat."
Catherine McKinley

It took me eight months to conceive. Then suddenly I was having my encounter with the magical: a routine 8-week sonogram where I expected to hear the baby's heartbeat for the first time. My ob-gyn tried to mask his concern as he moved the wand across my quiet belly. He was strangely nonchalant as he told me that the office equipment was not always able to get sensitive readings early in pregnancy. He wrote out a referral for a hospital sonogram, and I tried to brush off my anxiety.

The radiologist performing the sonogram was very pregnant. I laughed at her crankiness because she was so stunning, with a stomach so large her belly button was pointing toward the floor. But then her body almost seemed to be mocking me as she told me that she was unable to find a heartbeat. "You've miscarried," she said emotionlessly. It was difficult to process what she was saying. There had been no sign of blood; my body had not pushed out anything.

For weeks I'd felt this blooming feeling. But the night before, I had noticed that my skin had a funny new smell and I was suddenly feeling achy all over. Now I felt my body turning in on itself, betraying itself. I was admitted to the hospital for a D&C the next afternoon. That wait and the days after were some of the hardest moments of my journey to motherhood.

The loss roused old griefs: the eight months of wild fear that conception was impossible; the legacy of an illegal abortion, registered as a D&C while I was a college exchange student in Jamaica; birth family lost through adoption; and later the family I recovered whose inabilities rendered them as good as lost to me. An older friend who had had five children and twice as many pregnancies told me to embrace the heartache; I was being seasoned for motherhood. "You won't always get it easy," she said, "But the difficulty is what gives you the desire and the heart to mother better."

I got pregnant two months later and held my breath until the end of my first trimester. I was healthy and enjoying my pregnancy, but there was that lingering grief. I have come to like the idea of being seasoned. All of the trials have inscribed a kind of passion and will in my mothering.

loss, and support us in grieving, healing, and making decisions about future childbearing.

CAUSES OF CHILDBEARING LOSS

MISCARRIAGE

An estimated 15 to 20 percent of *known* pregnancies end in miscarriage, the loss of a pregnancy before the twentieth week.* Most clinically recognized miscarriages occur between the seventh and twelfth week after a woman's last menstrual period. The chances of miscarriage decrease significantly once a heartbeat has been detected on ultrasound or by Doppler stethoscope.

The vast majority of miscarriages cannot be prevented. Early losses often occur without a detectable embryo (sometimes there is just an empty sac or a "blighted ovum"). Up to 70 percent of first-trimester miscarriages, and 20 percent of second-trimester miscarriages, are caused by chromosomal anomalies from either the sperm or the egg cell.[1] Other known causes that are more likely to result in later miscarriages include infection, abnormalities of the uterus or cervix, smoking, substance abuse, exposure to environmental or industrial toxins, and autoimmune diseases. A serious physical trauma could cause a miscarriage. In rare cases, women miscarry after certain tests during pregnancy, such as chorionic villus sampling (CVS) or amniocentesis.

Many women learn about a miscarriage at a routine prenatal visit before experiencing any physical symptoms. The first symptoms of miscarriage are usually spotting or bleeding, followed by cramps in your lower back or abdomen. Other signs include fluid or tissue passing from the vagina.

Roughly two out of five pregnant women experience some vaginal bleeding or spotting during pregnancy, and only half of these women will miscarry.[2] If you have any vaginal bleeding during pregnancy, your health care provider can help determine if the bleeding is likely to result in miscarriage or if it has another cause that does not threaten the pregnancy. If you are miscarrying, bleeding will become heavier and cramping can be painful as the cervix dilates. A loss after 9 to 10 weeks' gestation may cause painful contractions.

If a blood test or sonogram indicates that you have had or are about to have a miscarriage, you may have a few options. Some women choose to allow the miscarriage to occur and complete itself naturally. Others find that scheduling a termination provides a sense of control and closure. There are several different ways to end the pregnancy. Medication treatment involves taking a drug, such as misoprostol, that causes uterine contractions and miscarriage, and can be used only early in the pregnancy. Other procedures (suction curettage, also known as *dilation and evacuation,* or D&E) use an aspiration technique to remove any remaining tissue. All of these are outpatient procedures. The aspiration technique may be performed on an outpatient basis in a clinic, obstetrical office, hospital, or emergency room.

If you miscarry naturally or with medication, you will probably miscarry at home. The process may be over quickly or may take several days. The fetus, amniotic sac, and placenta, along with a large amount of blood, will be expelled. If you are less than 8 weeks pregnant when the miscarriage occurs, the expelled tissue will look no different from heavy menstrual bleeding. If you have reached 8 to 10 weeks, more tissue will be expelled and miscarrying can be more painful. In this instance, if you have

---

* The actual number may be significantly higher because many miscarriages occur very early on, before a woman knows she is pregnant, and may simply seem to be a heavy period on or near schedule.

chosen to allow the miscarriage to occur spontaneously, try to arrange for a trusted, knowledgeable person to be with you through the process, throughout the night if needed. Think about where you will be most comfortable and what you will need, such as bed liners and sanitary pads, or hot water bottles and massage to comfort you and help with cramping. You may want to think and talk about what you would like to do with the remains. There will be some blood clots, and you may notice tissue that is firmer or lumpy-looking, which is placental or afterbirth tissue. You may or may not see tissue that looks like an embryo or fetus.

Once everything in your uterus has been expelled, bleeding will continue, lessening over several days. If bleeding increases or stays bright red, or if you have foul-smelling discharge or a fever, contact your health care provider. If fetal tissue remains in your uterus, your provider can perform a D&E to remove it and thereby prevent infection. A D&E involves dilating the cervix and using suction (aspiration) and/or a medical instrument to remove remaining fetal and placental tissue.[3]

Once bleeding has ceased and the cervix is closed, you can have sex (including penetration) without risk of infection. Since it is difficult to know when the cervix has completely closed, most providers recommend waiting two weeks. A repeat pregnancy test after a few weeks is important to make sure your hormone levels are normal. If you feel dizzy or tired, ask to be checked for anemia. If you do not know your blood type, you should have a blood test.

If your blood type is Rh-negative, you will need a shot within seventy-two hours of the miscarriage. (If you are Rh-negative and you were carrying an Rh-positive fetus, there is a small chance that you have been exposed to Rh-positive blood cells from the fetal tissue during the miscarriage. A shot of RhoGAM prevents your body from producing antibodies to Rh-positive blood that could harm a fetus during a future pregnancy. For more information, see "The Rh-Negative Mother," page 137.)

If you have a second-trimester miscarriage, or have had two or more earlier miscarriages, medical tests to help identify the cause are recommended. If you are at home when you miscarry, you may be able to collect fetal or afterbirth tissue in a clean container for examination at a hospital-based laboratory. Blood tests may identify or rule out hormonal, immunological, or chromosomal abnormalities in the parents or in any fetal tissue. Examinations of the uterus by ultrasound, hysteroscopy, and hysterosalpingography, or an endometrial biopsy, may also provide important information. Ask to see the pathology report, and ask for a full explanation of all terminology. Even if the cause cannot be determined—which is often the case—you will gain knowledge. You may be able to rule out likely causes of a repeat miscarriage and at least know that you have done all you can to get an answer.

Physical recovery from a miscarriage ranges from a few days to a couple of weeks. Your period will return within four to six weeks. Emotional recovery is likely to take longer. Give yourself time to grieve, search for medical explanations if there are any, and seek out other women who have miscarried.

Friends encouraged me to call their friends who had been through similar situations. This helped me tremendously. I loved talking to the woman in Oregon who had had four miscarriages before they discovered she had a blood-clotting disorder, or the woman in Boston who had three miscarriages and now had two small boys. These women became my friends.

ECTOPIC PREGNANCY

In an ectopic pregnancy, the fertilized egg implants outside the uterus, usually in the fallopian tube, where it cannot develop normally. This can be a life-threatening condition, requiring immediate treatment. Ectopic pregnancies occur in one in fifty to a hundred pregnancies. Most are caused by an infection or inflammation of the fallopian tube, scar tissue or adhesions from previous tubal or pelvic area surgeries, or a tubal abnormality. If you have had a previous ectopic pregnancy, pelvic surgery, or pelvic inflammatory disease, or if you conceived using assisted reproductive techniques, your risk may be higher. In addition, if your mother used DES while pregnant with you, your risk may be higher.[5] (DES, or diethylstilbestrol, is a synthetic estrogen that was often prescribed to help prevent miscarriage from 1938 until 1971, when the Food and Drug Administration advised against its use because of associated risks for vaginal cancer and other poor reproductive health outcomes in female offspring.[6])

If you have an ectopic pregnancy, you may have a positive pregnancy test and all the signs of early pregnancy. Vaginal bleeding, dizziness, weakness, and gastrointestinal discomfort are common early symptoms. As the pregnancy progresses, the pressure in the tube may cause stabbing pains, cramps, pain in your shoulder, or a dull ache that may vary in intensity, and come and go. It is critical to contact your provider if you have vaginal bleeding and/or sharp pain in the pelvic area, abdomen, and/or neck and shoulders. If an ectopic pregnancy is not diagnosed early, the fallopian tube can rupture, causing severe blood loss and shock.

If you have any of the symptoms of ectopic pregnancy, your health care provider will check your hormone levels every other day and do a vaginal ultrasound as early as possible (about 6 weeks). Ectopic pregnancy is occasionally misdiagnosed as an early miscarriage. This is why your provider may ask you to get a blood pregnancy test after a suspected miscarriage. The test can help confirm the presence or absence of fetal tissue in the fallopian tube.

When doctors detect an ectopic pregnancy, they will remove the embryonic tissue and try to save the tube. If the pregnancy is found early, physicians can give you the drug methotrexate, which dissolves the embryonic tissue. If your pregnancy is more advanced, you may need a laparoscopy, which requires small incisions in your abdomen to insert a fiberoptic light (laparoscope) and other instruments to view the pelvic area and to remove the embryonic tissue. If it is necesary to remove the whole tube or to have emergency surgery, a laparotomy can be performed to repair or remove the ruptured tube. Blood tests will be performed to check changes in your levels of HCG (human chorionic gonadotropin, the hormone produced by placental tissue) after any of these treatments in order to confirm that no ectopic tissue remains.

The loss of an ectopic pregnancy may bring on feelings like those that follow miscarriage, including fear that such a pregnancy could happen again. If you have had internal bleeding or a traumatic emergency surgery, talk with your provider about how this may affect future conception and pregnancies, and how to minimize your future risks.

MOLAR PREGNANCY

Molar pregnancies (also called *gestational trophoblastic disease* and *hydatidiform mole*) happen when the cells that are supposed to develop into the placenta instead develop into a tumor made of trophoblastic (placental) cells. The growth must be removed so that it does not spread. The chances of a molar pregnancy are very small (one in every one thousand to twelve hundred pregnancies).[7]

Signs and symptoms, usually identified through routine pregnancy visits, include first-trimester vaginal bleeding and a uterus that is too large for the gestational age. Molar pregnancies are treated by a D&C to remove the abnormal tissue and, in rare cases, by chemotherapy to treat any remaining abnormal cells. Close follow-up after a D&C is very important to ensure that no more abnormal tissue remains. A molar pregnancy does not affect your chances of having a subsequent normal pregnancy, but like any other pregnancy loss it is likely to bring grief, fears, and questions.

The news of the trophoblastic tissue put me into high gear. Keep busy. Or sleep. Can't stop to think, can't stop to cry. I feel driven. I need to stop and mourn, but how can I feel it necessary to mourn when there wasn't even anybody in there!?

MULTIPLE GESTATION PREGNANCY

Pregnancy loss and complications are more likely in multiple gestation pregnancies, in which there are two or more embryos or fetuses. There has been a dramatic increase in the number of multiple gestation pregnancies in the United States over the past twenty years. More women are conceiving after age thirty, which naturally increases the chance of multiples, and more women are using infertility treatments that increase the chance of having a multiple gestation pregnancy.[8]

At my 8-week ultrasound we were told that Twin B wasn't developing at the rate of Twin A, and that we were most likely going to lose the baby. They were confident that Twin A would continue to develop normally, and that my body would simply expel the dying twin.

Rarely, very early in pregnancy, one twin will die and the other will be fine. This is called "vanishing twin syndrome" and may be associated with some vaginal spotting during the first months.[9] If one fetus dies later in pregnancy, the surviving fetus or fetuses will need to be closely monitored.

LOSS AFTER PRENATAL DIAGNOSIS

Some of us choose to end a pregnancy after discovering that we are carrying a fetus with severe impairments. Loss from terminating a pregnancy is different from other childbearing losses because it arises out of our own decision, but it can be just as painful and difficult.

Religions, subcultures, communities, and individuals vary widely in their beliefs about the ethics of ending a pregnancy because of a diagnosed impairment. Those of us who experience this kind of loss may not speak openly about it for fear of being judged. Support from those around us, accurate and adequate information about the diagnosed disability and its potential impact, and support from other women with similar experiences can help many of us come to terms with our decision. (For more information, see Chapter 7, "Prenatal Testing.")

STILLBIRTH

"Stillbirth" refers to fetal death after 20 weeks' gestation. It occurs in one in two hundred pregnancies and often involves apparently healthy fetuses.[10] The most common known causes of stillbirth are maternal diabetes, bacterial infection, high blood pressure, placental problems, growth restriction, and umbilical cord accidents. But in over half of stillbirths, a cause cannot be determined even after extensive testing.

Most fetal deaths are detected before labor begins,[11] usually at a routine prenatal check, or when a woman notices an absence of the usual kicks and movement. An ultrasound and fetal heart monitor will confirm that the baby has died. If there is no medical need for immediate delivery, you will be able to decide whether to wait for labor to come naturally or to have labor induced. Having the chance to prepare yourself for the experience may help you manage the physical and emotional pain.

Emilio III was stillborn at almost 24 weeks. I was going to go through labor knowing that I wouldn't have a new life in my life. It was the worst eight hours of my life. The labor was painful both physically and emotionally. In the end we delivered a beautiful baby boy. At the nurses' urging, we agreed to see and hold him. We got to hold him for a long time. We have pictures of him and share them with our daughter who was born a little over a year later. She talks about her big little

brother all the time, which reminds us that he is a part of our family.

Once the baby is born, you will need to decide whether you want to see and hold her or him. You may want to name the baby if you haven't already done so, take photos, and take some time to say your goodbyes. It may seem at first that seeing or holding the baby will be too much to handle, but many women later feel grateful that we did this. Such acts help to acknowledge the infant's existence and to preserve her or his memory. Some hospitals now offer a "memory box" to bereaved parents; it can include footprints and handprints, along with any items that were in contact with the baby, such as a blanket.

You will be faced with a number of difficult and pressing decisions, including how you wish the baby's remains to be handled and whether you want to have an autopsy performed. The thought of an autopsy can be painful, and in many cases there is no conclusive answer. Yet an autopsy could provide important information about the cause of the stillbirth, which may help with closure and provide information for future pregnancies. If you choose to have an autopsy done, the person performing it should be a pediatric or neonatal pathologist, or working with one. If the person is not, you may want to ask for a referral to a pathologist with the necessary expertise to review the findings.

INFANT DEATH

In 2002, the rate of deaths in infants under one year old rose for the first time in forty-four years (seven out of every one thousand infants born in the United States died before their first birthday).[12] The increase was linked to a rise in neonatal deaths (death within the first twenty-eight days of life) due to an increase in births of extremely low-birth-weight infants and of multiples, who are often born prematurely and at lower birth weights.[13] Improved technologies that enable intensive monitoring of high-risk pregnancies are allowing for the emergency delivery of more preterm babies, but these babies are at increased risk of early death.[14]

While more recent data suggest that the infant mortality rate is declining again, large disparities persist between different racial and ethnic groups. African-American women remain at highest risk for childbearing loss and, along with women who are American Indian or Alaskan Native, Puerto Rican, or Hawaiian, are more likely than white women to lose an infant under one year old.[15] Race and ethnicity are not the only factors: access to good-quality prenatal care and health care in general, age, education, economic and health status, substance abuse, and the environment all play a role. Smoking during pregnancy—by itself—increases the risk of loss by over 60 percent.[16]

Congenital anomalies, low birth weight, and *sudden infant death syndrome* (SIDS) are the leading causes of infant death in the United States.[17] Most infant deaths happen in the first month of life.[18] While SIDS accounts for approximately two of every twenty-five infant deaths, it is the leading cause of death in infants over one month old.[19]

Each year, about twenty-one hundred apparently healthy infants die in their sleep in the United States.[20] These infants may lack the arousal mechanism that would cause them to wake up and shift their position if their breathing was somehow blocked. Most babies in such conditions would wake up and cry, enabling them to take in fresh air and bring their oxygen levels back to normal.

Why some infants lack an awakening response and why some populations are more vulnerable to SIDS than others remain subjects of continuing study. Male SIDS cases outnumber females by two to one, while African-American and Native American infants are more than two times more likely to die of SIDS than white infants.[21] The period of greatest vulnerability for all infants is the first six months of life.

SIDS cases have declined over the last decade due to a vigorous "Back to Sleep" public education campaign. The campaign has publicized that it is risky to put babies to sleep on their stomachs or sides, use soft bedding, overheat babies, and expose infants to secondhand smoke. Research suggests that a biological predisposition may interact with these risk factors to affect an infant's ability to detect or respond to reduced oxygen or increased carbon monoxide levels.[22] A recent study, which compared white and Hispanic babies who died of SIDS to those who died from other causes, identified specific abnormalities in how the neurons in the brains of the babies who died of SIDS processed serotonin.[23] Serotonin regulates breathing (including upper-airway reflexes), body temperature, mood, and arousal or awakening.

The latest research may lead to the development of a diagnostic test and preventive treatment for SIDS. However, more research is needed among African-American and Native American infants to understand the significant racial and ethnic disparities of SIDS.[24] The Back to Sleep campaign remains critical to continued prevention.

COPING WITH LOSS

Childbearing loss evokes many emotions. You may feel buffeted and torn by confusion, relief, shame, anger, sorrow, fear, powerlessness, or despair. You may need to withdraw at first and you may feel numb about a reality that seems to be too much to bear. You may want those around you to comfort you physically and listen empathetically. Some of your friends and family may not be able to handle the loss. Others may offer platitudes such as "You'll have another baby" that can fail to comfort you or to acknowledge the importance of your baby's existence. Thoughtful compassion from family, friends, and health care practitioners—and from yourself—is what you need most.

A tremendous void and a sense of loneliness often follow a loss. If you have a partner, your feelings may differ from his or hers in strength or content. Grief may be mixed with guilt; both can cause tension between you. You may blame yourselves and wonder if either of you did something "wrong," but this is rarely true. For some of us, it helps to talk about our feelings and to seek out a bereavement counselor and/or a support group.

In addition to these emotional responses, your body will be going through changes. It is important to have a follow-up visit with your provider not only for physical reasons, but as an opportunity to ask questions that may come up. Ask for the first appointment of the day or for one before the day officially starts, so that you don't have to face a room full of pregnant women. Bring your questions with you in writing, and take notes, since you may have trouble focusing. Ask a support person to go with you if you think that this might be helpful.

The depth of grief is not simply related to the duration of the pregnancy or age of the infant. Unexplained loss can be especially hard to accept, and healing from the loss can be a long process. You may feel a strong resurgence of grief on the date when your baby would have been born, or when you see children the same age as your child would have been.

Our society has few formal ways of dealing with childbearing loss. Some kind of ceremony may help recognize the significance of the loss and honor the memory of the one who died. The ceremony can be performed immediately after the loss or whenever you are ready, such as at a one-year mark. Some women find that giving to a favorite charity on an annual basis or planting a tree offers comfort over time.

This summer we will be planting a tree in front of our house in memory of Kyle. Summers will forever bring mixed emotions for us, July especially. Growing up in Brazil, summers were such a highlight of our lives. I like to think that there is a reason why we lost Kyle in the summer. Perhaps slowly we will be able to hold his memory as one of those forever-treasured childhood memories of joyful and innocent summers. With time, we are better able to embrace the full cycles of life even when it feels unnaturally "wrong" that some life cycles are not as long as we expect.

You may find healing in creative expression—a memorial quilt, artwork, or writing about your loss. Some women choose to mark the anniversary of important days in the lost baby's life—such as the date of conception or her or his birthday—in order to acknowledge the baby's existence and place in the family.

Some of us heal by working to improve the way that women who experience childbearing loss are treated by hospitals and providers, or by creating resources on childbearing loss. As a result of such efforts, many hospitals now have bereavement teams and organize pregnancy-and-infant-loss support groups. There are also a number of support organizations and books on childbearing loss—most formed or written by women with personal experience of it—that offer guidance on grieving as well as on coping during future pregnancies. One such group, Share Pregnancy & Infant Loss Support, Inc., has articulated a set of rights for parents who experience the loss of a pregnancy or a baby, for the baby, and for siblings (see www.national shareoffice.com). You may be the beneficiary of such work; or, if you experience loss, you may also feel moved to use your sorrow, anger, and determination to help others.

While some women cope best by trying to get pregnant again as soon as possible, other women need more time. Others may decide not to try again. There is no "right" decision; there is only a decision that feels right for you.

SUBSEQUENT PREGNANCY

The vast majority of women are able to have a baby after a childbearing loss. However, future pregnancies may be emotionally challenging. They also may be physically difficult if you are now considered "high risk." And the fears, anxieties, and joys that we all experience during pregnancy are likely to be more intense, especially if the loss was unexplained.

Depending on your experience, you may want to remain with your health care provider or find a new one. Either way, talk with your provider about her or his policy for dealing with pregnancy loss and monitoring a woman who has had a prior loss. If the provider brushes off your questions or does not respond compassionately to your concerns, she or he may not be right for you.

You are likely to feel most anxious around the time in the pregnancy that the previous loss occurred. It may help to remind people around you as you approach that point, so that they are prepared to support you or give you the space you need—and to celebrate with you when you pass that point, while recognizing that fears remain. And you may experience a resurgence of grief around the time of childbirth. Being aware of these emotions, letting them happen, and talking about them may help you to work through them during the subsequent pregnancy and into motherhood. Therapists or pregnancy-after-loss support groups can be especially helpful. If possible, talk with women who have had the same experience to learn how they managed their feelings and found the courage and optimism to try again.

It was six months after the second miscarriage before we felt ready to try again. We became pregnant easily. Understandably, we were terrified. We tried to face every test with guarded optimism. Pregnancy test, hormone levels, first sonogram, heartbeat, nuchal translucency, amniocentesis. By the time we made it through the 20-week sonogram I believed we were actually going to have a baby. I never complained about any of the discomforts of pregnancy. I didn't want to jinx it. I loved being pregnant, loved giving birth. . . . I felt and still feel such gratitude for our two sons. Because the path to motherhood was more bumpy than I imagined, it feels especially miraculous, especially precious.

NOTES

1. March of Dimes Defects Foundation, Quick Reference and Fact Sheets, "Miscarriage" (2004), accessed at www.marchofdimes.com/professionals/681_1192 .asp on July 10, 2006.
2. Mayo Foundation for Medical Education and Research, "Miscarriage" (2004), accessed at www.mayo clinic.com/health/miscarriage/PR00097 on July 10, 2006.
3. Ibid.
4. March of Dimes Defects Foundation, "Miscarriage" (2004), accessed at www.marchofdimes.com/ professionals/681_1192.asp on July 10, 2006.
5. B. E. Seeber and K. T. Barnhart, "Suspected Ectopic Pregnancy," *Obstetrics & Gynecology* 107, no. 2 (February 2006): 399–413; and see review, erratum in *Obstetrics & Gynecology* 107, no. 4 (April 2006): 955. See also March of Dimes Defects Foundation, Quick Reference and Fact Sheets, "Ectopic and Molar Preg-

nancy" (1999), accessed at www.marchofdimes.com/professionals/14332_1189.asp on September 20, 2006.

6. Centers for Disease Control and Prevention, "DES Update: Consumers" (2006), accessed at www.cdc.gov/DES/consumers/about/index.html on August 7, 2006.

7. American College of Obstetricians and Gynecologists, "Early Pregnancy Loss: Miscarriage and Molar Pregnancy" (2002), accessed at acog.org/publications/patient_education/bp090.cfm on July 10, 2006.

8. J. Martin et al, "Births: Final Data for 2000," *National Vital Statistics Reports* 50, no. 5 (February 12, 2002). See also March of Dimes Birth Defects Foundation, Quick Reference and Fact Sheets, "Multiples: Twins, Triplets and Beyond" (2006), accessed at www.marchofdimes.com/printableArticles/14332_4545.asp on August 7, 2006.

9. Pamela Prindle Fierro, "Vanishing Twin Syndrome," *Parenting of Multiples* (April 2006), accessed at http://multiples.about.com/cs/medicalissues/a/vanishing twin.htm on August 25, 2006.

10. March of Dimes Birth Defects Foundation, Quick Reference and Fact Sheets, "Stillbirth" (2006), accessed at www.marchofdimes.com/professionals/14332_1198.asp on July 10, 2006.

11. Ibid.

12. National Institute of Child Health and Human Development, "Federal Interagency Forum on Child and Family Statistics" (July 2004), accessed at www.nichd.nih.gov/new/releases/americas_children.cfm on August 25, 2006.

13. National Center for Health Statistics, *Chartbook on Trends in the Health of Americans* (2005), Hyattsville, MD. See also Centers for Disease Control and Prevention, "Infant Mortality Statistics from the 2002 Period Linked Birth / Infant Death Data Set," *National Vital Statistics Reports* 53, no. 10 (2005): 1120.

14. National Center for Health Statistics, "Explaining the 2001–02 Infant Mortality Increase: Data from the Linked Birth / Infant Death Data Set," *National Vital Statistics Reports* 53, no. 12 (2005): 1120.

15. American Public Health Association, "Fact Sheets: 'Disparities in Infant Mortality,' 'Eliminating Health Disparities: Communities Moving from Statistics to Solutions'" (April 2004), accessed at www.nphw.org/2005/facts/InfantMort-PHW04_Facts.pdf on January 26, 2007.

16. National Center for Health Statistics, "New CDC Report Confirms Increase in 2002 Infant Mortality Rate," news release, November 24, 2004; accessed at www.cdc.gov/nchs/pressroom/04facts/infant.htm on July 10, 2006.

17. Laurie Cawthon, "Infant Mortality and SIDS," First Steps Database, Washington State Department of Social and Health Services (May 2002), accessed at www.dshs.wa.gov/pdf/ms/rda/research/9/62.pdf on September 1, 2006.

18. March of Dimes Foundation, News Desk, "U.S. Infant Mortality Rate Fails to Improve," May 2006; accessed at www.marchofdimes.com/aboutus/15796_19840.asp on September 1, 2006.

19. March of Dimes Birth Defects Foundation, "Infant Deaths Due to Sudden Infant Death Syndrome: US, 1996–2002," accessed at www.marchofdimes.com/peristats on July 10, 2006. See also National Institutes of Health, National Institute of Child Health & Human Development, "Research on Sudden Infant Death Syndrome" (2005), accessed at www.nichd.nih.gov/womenshealth/research/pregbirth/sids.cfm on July 10, 2006.

20. D. L. Hoyert, M. P. Heron, S. L. Murphy, and H.-C. Kung, "Death: Final Data from 2003," *National Vital Statistics Reports* 54, no. 13 (2006): 99.

21. National Institutes of Health, National Institute of Child Health & Human Development, "Research on Sudden Infant Death Syndrome" (2005), accessed at www.nichd.nih.gov/womenshealth/research/pregbirth/sids.cfm on July 10, 2006.

22. Debra Ellyn Weese-Mayer, "Sudden Infant Death Syndrome: Is Serotonin the Key Factor?" *JAMA* 296, no. 17 (November 1, 2006): 2,143–2,144.

23. David S. Paterson et al., "Multiple Serotonergic Brainstem Abnormalities in Sudden Infant Death Syndrome," *JAMA* 296, no. 17 (November 1, 2006): 2,124–2,132.

24. National Institutes of Health, National Institute of Child Health & Human Development, "Research on Sudden Infant Death Syndrome" (2005), accessed at www.nichd.nih.gov/womenshealth/research/pregbirth/sids.cfm on July 10, 2006.

Giving Birth

CHAPTER 10

Labor and Birth

Women's experiences with labor and birth vary widely, from woman to woman, from one phase of labor to another, and from one labor to the next. Your labor will be unique, influenced by many factors: the size and position of your baby, your health and medical history, your expectations and feelings, the people who surround and support you, your professional attendants, and the place you labor and give birth.

But despite the variations, there is a common theme: the natural flow of labor. This process involves an interplay between your body and your baby, as your baby moves lower down in your uterus and your cervix changes in preparation for birth. During your pregnancy, your body has held and protected your baby. Your cervix has been firmly sealed with a plug of mucus and the baby has grown within the protective amniotic sac. Now your body needs to soften, open, and yield to allow the baby to pass through. Labor contractions will firmly squeeze and push the baby down and the baby will rotate to navigate the birth canal. The birth process progresses from the opening (dilation) of your cervix to your baby's descent and birth, to the delivery of the placenta.

Most women experience the signs of approaching labor and the latent phase of labor at home, using comfort measures that do not include pain medication. But by the stages of active labor and pushing, women follow different paths, at home, in birthing centers, and in hospitals.

Giving birth was life-changing for me and for many of the women I have attended as a midwife. In a world in which we may often feel ineffective and pessimistic, working through labor under our own power can transform our sense of self. We experience ourselves as strong, sturdy, resilient, and able. We tap on inner strengths we may never have tapped before, and are amazed by what we are able to accomplish. Once we become aware of how powerful we can be in giving birth, we can call

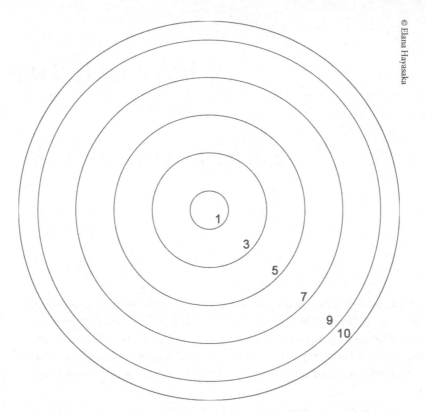

Cervical dilation shown in actual size (in centimeters). When you reach about 10 centimeters, you will be ready to push.

on this throughout our lives, in all sorts of situations.

SIGNS OF APPROACHING LABOR (PRE-LABOR)

Labor continues the process begun at conception. The finely tuned biological system that nurtures developing babies guides labor as well. Just before labor begins, your body readies itself. The joints in your hips and pelvis relax and open, ligaments soften, and the baby may drop deeper in your pelvis. Toward the end of pregnancy—for some women, even earlier—you may occasionally feel a painless tightening of your uterus, the *Braxton-Hicks contractions.*

These normal "practice contractions" do not cause your cervix to dilate, or open (something it will do to about 10 centimeters—about 3.5 inches—by the time you push the baby out into the world). You may also feel increased pressure in your pelvis and on your bladder as the baby drops lower, settling deeper into your pelvic cavity. This process of *dropping*—or "lightening," as it is also called—is not an indication that labor is about to start. If you are a first-time mother, you may still be a month away from delivering your baby, but dropping is one sign that your body is preparing for childbirth. After dropping, you may find it easier to breathe, but at the same time, you may have to urinate more often (because the baby is resting closer to your bladder) and walking can become painful.

Toward the end of my pregnancy I had to urinate so often that I developed a sixth sense about where a restroom might be. Some were obvious, such as at a movie theater, but others, like at the dry cleaner, were much more obscure. Fortunately, people were always willing to accommodate the pregnant lady in obvious need of a pit stop.

Although you won't feel this, during the last few days before labor starts, your cervix will likely change from firm to very soft, and then become flatter and thinner (see illustration, page 166). The process of flattening is known as *effacement*. It is frequently measured in percentages from zero to 100. Some women start labor at zero percent effacement, which means the cervix is still long. At 50 percent effacement—which can occur days or just hours before your baby is born—your cervix is half its original length. When you are 100 percent effaced, your cervix is completely flat.

As your cervix flattens, it will also *dilate*, or open up. This process is the result of subtle uterine contractions that you may feel in the days leading up to delivery. Dilation is measured in centimeters. In the early stages of labor, also called the "latent" stage, your cervix may dilate from 1 to 4 centimeters. By the end of active labor, repeated uterine contractions will widen your cervix to about 7 centimeters.

As your cervix starts to ripen, the mucous seal may begin to come out, tinged pink or streaked with blood ("bloody show"). It may come out as a clump all at once. Or it may come out over several days, so you might notice more discharge or spots of blood but won't see an obvious mucous plug. (Actual bleeding like your period may be cause for concern at this stage; you should call your midwife or doctor if it occurs.)

You may experience contractions, especially at night. Contractions gradually shorten uterine muscles and pull up on your cervix, moving your baby down. This pressure can feel like gas pains, menstrual cramps, backache, or painful throbbing in your thighs or pelvis. Early on, contractions may vary, occurring regularly or irregularly. They may be inconsistent, widely spaced, or short-lived. Frequently, they will come regularly for a few hours and then stop—sometimes even for a few days. Regular contractions can happen for several days without dilating the cervix.

Other signs of approaching labor may include loose stools, more mucous discharge, or crampiness. Many women have a strong burst of energy at this point, a nesting impulse that compels us to cook, clean house, or become more organized. Some women feel clingy, uncharacteristically needing to be close to loved ones. Most of these signs of impending labor are not specific enough to be obvious, but in retrospect, you may recognize them as signals that your body and mind were gearing up for labor.

During my pregnancies, I always tried to take a walk during lunch. The bigger I got, the shorter my walks became, and in retrospect, they also became more focused. In the days leading up to my daughter's birth, I went like a homing pigeon to a local bookstore that always seemed to have some must-have cookbook on sale. The Food and Cooking of Thailand; The Complete Spanish Cookbook; One-Pot, Slow Pot, and Claypot Cooking; Slow Cooker; *and* Russian, German & Polish Food & Cooking—*I simply had to have them all. These books are now fondly known as my "nesting collection."*

WHAT CAUSES LABOR AND WHEN LABOR BEGINS

The biological mechanisms that cause labor to begin are not well understood. The best gestational length for a particular baby also is not

THE STAGES OF LABOR

Stage/ Phase	How long will it last*	How dilated will my cervix be?	What will my contractions be like?	What else might be happening?
Warm-up labor (Prelabor, prodromal labor)	On and off for days or weeks	0 to 3 cm	Vary greatly in length and intensity.	Mucous discharge, backache. It's hard to tell when you move from this into latent-phase labor.
Stage 1: Latent Phase	A few hours to a day or more	0 to 4–5 cm	Vary widely. Usually short (about 30 to 60 seconds), spaced relatively far apart (anywhere from 5 minutes to over 20 minutes apart). You may be able to ignore or distract yourself from them.	Mucous discharge (with "bloody show"), backache, upset stomach.
Active Phase	Between 2 and 10 hours	4–5 to 7–8 cm	Last about a minute or more, spaced regularly. You probably will not be able to walk, distract yourself	May feel tired or discouraged, wondering if you can do it. Pressure in your lower back, need to change positions often.
Transition	A few contractions to 1 to 2 hours	7–8 cm to full dilation (about 10 cm)	Occur about every 2 minutes, and last about 60 to 90 seconds, so you have only short rests in between. Very intense.	Intense emotions and physical sensations. You may feel restless, irritable, exhausted. Trembling, nausea, and vomiting are common.

* Many factors can affect how long a stage or phase of labor can last. Labor tends to last longer for first-time mothers than for women who have previously given birth vaginally.

Stage/ Phase	How long will it last*	How dilated will my cervix be?	What will my contractions be like?	What else might be happening?
Stage 2: Pushing, giving birth	A few contractions to over 3 hours	Fully dilated 10 cm ("complete")	Powerful contractions about every 3 minutes.*	Pain lessens, and you may be able to rest. You may also become more clearheaded and energetic. As baby descends, you will feel strong pressure in the vaginal and rectal areas, resulting in a strong urge to push. Stinging, burning sensation as baby's head crowns.
Stage 3: Delivery of placenta	5 to 30 minutes		No contractions, then one to several strong cramps	Provider may massage uterus to cause it to contract and reduce bleeding—this can be painful.
Stage 4: Recovery	May last 1 or 2 hours if birth was unmedicated and not prolonged or difficult; longer if otherwise		Mild cramps as uterus contracts	Thick bloody vaginal discharge (lochia) may last 2 to 4 weeks. Uterus will tighten to prevent bleeding. Swelling and discomfort in your perineum. Trembling legs.

* Some women experience a break in contractions for 10 to 25 minutes once the cervix is fully dilated, before feeling the urge to push.

known. Therefore, no one can predict or determine exactly when your labor will start. The baby's size and maturity, as well as multiple hormonal and placental changes, affect the onset of labor.

Normal-term pregnancies range from about 37 to 42 weeks; a due date marks the midpoint in this window of time (for more information, see page 47). Inductions are increas-ingly common, but as long as mother and baby are healthy, and you are not more than two weeks beyond your known due date, there is no physiological reason or benefit to forcing or rushing the process. (For information on labor that begins before 37 weeks, see page 134. For information on pregnancies that extend beyond the due date and medical reasons to induce labor, see page 146.)

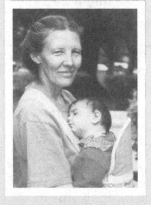

"Women in early labor are left alone or with an inexperienced partner, just when they need help the most."

Faith Gibson

The early phase of labor is often where the trolley goes off the track, so to speak, triggering a cascade of obstetrical interventions that can interfere with the progress of labor and lead to an operative delivery.

During this phase of labor, women need to understand what is happening in their bodies, to know that what they are experiencing is normal, and to get concrete physical and emotional support from a skilled and experienced labor attendant. Yet the typical "obstetrical package" offers little of this.

Healthy women who are planning a hospital birth are rightly advised by their doctors to stay home until they are in active labor, to decrease the chance of interventions. But most of the time, this means women in early labor are left alone or with an inexperienced partner, just when they need help the most. Obstetricians don't make house calls. Unless a woman is accompanied by a doula or has a midwife who will come to her home, she likely has no skilled support.

A woman may be excited and committed to staying home and avoiding obstetrical interventions, but her confidence and endurance often ebb as the hours pass and contractions continue. She doesn't know how far she has progressed or how long she can keep going. If a woman experiences a particularly long, hard, or stalled early labor, she may panic as she finds herself gripped by the five-hundredth labor pain—with no end in sight, no help, no hope. Midwives call this the "Kill me now" phenomenon. At this point, women will agree to anything.

Going to the hospital may seem like the solution. But getting obstetrical care too early in labor can lead to unwanted interventions.

Having a midwife or doula present during early labor can make all the difference. She can address and defuse the mother's fear and anxiety. She can also provide effective nondrug methods to manage the mother's pain and reduce it to a tolerable level. This usually includes providing touch relaxation; helping the mother walk around, be upright and mobile, and to make the right use of gravity; using a hot shower or warm, deep-water tub; and giving lots of encouragement. If a woman is exhausted, the midwife or doula may prop her up so she can take micro-naps between contractions. When the going gets tough, it usually helps if someone—midwife, doula, husband, partner, or family friend—breathes with the woman through *each and every* contraction.

I often tell women to do labor a half hour at a time. It helps everyone to keep focused on the moment and away from the what-ifs: "What if something is wrong?" "What if this goes on all night?" "What if I can't take it anymore?" During the crucial period of early labor, women need this kind of face-to-face, one-on-one support.

LABOR BEGINS
(STAGE 1, LATENT PHASE)

The latent phase of labor may feel much the same to you as pre-labor, but during this time your cervix will open up (dilate) to 4–5 centimeters and will usually completely flatten (efface). Labor contractions will be short and spaced relatively far apart (from 5 to 20 minutes apart). During the latent phase, your contractions will become longer, more painful, and more regular. This is not yet the time to go to a hospital or birthing center. However, most women at this stage want some kind of care, such as the reassuring presence of a partner or close friend or regular phone check-ins with a provider or other guide familiar with birth. Some women say that this phase of labor is the hardest psychologically, because no one can predict how long it will last. One midwife explains:

It's like starting a hike and no one is telling you how long it is. The trail has lots of meandering switchbacks and hills, and you don't know where you're headed or how long it will take to get there, but you just keep going. Later, it may get physically more difficult, but at least then you can see the end in sight, the peak of the mountain, and you can push on.

Contractions will start, or continue, and become more regular. Sometimes a hot bath or shower will make you more comfortable, enabling you to rest. If you feel contractions during the day, go about your usual routine if you can, but take time to eat and rest. Drink frequently.

Sometimes contractions build up gradually, starting with any of the signs mentioned above, with crampiness evolving into stronger contractions that grow closer together over a long period of time, even over a period of days. At the other extreme, labor can begin abruptly, with strong regular contractions no more than 5 minutes apart, causing you to stop everything you are doing and concentrate.

Everyone responds differently to early labor. Walking, showering, taking long baths, or cuddling with loved ones can relax you and help labor progress. These early hours may be sweet as you lie with your partner or sit alone, the baby still within you in the quiet of your home. Some women are too excited or apprehensive to sleep. You might want family and friends to come early on. Save your energy for active labor. Don't worry if contractions slow down when you lie down to rest.

For some women, this latent phase of labor lasts for many hours or up to two days, with regular strong contractions that slowly efface the cervix and open it to 4 centimeters. First labors can vary greatly in the early/latent phase. When you hear of labors that lasted for days, the women involved spent the bulk of that time in latent-phase labor, not active labor. If you have a very long latent phase and have missed more than one night of sleep, your provider may suggest taking sleep medication to help you rest and regain your energy.

LABOR PROGRESSES
(STAGE 1, ACTIVE PHASE)

For many first-time mothers it can take a day or more to get to 3 or 4 centimeters dilation, which signals entry into the active phase of labor. When you feel strong, wavelike, regular, rhythmic contractions that are 2 to 3 minutes apart, that last 45 to 60 seconds, and that are so intense you can't talk or walk while you are having one, you are most likely in active labor. The contractions may begin in your back, or

WATERS BREAK

The sac containing the amniotic fluid that surrounds your baby (the membranes, or "bag of waters") usually breaks either shortly before contractions start or during labor. In a small percentage of women, though, the waters can break many hours or days before labor starts. This causes the fluid to leak out before contractions begin. You may experience a large gush of fluid, followed by continuous leaking.

At first it was kind of a trickle and I wasn't totally sure if this was it, but then it was a huge gush and I had to run to make it to the toilet. I couldn't really get up from there for a while as I was just dripping. Soon after that the surges started and they were pretty regular . . . every 5 minutes or so. Nothing intense, but they were there. . . . It was really late, so I thought I would try to get some sleep, since I had no idea how long the whole thing would be. So I lay down and just as I was falling asleep, had another HUGE gush of fluid—I'm talking like a half inch on the bed in a puddle.

If the sac breaks on its upper side, the fluid may trickle out slowly. A slow leak may be confused with urine leaking or with discharge of mucus.

Call your midwife or doctor to make a plan when your bag of waters breaks or if you think you are leaking amniotic fluid. Notice the color of the fluid and tell your provider if there's any brown or green staining, a sign that meconium, the first stool in your baby's bowels, has been squeezed out and has colored the amniotic fluid. Some providers routinely have women head to the hospital once the bag of waters breaks, but this is not always necessary.

If your bag of waters breaks before your labor contractions begin, your provider will probably want to see you to confirm that the bag has broken and to check the baby's position and heartbeat. At this time there will likely be a discussion of the pros and cons of waiting for labor and inducing labor. Health care providers have different opinions about how long to wait for labor to start after the bag of waters has broken.

If you have tested positive for Group B strep (GBS) during the last four weeks of your pregnancy, your provider will probably advise that labor be induced. (For information about testing for GBS, see page 61.) However, if you have not tested positive for GBS and there is no sign of infection (fever, chills, smelly discharge) or other problems (such as a fetal heart rate that is too fast or too slow), it may be all right to wait for labor to begin on its own, while taking certain precautions.

The risk of infection for the mother and the baby increases with the amount of time since the membranes ruptured. The policy in most institutions is to suggest induction at twelve to twenty-four hours after the rupturing of the membranes. However, eight out of ten women begin labor naturally within twenty-four hours once membranes have ruptured.[1] There is no clear justification for routine induction before twenty-four hours. (For more information on induction, see page 146.)

If you wait for labor contractions to start spontaneously, you will be less likely to receive unnecessary interventions or to develop the complications that can result from inducing labor. If you and your provider agree that it is safe for you to wait for labor to begin, avoid vaginal exams except when absolutely necessary and make a plan for when to induce labor if it does not begin on its own. To reduce the risk of getting an infection, do not have intercourse and do not put anything into your vagina. It is okay to take a bath if you want to; bathing does not increase the risk of infection.[2]

Most women in labor experience an intensification of contractions after the bag of water breaks.

you may feel them only in the front. Your uterus feels hard to the touch.

I spent most of the night laboring alone in the dark, like a cat. It was marvelous. Not easy—it's hard work; that's why it's called LABOR. It was intense. Not painful—I can't call it painful. But it's . . . inevitable. Unescapable. Uncontrollable. You can't get away. I kept thinking of that kids' game, "Going on a bear hunt": "Can't go over it, can't go around it, have to go through it!"

This is the time to gather your support people, to call your provider if you are having a home birth, or to prepare to go to the birth center or hospital. Travel can be an uncomfortable challenge at this point, but you can regain your rhythm once you are settled in your chosen birth setting.

I couldn't wait for the traffic to move so we could get to the hospital where I could labor in full, open glory. And I'm sure the taxi driver couldn't, either! I was writhing and rocking in the back seat, trying not to look at my husband's face because his . . . concern escalated my own. In my

first pregnancy, it took about twenty hours to get to this "It's happening!" stage, so I didn't even think we needed to call a taxi so soon after my waters broke in my second pregnancy. But the second time, my labor went right there. We did make it to the hospital with about an hour to spare, but only because William insisted on calling the taxi pretty much right away.

In the active phase of labor, there is an expected pattern of progress in cervical dilation. This can vary for first-time mothers and also for women who have given birth before. Your midwife or doctor will check on your progress. If it does not fit expectations, your provider will try to figure out why and what to do about this.

One woman describes her experience of getting "stuck" temporarily at a certain point in active labor:

I got stuck at about 8 to 9 centimeters for a really long time. I wasn't aware how long, except that it was hours. [The doctor] who was on call suggested Pitocin to speed things up, but I refused. Part of my concern was that the contractions were already so intense that I felt if they were stronger and closer together I wouldn't be able to cope, and I did not want to do anything that put me at risk for a C-section. . . .

. . . In the end, I realized that though it was hard it was never more than I could take, and I had been prepared to keep pushing for even longer if necessary. I had not reached the end of my strength. We never would have been able to do it without our doula's help—she was worth her weight in gold.

Women describe the sensations experienced in labor in many ways: shocking, powerful, intense, painful, uncontrollable, difficult but doable, overwhelming. All the sensations you experience in labor are *making it happen,* moving toward a goal—the birth of your baby. Many women find it helpful to change positions, walk, soak in water, rock on a birthing ball, or focus on breathing to manage and ease the experience of labor. Relaxing deeply between contractions renews your energy, allows contractions to work effectively, and helps reduce the intensity and pain. Breathing deeply and focusing your energy can help you relax. Some women become quiet and focus inward. Others moan, hum, chant, or sing to match the intensity of active labor. In between contractions, rest, sleep, walk, or talk.

During active labor and pushing, women follow different paths, at home, in birthing centers, and in hospitals. The differences are determined partly by individual preferences, partly by routines and requirements of the various birth settings, and partly by how each labor proceeds. Some women who give birth in hospitals choose to use pain medication during part of labor. (For more information, see Chapter 11, "Coping with Pain.") Sometimes women who have planned to have an epidural are surprised by fast labor and arrive at the hospital too late to receive one. Hospitals may not administer an epidural if you are nearly 10 centimeters dilated or the baby is "crowning," which means that the head is visible. In some hospitals, there may not be an anesthesiologist immediately available to administer an epidural.

FETAL MONITORING

Whether you have your baby in a birthing center, in the hospital, or at home, your provider will monitor your baby's heartbeat to see how

WHEN TO CALL

Call your provider if:

- your bag of waters breaks (membranes rupture),
- you experience strong contractions every 2 to 3 minutes for an hour (if this is your first baby),
- you are experiencing severe pain,
- you think that your labor has started and you are less than 36 weeks pregnant,
- you experience bleeding that is as heavy as a period, or
- you have any questions or concerns.

the baby is tolerating labor. Your baby's heart rate will generally range between 110 and 160 beats per minute. During a contraction, the flow of blood to the baby is reduced, and as a result, the baby's heart rate may temporarily go down.

Your provider can listen to the heart rate intermittently or continuously. Most hospitals will require 30 minutes of external fetal monitoring to obtain a baseline reading of your baby's heart rate and response to contractions. From there, your baby's heartbeat can be monitored periodically. Continuous fetal heart rate monitoring is not necessary in most births.

Intermittent Monitoring

Intermittent monitoring can be done with a fetoscope (a special stethoscope), or with a Doptone, a handheld device that uses ultrasound to detect and transmit the baby's heart rate. Intermittent fetal heart rate monitoring is done by listening to the baby's heartbeat through and right after a contraction for about 2 minutes every 5 to 30 minutes during labor, depending on the stage of labor you are in.

Continuous Monitoring

Continuous external electronic fetal heart rate monitoring involves placing two recording devices, held by soft belts, on your abdomen. One device detects the fetal heart rate and the other detects the uterine contractions. The baby's heart rate and your contractions show up as peaks and valleys on a screen and on a paper printout, called the *fetal heart rate tracing.*

Usually, continuous fetal monitoring is done externally. If the external monitoring is not adequate or there are special concerns about the baby, internal monitoring is used. Internal monitoring is most often used to measure the baby's heart rate, but sometimes a different kind of internal monitoring is used to measure the strength of your contractions.

To monitor the baby's heartbeat internally, a small flexible wire, known as a *fetal scalp electrode,* is inserted through your vagina and attached to the baby's scalp. The other end of the wire is attached to the monitor to provide a continuous recording of the baby's heart rate.

An *internal fetal monitor* (IFM) produces the most accurate reading of your baby's heart

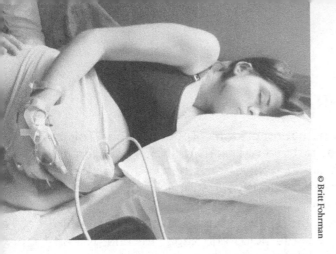

© Britt Fohrman

rate and response to contractions during labor. If an IFM is used, the newborn baby may have a small scab at the spot where the electrode was attached. This generally heals quickly and is not noticeable in a day or two.

Occasionally, your provider may want to measure internally the strength of your uterine contractions. To do this, a small catheter is inserted into the uterus through the vagina and the cervix and left in place. This pressure sensor is more accurate than the external monitor at measuring the intensity of the contractions.

Continuous monitoring usually limits a laboring woman's ability to move, although in some instances a technique known as *telemetry*

can allow a woman to walk while the fetal heart rate is being monitored continuously.

Intermittent Versus Continuous Monitoring

There is good evidence that continuous fetal monitoring in uncomplicated pregnancies has done nothing to improve outcomes for babies and mothers but has dramatically increased the cesarean section rate.[3] Unfortunately, for a variety of reasons, continuous fetal monitoring has become the norm in many hospitals. (For more information on why this is so, see "Why Is Maternity Care Like This?" (page 305).

Continuous fetal heart rate monitoring should be reserved for situations in which epidurals or Pitocin are being used and for women who have certain complications. If you are having a hospital birth and there is no clear-cut medical reason for you to have continuous monitoring, ask your provider to consider intermittent monitoring. (For more information on the limitations of continuous fetal heart rate monitoring, see "Variations in Fetal Heartbeat," page 216.)

MYTH OR REALITY?

Continuous fetal monitoring can compromise labor for both mothers and babies.
- Reality. Although some monitoring is good, it does not necessarily follow that more monitoring is better. Many hospitals use continuous electronic fetal heart rate monitoring to ensure that your baby's condition is being evaluated, even if your doctor, nurse, or midwife leaves the room. However, continuous monitoring restricts your movement, which can make labor more challenging, and leads to higher rates of cesarean section.[4] If you are in a hospital and you enter labor without any pregnancy complications, ask for intermittent monitoring of your baby's heart rate by Doptone.

INTRAVENOUS INFUSION OF SALINE OR FLUIDS (IV)

Many hospitals routinely insert IVs in laboring women, just in case of emergency and for delivery of pain relief medication. Intravenous fluids are not necessary in normal labor. Instead, it is important to eat and drink to keep up your energy. Bring tea, juices, and other nourishment that you find appealing. Many hospitals have policies that limit food and drink intake, so discuss the situation with your provider ahead of time.

An IV restricts your freedom and ability to move about. If you agree to have an IV to accommodate hospital routines, ask for a saline lock (or heparin lock) taped to your wrist but not attached to a pole, so that the IV line from the bag of saline can be attached only if you need the fluids. An IV can be used for a short period of time to rehydrate you and give you energy. An IV will be used continuously if your labor is induced or you have epidural anesthesia. You will likely have a heparin lock if you are laboring after a previous cesarean section.

POSITIONS FOR LABOR

I found many positions which helped pass the time as I dilated. . . . My favorite positions were straddling the birth ball holding on to a solid chair back in front of me and lying on my side on the bed. [My midwife] Sandra sometimes just put her warm hands against my back, sending warm calming forces through me. Sometimes my mom sat by me and just kept me company. Sometimes we chatted until my breath and mind were taken away by a contraction.

Women labor in all sorts of ways: squatting, sitting on the toilet, side-lying with one leg supported, reclining in a tub for a water birth, rocking on hands and knees. When you want to rest, lie on your side. Lying flat on your back is generally not recommended, as it is often painful and may make labor less efficient. It is also not good for the baby, as the blood flow to the baby may be diminished. Experiment with other positions until you find ones that are comfortable for you. Changing positions helps manage pain.

Most birth centers have stools, birthing balls, or squatting bars to hold on to. Some hospitals may have birthing equipment, too, but your choice of positions may be more limited. Even if you have an IV or an external monitor, your provider and birthing partner can help you find a comfortable position or place in the room.

Some hospitals also have regular-sized tubs that you can use during labor, and many birthing centers have large tubs where you can labor or give birth, with your partner in the water beside you. You can also have a birthing tub brought into your home. Water can help reduce pressure by supporting your weight, and some women feel more relaxed in the water. (For more information on laboring in water, see page 201.)

THE SHIFT TO PUSHING (STAGE 1, TRANSITION PHASE)

Transition can be the most intense phase of labor, but it is also usually the shortest. In first pregnancies, transition generally lasts no more than a couple of hours. Transition is when many women will consider having an epidural, so it is important to keep in mind that this is the home stretch, with your body having already accomplished most of the difficult work. During this phase, contractions are stronger, longer, and more frequent as they dilate your cervix and move your baby down the birth canal. Contractions may come so close together

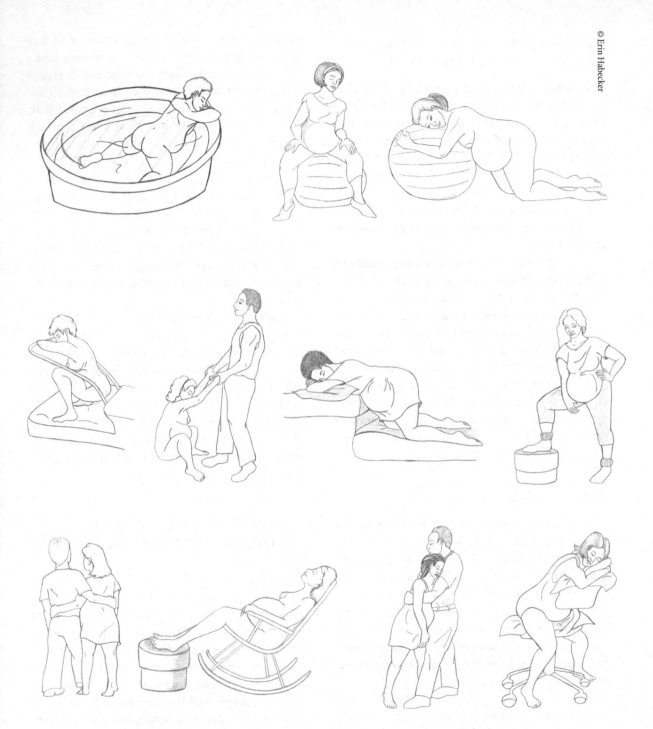

Trying different positions for pushing and giving birth may help make the process faster and more comfortable.

LABOR AUGMENTATION

Augmentation strengthens contractions that are not strong enough to cause the cervix to dilate and/or the baby to descend through the pelvis. Augmentation can prevent the need for a cesarean section if your contractions are not forceful enough on their own.

Walking and nipple stimulation can help labor be more efficient if it's not progressing. If these strategies don't work and you are having contractions but your cervix is not dilating, breaking the membranes of the amniotic sac, or "bag of waters (amniotomy), and/or having Pitocin through an IV may be the appropriate next steps to help you progress through labor. Having labor augmented with amniotomy or Pitocin is more common if you have an epidural.[5]

Artificial Rupture of Membranes (Amniotomy)

If you are in active labor with a bulging sac of water in front of your baby's head, and the baby is deep in your pelvis, your doctor or midwife may rupture the membranes to strengthen contractions or to speed up a prolonged labor. This procedure, known as *amniotomy,* may also be done to check for meconium (the baby's first bowel movement) in the amniotic fluid.

Amniotomy does not need to be done routinely if your labor is progressing normally. Most women's membranes rupture spontaneously during pushing, if they haven't ruptured earlier in labor. Artificially rupturing the amniotic sac carries some risks: cord compression can cause decelerations in the fetal heart rate; the baby's head may be poorly positioned because the water is not buffering the turns a baby's head normally makes during labor; the risk of infection increases over time after the membranes are ruptured; and, very rarely, the umbilical cord can *prolapse* (be pushed down below or next to the baby's head).

Pitocin

Pitocin (synthetic oxytocin) is given through an IV to make labor progress better by making contractions more frequent and forceful. Use of Pitocin requires continuous fetal heart rate monitoring. Pitocin is begun at a low dose and the dose is gradually increased to achieve contractions that are closer together.

Negative consequences to having labor augmented with Pitocin include being attached to an IV and the fetal monitor, which limits your freedom to move in any position. With Pitocin, contractions may reach their peaks more rapidly. If this occurs, the contractions may be more painful.[6]

(continued)

Since using Pitocin requires continuous fetal heart rate monitoring, there is a greater likelihood that fetal heart rate changes that are not reassuring will be noted. The interpretation of these changes may lead to other interventions. In addition, you may get too much medication for a short time if your body is producing more oxytocin as well, and this can cause contractions that come too close together. This situation can be quickly remedied by turning the medication off, having you lie on your side, and/or giving you extra IV fluids.

that they seem to merge into one long one with an overwhelming urge to push. Do whatever makes you feel more comfortable and helps you handle the intensity of labor.

At this point, comfort items such as mood music, a favorite pillow, or a photograph of your dog may become distracting and annoying, and even words of encouragement from your birthing partner may grate on your nerves. You may be irritable, nauseated, or shaky, with trembling thighs and knees. You may vomit, panic, or feel out of control.

One woman recalls how she shed her usual inhibitions:

The hospital's Birthing Pavilion was like a good hotel. But I didn't get to kick back with a book and some room service. All through the night, I heaved around on the floor in a variety of positions—on my side Jane Fonda aerobics style, on all fours with ass and yoni to the wind, on the floor, and then up on the bed. I was desperate for comfort, relief, and a baby in my arms.

Shift changes were going on, and people were coming and going. It was like Grand Central Station. . . . They asked me if I minded having a nursing student watch the birth. By this time, I didn't care if the security guard from the parking lot brought in popcorn and Raisinettes to watch the event.

A woman who had an unmedicated birth in a birth center says:

The peak of each contraction was such that I needed to close my eyes and really concentrate on the number of deep breaths I was taking, knowing that at the count of 5 or 8, depending on the length of the sensation, it would start to ease up. There's a sureness in numbers—the logic overwhelmed the raw wildness of the sensation. I knew time was my only ally in dealing with the pain. With time each contraction would be over, with time the baby would be born.

PUSHING (STAGE 2)

The active phase of labor is complete when your cervix is 10 centimeters, or "fully," dilated. With your cervix now open wide enough to accommodate the baby's head, you can begin pushing your baby out the final few inches.

The contractions were coming hard [but] I could actually sleep between them. It was all very surreal and otherworldly. Immense pain and then total relaxation. I felt like I was in a scene from The Red Tent [a novel set in biblical times; the title refers to a tent where women gave birth]. I pushed from somewhere buried inside me. Deep guttural, almost animal-like noises came from within me. Loud noises. Noises I soon had no control over. My body was pushing out my baby and I was merely providing the sound track.

More rapid, intense contractions; a powerful "opening up" feeling; and rectal pressure are signs that you are completely dilated and ready to push your baby down through your vagina (birth canal) and give birth. You may urinate or defecate involuntarily. Often just before you feel like pushing or bearing down, contractions space out to provide a resting period that can last for a brief time, allowing you to rest, even to doze.

If you have had an epidural, be patient after you are fully dilated. You can increase your chance of avoiding a vacuum or forceps delivery or a cesarean by not pushing immediately when your cervix is completely dilated. If you wait until you feel the urge to push, or your baby's head is descended further, you will have more energy and will be able to push more effectively. Research suggests that the length of time before the baby is born is the same if you allow one hour of "passive descent" of the baby (when you relax and don't consciously try to push) or you start pushing immediately after you are fully dilated.[7]

When I started pushing it was more like grunts and it just felt like I had to have a bowel movement. I didn't really feel any intense urge to push or pressure, as most people will talk about. I just had a few grunts every so often. . . . [Later, my] groans/screams when I pushed felt so loud that I was sure the whole neighborhood could hear me. . . . My mother sat behind me while I was on the stool and I was able to lean back onto her thighs and push off. . . . At first it felt like my pushes weren't doing anything, but then they put a mirror under the stool so that I could see my baby's head crowning and watch what happened as I pushed. This really helped me to focus my pushing.

Pushing can be a great relief because it requires you to become an active participant, in contrast to the yielding and letting go necessary for opening the cervix. In fact, most women feel better when we move from the transition phase into pushing.

Pushing your baby out works best when you do just what your body wants, without external direction. Bear down when you feel the urge. Your pushing efforts will be more effective and powerful if you push when your urge is the strongest. If you have an epidural and cannot feel the contractions well, your care provider and support people can help you identify when to push down.

In the past, women were taught to hold their breath and push during each contraction. Many providers or nurses may still tell you to hold your breath and push down as hard as you can for a count of ten. But breath holding and sustained, directed bearing down can be exhausting and frequently are counterproductive. Studies of women in labor have shown that holding your breath can do more harm than good and keep you from pushing effectively.[8] Just push the way you push when you have a bowel movement and don't worry about your breath. You will be less tired and your baby will tolerate this stage of labor better.

Progress in this phase of labor is measured in terms of the descent of the baby's head. If the baby is descending, you don't have to do anything differently; but if not, you and your provider can find ways to change what you are doing. It's common for a baby's heart rate to drop while you are pushing. As soon as each contraction is over, the baby's heart rate should return to normal. (If it doesn't, those assisting you may ask you to change your position or breathe in extra oxygen through a mask, or they may start an IV.)

Pushing has a rhythm of its own. Each woman generally finds her own most comfortable ways of pushing within the first thirty minutes. At the beginning, your baby's head moves down with a contraction, then retreats a little; down again during the next one, and back again. This to-and-fro stretches your vaginal tissues, and the architecture of your pelvis molds the baby's flexible head bones to fit through it.

Depending on the baby's position, pushing can sometimes be very painful and very hard work. Change positions to relieve pressure points and to find positions that are more comfortable for you at this time. Being upright (leaning, squatting, hanging from something or someone) helps you and your baby and often

lessens pain and backache. These positions help align the baby in your pelvis better and they open the pelvic bones a bit to give the baby more room, which allows the baby to navigate through the birth canal better.

At some point . . . I realized I was starting to push with each contraction. "Can't be," I told myself. "It's too soon! I'll swell my cervix shut!" But I couldn't help it—I was pushing. Rather, my body was pushing, with me along for the ride! . . . Surge. Roar. PUSH! Breathe. Again. And again. And again . . . and again . . . again . . . I didn't feel I was making any progress (although it looked much different from John's point of view, he tells me!). I started crying. "I can't," I wailed. "No more. I can't do it anymore." "Yes, you can," he said firmly. "You can. You ARE. You're almost there."

With the next contraction, I felt some burning—ring of fire? That's a sign that baby is crowning, that the head is almost out. Oh, surely not . . .

I reached down—and stared at John. "There's a head there! Right there!!"

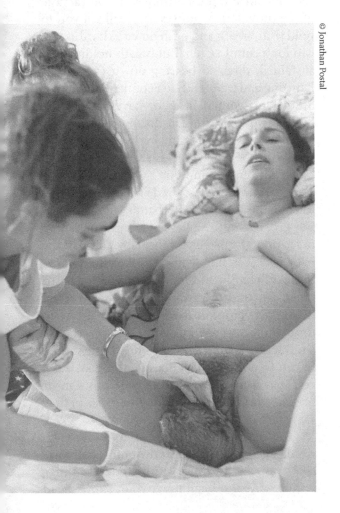
© Jonathan Postal

Between pushes, breathe slowly and deeply and rest. You might even fall asleep for a few minutes. Remember that—just as in earlier phases of labor—your uterus works involuntarily to move the baby down and out. Work with it, and give it time. Your labor may not progress as quickly as you had imagined, or as others around you expect.

Direct your energy downward and outward. Some women make deep, loud sounds as we push, while others simply "breathe" our babies out, concentrating intensely and making no sound at all.

It may take only one or two pushes, or a few hours of pushing during contractions, to birth your baby. As long as both you and your baby are doing fine and the baby is moving down, there's no reason to limit this phase of labor.

As your baby's head moves back and forth, it slowly stretches the tissues of your perineum, the area between the vaginal opening and the rectum. The perineum can stretch and expand to accommodate your baby. Hormones cause your tissues to stretch and soften. Techniques such as gentle guidance, touch, hot compresses and warm oils for comfort, and encouraging favorable positions all work with this process and may prevent or minimize tearing.

A midwife who gave birth at home says:

I often tell women in labor that they will feel a second wind—a surge of energy—when it is time to push. I found that this didn't really happen when I started pushing. But I definitely felt this when I started feeling the stretching and knew [my baby] would be born soon. It was like the only thing I needed to do in the world was push with all of my might. And that was true! It was the only thing I had to do. All the wonderful people supporting me were taking care of every single other thing.

I pushed and the burning peaked and then all of a sudden, nothing. [My baby's] head was out. It is truly amazing how quickly you can go from the most intense pain imaginable to no pain at all.

EPISIOTOMY

An episiotomy is an incision made along the perineum, which is the area between the vagina and the rectum, to allow more room for the baby. Episiotomy can speed delivery by a few minutes, but normally there is no need to hurry the process. An episiotomy may be necessary in rare circumstances, if there is concern about the baby's condition.

Episiotomies increase the chance that you will have a more severe tear that extends into the rectum; in general, naturally occurring tears are less extensive and not as deep. Despite extensive, well-documented evidence that routine episiotomy does more harm than good,[9] some obstetricians in the United States still do the procedure at all or almost all births. Ask your provider during prenatal care what her or his group usually does, and discuss your thoughts about it. Since episiotomy is a surgical procedure, practitioners should obtain consent from the woman involved. If you are

MYTH OR REALITY?

A spontaneous tear in the perineum may heal better than an episiotomy.
- Reality. Episiotomy, which is an incision made between the vagina and the rectum to allow more room for the baby, is no longer routinely recommended. Most women who do not have an episiotomy will have a small or superficial tear in the vagina or perineum. Such tears are easy to repair and do not cause more pain than an episiotomy. An episiotomy will shorten the time to birth by a few minutes, but women who have an episiotomy are more likely to have an extended tear near the rectum.

TWO MECHANICAL WAYS TO ASSIST BIRTH

The vacuum extractor and forceps can help when babies need to be born quickly. They are important tools in skilled hands. They can be used only when the cervix is fully dilated and the baby has descended well into the birth canal. With both vacuum extractors and forceps, the mother must continue to push with contractions. In most instances, anesthesia is given prior to the use of these instruments.

The ***vacuum extractor*** is a small, flexible suction cup that fits on the baby's head when she or he is still in the vagina. Use of the vacuum extractor will result in an exaggeration of the natural elongation of the baby's head caused by labor. Even when done properly, it can cause a blood-filled swelling (cephalohematoma) on the baby's head.

Forceps resemble hinged salad tongs with long spoons curved to fit the shape of a baby's head. They can cause serious damage to babies and mothers when used inappropriately or by unskilled providers.

The use of vacuum extraction has increased. A number of factors account for this, including (1) the increase in the use of epidural anesthesia, which lengthens the pushing stage, (2) a maximum time limit for pushing allotted to women in some hospitals, (3) hospital efforts to lower the C-section rate, and (4) reduction in the use of forceps. Vacuum extraction is often used with epidurals because epidurals can interfere with pushing.

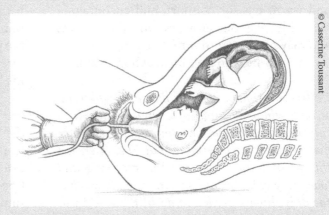

Vacuum Extractor

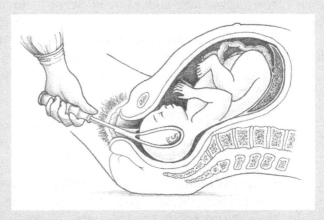

Forceps

© Casserine Toussant

Before using an extraction delivery method, if there is no immediate emergency, move into different positions that open your pelvis. Try squatting to make your pushing more efficient or nipple stimulation to increase the strength of contractions.

having an unmedicated birth, your perineum can be numbed with a local painkiller such as Novocaine so that you do not feel the incision.

BIRTH COMPLICATIONS

If your baby is not descending through the birth canal as expected despite all your efforts, or if your provider notes signs of fetal heart rate abnormalities, you may need certain medical interventions, including a cesarean section. (For more information, see Chapter 12, "Special Concerns During Labor and Birth" and Chapter 13, "Cesarean Births.")

GIVING BIRTH

When the baby moves under your pubic arch, your perineum stretches slowly to accommodate the head. When you feel a burning sensation, breathe lightly so as not to push too rapidly and risk tearing. Reaching down to touch your baby's head for the first time often produces an "Ahhhh" that opens you up even more.

Usually, the baby of a first-time mother takes longer to be born: The head emerges first, then the body follows, sometimes slowly, inch by inch. In subsequent pregnancies, the baby may be born in one continuous motion.

A woman who gave birth in a hospital, without pain medication and with the support of a doula, recalls her daughter's birth:

The sensation of her coming out was like nothing else I've ever experienced. It was cool (as in temperature, not like nifty-keen) and smooth. The sensation of her sliding out lasted longer than I'd expected and was a total shock. I had no idea she was going to come out when she did. When she was out pretty much all of the pain disappeared.

The contractions stopped, and other than a general stinging it didn't really feel like anything had happened.

Another woman, who gave birth to her son in a birthing center when she was seventeen, describes the moment:

When he had descended far enough, [the midwife] asked me if I wanted to feel his head, so I reached down to feel his head. That was when it really hit me that I was having a baby. Until then it had all been personal. "I" was pregnant, "I" was in labor, and "I" was having this baby. Now here the baby was, its own little being separate from me. When I touched his head I couldn't feel it, he felt it. I felt his fuzzy hair and realized that inside me right now was a human being that I created with my husband.

A woman in her thirties who gave birth to her third child at home, after having her first baby by cesarean section and her second vaginally in a hospital, describes the arrival of her third child:

I got on my knees and put my hands on a chair to steady myself. I kept my left knee on the floor, and put my right foot on the ground and pushed. It hurt so much that I started to climb up on the chair, trying to get away from the pain. Something went off in my head that told me if I didn't push the baby out, I was going to be feeling this pain forever! I pushed as hard as I could and felt his head start to crown. I think I yelled something, and then he came out! All of a sudden, the pain was gone and he gave a cry.

YOUR BABY IS BORN

Some babies breathe as they are being born, and look pink immediately. Others are still and

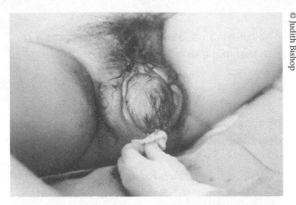

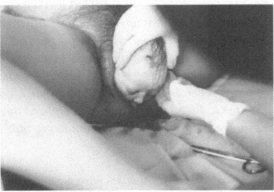

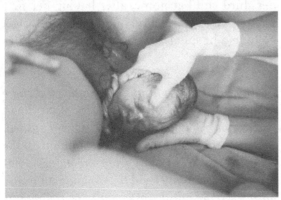

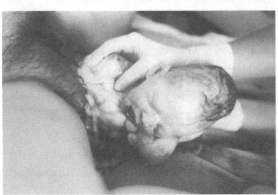

respond well if you rub their backs until they are breathing in a regular, sustained way. Healthy babies are usually able to clear their own airways of fluid and mucus. If a baby's breathing is a little difficult at birth, or there is a lot of mucus, gentle suctioning may be helpful. In these cases, midwives and doctors suction amniotic fluid and mucus out of the baby's mouth and nose. If there was meconium (the baby's first bowel movement) in the amniotic fluid, the baby may need additional deeper suctioning right after birth to prevent the fluid from getting into her or his lungs.

Not all newborns cry. Some do for a moment, then stop. Often they breathe, blink, and look around, or cough, sneeze, and snuffle. Your baby's head may appear oddly shaped, having been temporarily molded by coming through the birth canal. Her or his body may be covered with patches of vernix, a white, waxy substance that coats and protects the baby's skin inside the uterus. All babies arrive wet with amniotic fluid.

Mothers and babies belong together during this precious time. When you feel ready, hold your baby naked against your belly and breasts, near the familiar sound of your heart, so that she or he can touch your skin and smell, hear, and see you. Laying the baby on your naked body and covering the baby with a blanket will help stabilize her or his temperature.

Writing to her child, one woman recalls:

You were perfect, of course. Sue caught you and placed your warm, wet body on my chest. You immediately gave out a healthy, albeit short, cry, and then just looked around and took it all in. The three of us just sat there getting to know each other. We were so in awe and in love with you that we forgot to check to see whether you were a boy or girl!

CUTTING THE CORD

After birth, your baby is still attached by the umbilical cord to the placenta inside you. There's no medical reason to cut it immediately. In hospitals, many providers cut the cord as soon as the baby breathes. Let your provider know what you want. If you wait until the cord stops pulsating, the baby receives up to 50 milligrams of iron to add to her or his reserves, which helps prevent anemia. The cord is clamped or tied off a short distance from the baby's navel. If you have decided to save cord blood for storage (see page 41), your provider will collect it now. You may want your partner or family member to cut the cord. The bit of cord left on the navel will dry up and usually falls off within ten to fourteen days.

DELIVERY OF THE PLACENTA (STAGE 3)

Delivering the placenta, or afterbirth, completes the birthing process. At some time between five and thirty minutes or so after the baby is born, the placenta may be ready for delivery. A gush of blood will leave your body and the umbilical cord will seem to lengthen.

Women usually feel a contraction or a cramping sensation at this time. You may need to push again to expel the placenta, which has separated from the uterine wall. Since the placenta is soft, it will feel easier to push out than the baby's head. It's important that your provider not pull on the placenta before it has separated from the uterine wall.

Once the placenta comes out, blood vessels close off. Your uterus contracts and begins to shrink. Early breast-feeding helps with this process: Your baby's sucking stimulates oxytocin, which causes your uterus to contract to expel the placenta and to stay contracted afterward, reducing any bleeding.

Some people view the placenta as a beautiful organ, with its pattern of blood vessels resembling a tree of life. Many cultures have rituals surrounding the afterbirth, including planting trees or flowering bushes above it. If you want to see and/or keep the placenta, let your birth attendants know in advance, and find out about any necessary procedures.

MEETING YOUR BABY

Suddenly, months of waiting and wondering are over. You can actually see your baby's face

---

MYTH OR REALITY?

My doctor should cut the umbilical cord immediately after my baby is born.
- Myth. It has been routine medical practice to cut the cord as soon as the baby breathes. But there is evidence that it is better to place the baby on your abdomen or chest and wait until the blood stops pulsing before cutting it.[10]

  If you wait to cut the cord, your baby receives additional blood from the placenta that can protect her or him against getting anemia in the first few months of life.

rather than just imagine it. You can stroke his hair or count and kiss her fingers and toes. You can watch her drift in and out of sleep or whisper his name into his ear.

You and your new child need as much peace and quiet time together as you can create. In any setting, well-meaning providers and others can interrupt this important personal time because they want to know how you and your baby are doing. In a hospital, medical personnel may have their own schedules for evaluations. Providers often can unobtrusively examine your baby in your arms. It is usually not necessary to have tests done right away. If there is a medical reason to take your baby away from you for a short time, your partner or support person can accompany the baby.

The first few hours of a baby's life are a time of heightened awareness. Breast-feeding will be easier to establish if your baby nurses within the first hour or two after birth. Babies have an instinctive sucking reflex but show varying degrees of interest and take different amounts of time to nurse. Some latch on to the breast immediately; others learn to do so more gradually over a period of hours. Smelling, licking, and exploring your breasts are part of the process. Allowing your baby to suckle, even if you don't plan to breast-feed, will give her or him the benefit of antibodies and nutrients from colostrum, the first "milk."

You might want to ask your midwife or doctor in advance if she or he will help you start breast-feeding by placing your baby onto your chest, skin to skin, right after birth. Also, if you are planning to breast-feed, insist that the baby not be given any water or formula without a clear medical need. (For more information on the period immediately after birth, see Chapter 14, "Your Physical Recovery and Your Newborn." For more on breastfeeding, see Chapter 15, "Feeding Your Baby.")

Finally, the head was out, and another push or two later, the body came out. Just like that, it was over. The pain, the hard work, the exhaustion. It was all over. I was wide awake, full of energy, and over the moon to be holding our new baby in my arms. We had a baby!

NOTES

1. F. Zlatnik, "Management of Premature Rupture of Membranes at Term," *Obstetrics and Gynecology Clinics of North America* 19 (1992): 353–364.

2. Patricia A. Robertson, Lily J. Huang, Mary S. Croughan-Minihane, and Sarah J. Kilpatrick, "Is There an Association Between Water Baths During Labor and the Development of Chorioamnionitis or Endometritis?," *American Journal of Obstetrics and Gynecology* 178 (June 1998): 1215–1221. See also M. Eriksson, L. Ladfors, L. A. Mattsson, and O. Fall, "Warm Tub Bath During Labour: A Study of 1385 Women with Prelabor Rupture of the Membranes After 34 Weeks of Gestation," *Acta Obstetricia et Gynecologica Scandinavia* 75 (1996): 642–644.

3. Z. Alfirevic, D. Devane, and G.M.L. Gyte, "Continuous Cardiotocography (CTG) as a Form of Electronic Fetal Monitoring (EFM) for Fetal Assessment During Labour," *Cochrane Database of Systematic Reviews* 2006, Issue 3. Art. No.: CD006066. DOI: 10.1002/14651858.CD006066.

4. Z. Alfirevic, D. Devane, and G.M.L. Gyte, "Continuous Cardiotocography (CTG) as a Form of Electronic

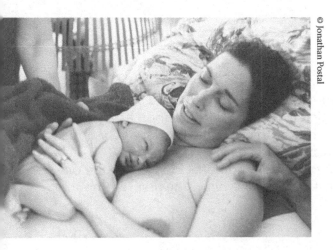

© Jonathan Postal

Fetal Monitoring (EFM) for Fetal Assessment During Labour." *Cochrane Database of Systematic Reviews* 2006, Issue 3. Art. No.: CD006066. DOI: 10.1002/14651858.CD006066.

5. Joey F. Minato, "Is it Time to Push? Examining Rest in Second-Stage Labor," *AWHONN Lifelines* 4, no. 6 (2000): 20–23. See also Susan L. Hansen, Steven L. Clark, and Joyce C. Foster, "Active Pushing Versus Passive Fetal Descent in the Second Stage of Labor: A Randomized Controlled Trial," *Obstetrics & Gynecology* 99, no. 1 (January 2002): 29–34.

6. L. Mayberry, "Epidural Analgesia Side Effects Co-interventions and Care of Women During Childbirth: A Systematic Review," *American Journal of Obstetrics and Gynecology* 186, no. 5 (2002): s81–s94.

7. Judy Lothian, Debby Amis, and Jeannette Crenshaw, "Care Practices That Promote Normal Birth No. 4: No Routine Interventions," *Lamaze International,* accessed at www.lamaze.org/institute/CarePractices/documents/4NoRoutineIntervention.pdf on August 23, 2006.

8. J. Roberts and L. Hanson, "Best Practices in Second Stage Labor Care: Maternal Bearing Down and Positioning," *Journal of Midwifery & Women's Health* 52, no. 3 (2007): 238–245.

9. K. Hartmann, M. Viswanathan, R. Palmieri, G. Gertlehner, J. Thorp, and K. N. Lohr, "Outcomes of Routine Episiotomy: A Systematic Review," *JAMA* 293 (2005): 2,141–2,148.

10. Judith Mercer and Debra Erickson-Owens, "Delayed Cord Clamping Increases Infants' Iron Stores," *Lancet* 367 (June 2006): 1,056–1,958.

CHAPTER 11

Coping with Pain

When we are pregnant, most of us wonder how we will cope with the intensity and pain of labor and birth. It is useful to learn about the pros and cons of different comfort measures, coping strategies, and medications. This helps us be better prepared for decisions we will make before and during labor and birth.

Pain can vary during different times in the same labor and during different births by the same woman. Many techniques are available to ease labor pain and to help you cope with it. The techniques range from comfort measures such as walking or touch or relaxing in water, to mental strategies such as focused breathing or hypnosis, to medication such as narcotics or epidurals. This chapter covers the whole range, starting with the least invasive, nondrug approaches and ending with medication.

PLANNING AHEAD

The pain relief methods you choose to use can affect your experience and memories of labor. Learning about the potential advantages and disadvantages of different methods, thinking about your preferences with regard to pain control, and talking with your provider and support people about what you want before you go into labor will help you make sound decisions. Many midwives, childbirth educators, and other health care professionals are skilled at helping women sort through culturally prevalent notions about pain during labor and birth, some of which are misleading and unnecessarily frightening.

While preparing is important, labor itself is unpredictable. You can't know in advance what you will experience or what you will want or need. Your labor may be easier or more complicated than you imagine. You might plan to give birth without medication and find yourself needing greater relief, or you might plan on an epidural but find you don't need one. A good guiding principle is to know what your options are; choose the simplest, least invasive option first; and progress to more complicated approaches only if you need them. It's also helpful to rest as much as possible during early labor and conserve your energy, as exhaustion can diminish your capacity to tolerate pain and thus increase the need for pain medication. The support of trusted individuals throughout your labor is key to making good decisions along the way.

I was open to pain meds if I needed them, was a bit squeamish about getting an epidural, but was aiming for a nonmedicated birth if possible. At one point I did ask about narcotics, but when we checked, I was ready to push . . . so I didn't need them!

I was determined to have a total "medical buffet" during my delivery. I'd start with Nubain and then move to an epidural and be blissfully pain free. However, when I arrived at the hospital, my OB told me that it was too late for any medical intervention and it was time to push. In fact, I had been lucky not to have had him in the car on the way. I swore at my OB so atrociously that when I returned to the same hospital three years later for baby number two, the nurses remembered me. I had to throw my "imagined delivery" out of the window and have this baby. I labored for 64 minutes in the hospital and he was born. I was swearing like a sailor and yelled at everyone within a two-foot radius, including my husband. At one point my OB nonchalantly said, "If you focused that energy on pushing, instead of yelling at us, you'd have a baby by now." I got all huffed up at her and my husband and then my son crowned. She smiled and said, "I told you." It was the most powerful moment of my life; I delivered him, cut the cord, and held him in my arms . . . all before breakfast.

THINKING ABOUT PAIN

In everyday life, physical pain, especially intense pain, is usually a warning that something is wrong in our bodies. But the pain of labor and birth is not a sign of danger, nor is it a symptom of injury or illness. It is a sign that your body is working hard to birth your baby.

Labor pain is different from other experiences of pain in several ways. Labor pain is self-limiting—it will end when the baby is born. It is also intermittent, not continuous, which means you will usually have periods of less pain or no pain between contractions. In addition, labor pain intensifies gradually over time, and this allows your body time to adapt. These differences often make labor pain easier to cope with than other kinds of pain.

I could feel the contractions in front but the strongest pain was in my back. . . . It hurt! I spent most of this time . . . leaning on the rail . . . moaning loudly. I felt like I had to go to the bathroom with each contraction but I decided that must be birth-related, since when I tried to go nothing would come out. . . . During the contractions I needed Brian to press on my sacrum to ease the pain in my back. I also needed him to remind me that it was only pain, a physical sensation, and that it would end soon. Even more importantly, I needed him to remind me that this is what needed to happen for our baby to be born, that soon I would be holding our new baby in my arms.

PAIN VERSUS SUFFERING

Because pain and suffering often go hand in hand, we tend to think they're the same thing. But they're not. Pain is a physical sensation, while suffering is an emotional experience. We may suffer (feel helplessness, anguish, remorse,

WOMEN'S RIGHT TO PAIN RELIEF

Women's options for coping with pain during labor expanded in the late nineteenth and early twentieth centuries as doctors offered new methods to relieve labor pain, such as inhaling chloroform gas or ether. Another method, called "twilight sleep," used a combination of morphine, for relief of pain, and scopolamine, a sedative that reduced women's memories of giving birth. This method became popular among upper-class women, some of whom formed "twilight sleep societies" to promote its use.[1] The early suffragettes campaigned for the right to have medication in labor, along with the right to vote.

Yet many women who were given scopolamine and morphine became delusional, and some thrashed about so much that they needed to be restrained with leather straps while their babies were born. Babies were so sedated by the drugs that doctors held them upside down and slapped them to get them to breathe (a practice thankfully no longer necessary). In 1958, *Ladies' Home Journal* published an article titled "Cruelty in the Maternity Ward" and received a flood of letters from women, some of whom said they were drugged without consent and treated harshly, the skin worn off their wrists by arm restraints.[2]

In the 1960s and '70s, responding to the negative effects of previous medical approaches to childbirth, many women's health advocates campaigned for more natural childbirth. Like the first wave of feminists, those women believed that they could be empowered by choosing how they gave birth. And many in that generation wanted to do it consciously.

The medications available to women giving birth in the United States today are safer and more sophisticated than those of the past. They allow women to remain conscious while experiencing childbirth with less pain. Yet these medications can have adverse effects on mothers or babies, and many women still choose to avoid them for a variety of reasons.

fear, panic, or loss of control) even when there is *no physical sensation of pain.* And we may experience physical pain *without suffering.* As Penny Simkin and April Bolding, longtime advocates for birthing women, write, "one can have pain coexisting with satisfaction, enjoyment, and empowerment."[3] By the same token, they say, suffering can be caused or increased by factors other than physical pain: "loneliness, ignorance, unkind or insensitive treatment during labor, along with unresolved past psychological or physical distress, increase the chance that the woman will suffer."[4]

While it is commonly believed that a woman's satisfaction with her birth experience is linked to how much or how little pain she feels, this isn't typically so. Our satisfaction seems to be highest when we trust that we are getting good information, we are given opportunities to participate in decisions regarding our care, and our caregivers treat us with kindness and respect.[5] In the long run, pain and

WHAT DOES THE PAIN OF CHILDBIRTH FEEL LIKE?[6]

While women's experiences of pain during labor and childbirth vary widely, there are some commonalities. Nearly all of us experience pain in our lower abdomen during contractions. The pain may feel similar to menstrual cramps, but will likely be much more intense. Many of us also feel pain in our lower backs; generally this happens during a contraction, but occasionally it continues even after the contraction has ended. You may also feel pain in your hips, buttocks, and/or thighs. Sometimes you may feel the pain in only one area, while at other times you may feel it in several areas at once.

Pain generally increases as labor progresses. During the active phase of stage 1 labor, the intensity of the contractions increases. The final part of stage 1, called "transition," is the shortest but the most intense, as the last 2 or 3 centimeters of the cervix pull over the baby's head, much like a turtleneck being pulled over the head. Finally, during pushing, the sensations come from pressure on nerves in the vaginal area and the rectal area, which gets pressure through the thin wall between the vagina and the rectum.

There can also be pain related to what is called "back labor." Back labor can occur when the back of the baby's head is pressed against the inside of the mother's back. (For more information, see "'Back Labor'/'Posterior' Baby," page 215.) For some women, a baby in this position will result in a longer, slower labor in which the mother will feel more pain in her back than in her belly.

pain relief seem to have less effect on our overall satisfaction than the quality of support we receive from our caregivers. Whatever kind of pain relief options we choose to use during labor, it is important to remember that pain relief alone does not address our fears, worries, feelings of helplessness, or other emotions that might lead to distress or dissatisfaction. To prevent suffering, women need more than relief of pain. We need to trust in our strength and feel cared for as we respond to labor pain, and we need humane, nurturing, confident people giving us continuous support throughout labor.

My labor felt like a marathon that lasted over two days. There were easy periods, where I sailed along (I was even able to sleep), but there were stretches when it felt like a steep, uphill climb that would never end. But just like in a marathon, you just keep putting one foot in front of the other. You don't think about reaching the end, you just think about taking the next step. Having the support of a great midwife, my husband, and a few close loved ones made all the difference. I had such a HUGE sense of accomplishment when my daughter emerged and made her first tiny sounds. I was exhilarated by meeting such a great physical (and mental) challenge and felt I had earned a marathon "crown."

PREPARING TO MEET THE CHALLENGES OF LABOR AND BIRTH

Certain strategies lay the foundation to help you cope with the pain of labor. These include working with a provider you trust, knowing ahead of time what pain relief strategies are available in your chosen birth setting, and giving birth in a safe, comfortable space, surrounded by people who will provide you with good support. (For more information on the value of continuous support during labor, see page 32.)

Women labor best in a calm, nurturing environment. For instance, having privacy, dim lights, quiet voices, and/or music of your choosing can contribute to your sense of ease and safety.[7] (For a list of things to bring to a hospital or birth center that can help create a comfortable environment, see page 40.)

Your choice of provider and birth setting will affect what options are available to you in terms of both labor support and pain relief. For example, if you give birth in a hospital, you will have access to a range of pain medications, but you may have less support or help with medication-free methods of pain relief. However, hospitals vary in this regard. Some have birthing tubs and birthing balls or have doulas on staff; others have restrictive policies that will limit your options. Some hospital staff may regularly ask, "Are you ready for your epidural?" even if you have clearly stated your preferences for a nonmedicated birth. Some hospitals require an initial evaluation by an anesthesiologist when you arrive in labor; this information will be used to help take care of you if you decide to have an epidural or if you need a cesarean section. If you are planning to give birth in a hospital, ask about its policies and see what you can do to increase your own access to comfort measures (for example, by bringing in your own supplies and hiring a doula).

If you give birth at home or in a freestanding birth center, you will likely have access to many comfort measures and support with nondrug pain relief techniques as well as the support team of your choice. If you are having a complicated labor and need pain relief medication, you will be transferred to a hospital.

(For more information on choosing a provider and birth setting that are right for you, see Chapter 2. For more information on doulas, see page 33.)

NONDRUG STRATEGIES TO EASE LABOR

Coping strategies can be helpful for all women. Even if you plan to use pain medication, these approaches can help delay or decrease your need for it. Some of these strategies help reduce pain, while others can help you cope better with it.

Women's responses to these techniques vary; you may find that some techniques are more helpful for you than others. Your support team can help you try different strategies and see what works. An experienced midwife or doula will have suggestions for specific techniques to assist you, or your partner or other support person may want to read about them in advance in order to help you. You and those who will support you during labor can learn relaxation routines and other strategies from classes, books, or audio or video resources and practice them before you go into labor. In some cases, scientific evidence for a particular strategy is hard to find, but women describe it as helpful. (For more information, see "Resources.")

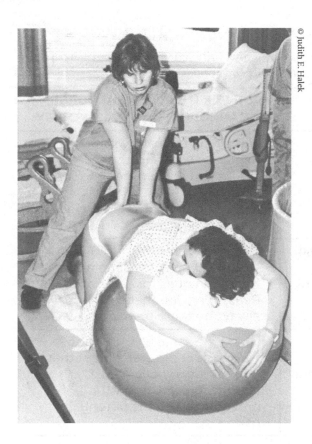

The two things that helped me through the labor were mooing and yelling at the top of my lungs. Mooing was the only sort of deep moaning noise that made my whole body feel good, but it did not fit into my mental picture of myself as a chic, polite woman, so I kept making myself laugh. I would do these big low bellows and then burst out laughing because I was so embarrassed, but then that felt really good, so I would just keep laughing.

MOVEMENT, POSITIONS, AND RHYTHMS

Movement

Having the freedom to move and change positions helps women cope with labor. Upright movements, such as walking, swaying, lunging,

and dancing, can help reduce the pain of labor and help move the baby down into a good position for birth.[8]

Many hospitals may restrict your movement, especially if you are alone, so try to have a support person with you and try to maintain your freedom to move during your labor. If you are encumbered with multiple attachments such as blood pressure cuffs, IVs, and electronic fetal monitoring equipment, it may be impossible to move freely. You have a right to refuse all these monitors. If you do accept them, you can adapt by standing by your bed, sitting in a chair, swaying in your partner's arms, and so forth. If you have an epidural or have taken medicines that make you feel dizzy, you will likely be restricted to bed.

Positions

Women often find it helpful to try different positions; different ones will work at different times. Upright positions include standing, sitting, semi-sitting (leaning back), kneeling, and squatting. Squatting and kneeling while leaning forward make the pelvic outlet bigger, so the baby has more room to come down during pushing.[9] Variations can include sitting on birth stools (specially designed stools that simulate squatting, but give support to the legs and

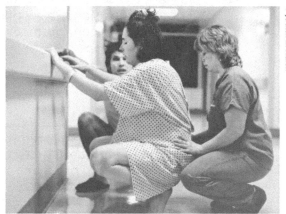

PAIN MEDICATIONS PREFERENCE SCALE

This table, created by childbirth educator Penny Simkin, can help you clarify your feelings about pain and pain management during labor. *Used with permission from Penny Simkin and Childbirth Graphics.*

NUMBER	WHAT IT MEANS	YOUR PARTNER, DOULA, NURSE, OR CAREGIVER CAN HELP YOU BY:
+10	I want to be numb, to get anesthesia before labor begins. (An impossible extreme.)	• Explaining that you will have some pain even with anesthesia. • Discussing your wishes and fears with you. • Promising to help you get medication as soon as possible in labor.
+9	I have a great fear of labor pain, and I believe I cannot cope. I have to depend on the staff to take away my pain.	• Doing the same as for +10 above. • Teaching you some simple comfort techniques for early labor. • Reassuring you that someone will always be there to help you.
+7	I want anesthesia as soon in labor as the doctor will allow or before labor becomes painful.	• Doing the same as for +9 above. • Making sure the staff knows that you want early anesthesia. • Making sure you know the procedures and the potential risks.
+5	I want epidural anesthesia in active labor (4–5 cm.) I am willing to try to cope until then, perhaps with narcotic medications.	• Encouraging you in your breathing and relaxation. • Knowing and using other comfort measures. • Suggesting medication when you are in active labor.
+3	I want to use some medication but as little as possible. I plan to use self-help comfort measures for part of labor.	• Doing the same as for +5 above. • Committing themselves to helping you reduce medication use. • Helping you get medications when you decide you want them. • Suggesting half doses of narcotics or a "light and late" epidural.
0	I have no opinion or preference. I will wait and see. (A rare attitude among pregnant women.)	• Helping you become informed about labor pain, comfort measures, and medications. • Following your wishes during labor.

NUMBER	WHAT IT MEANS	YOUR PARTNER, DOULA, NURSE, OR CAREGIVER CAN HELP YOU BY:
-3	I would like to avoid pain medications if I can, but if coping becomes difficult, I'd feel like a "martyr" if I did not get them.	• Emphasizing coping techniques. • Not suggesting that you take pain medication. • Not trying to talk you out of pain medications if you request them.
-5	I have a strong desire to avoid pain medications, mainly to avoid the side effects on me, my labor, or my baby. I will accept medications for a difficult or long labor.	• Preparing for a very active support role. • Practicing comfort measures with you in class and at home. • Not suggesting medications. If you ask, suggesting different comfort measures and more intense emotional support first. • Helping you accept pain medications if you become exhausted or cannot benefit from support techniques and comfort measures.
-7	I have a very strong desire for a natural birth, for personal gratification along with the benefits to my baby and my labor. I will be disappointed if I use medication.	• Doing the same as for -5 above. • Encouraging you to enlist the support of your caregiver. • Requesting a supportive nurse who can help with natural birth. • Planning and rehearsing ways to get through painful or discouraging periods in labor. • Prearranging a plan (e.g., a "last resort" code word) for letting them know if you have had enough and want medication.
-9	I want medication to be denied by my support team and the staff, even if I beg for it.	• Exploring the reasons for your feelings. • Helping you see that they cannot deny you medication. • Promising to help all they can but leaving the final decision to you.
-10	I want no medication, even for a cesarean delivery. (An impossible extreme.)	• Doing the same as for -9 above. • Helping you gain a realistic understanding of risks and benefits of pain medications.

© Erin Habecker

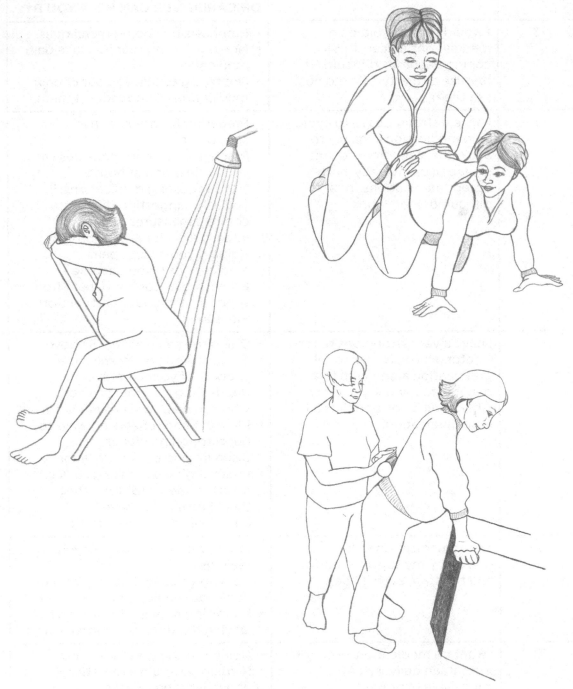

Having pressure or a massage on your lower back during labor may help make the process more comfortable.

have space in the center for the mother to give birth to the baby). "Birthing balls" are large physiotherapy balls that you can sit on, rock on, or lean over and rest your arms on. You may want someone with you to support you in getting on and off the ball for safety and balance. Another nice variation is to have a support person sit behind you in the bed, so that you can sit between the person's legs and be held in the person's arms. Any of these upright positions can support the descent of the baby.

If you need to give your legs and body a rest, side-lying is a great position. You can even push and give birth to your baby like this. The position you want to avoid is lying flat on your back. That position can decrease blood flow and oxygen delivery to your baby.

For "back labor" (when you are feeling the pain in your back), certain positions help take pressure off your back by bringing your belly forward. These include being on your hands and knees (either on a bed, or on the floor with lots of pillows under you), standing and leaning way over onto a pile of pillows on a bed, or kneeling and leaning onto a birthing ball. In a position called "the lunge," you stand with one leg elevated on a chair; this helps to tilt your pelvis, relieves some of the pressure, and encourages the baby to turn as well. Counterpressure may also be effective in relieving back labor discomfort. It can be provided by a partner who presses a firm ball, such as a tennis ball, into the area of the back where you are experiencing discomfort.

Rhythm

In active labor, you turn inward, and a rhythm develops. You may rock back and forth, moan, curl around a partner's hand during each contraction, and then want massage or total silence in between. You may experience a three-part cycle: relaxation between contractions, rhythmic movement during each contraction, and a ritual (such as vocalizing or rocking) that helps repeat and maintain the rhythm.[10] The pattern that works for you will be uniquely yours. While the woman is in this "zone," she can benefit when her support team reinforces her rhythm/ritual and keeps interruptions to a minimum.

TECHNIQUES OF BREATH AND FOCUS

Techniques that help us to feel relaxed and at ease can reduce the amount of pain we feel.

Breathing

While many breathing techniques are taught in classes and books, there really is no one special way to breathe that works best during labor. The truth is, we all know how to breathe, and for the most part, breathing in labor takes care of itself. Focusing on your own natural rhythm can center you and help you work with your labor. You can pay attention to your breath, letting it anchor you to the moment as your contraction begins, breathing along with the contraction, matching your breathing to the rise and fall of the contraction as it becomes stronger, peaks, and subsides. Focusing on breathing out slowly between contractions as you relax muscles and get rid of tension can help. Remember, each breath brings you closer to when your baby will be born.

In addition, there are several kinds of patterned breathing techniques that can best be learned through classes and/or videotapes or DVDs. Counting breaths or changing your breathing pattern can be a welcome distraction. These strategies can be especially useful if you start to feel "out of control" and need help to focus during an intense part of labor. A partner, family member, or doula can assist you with patterned breathing techniques.

Hypnosis

The use of hypnosis in labor has undergone a recent renaissance. Self-hypnosis involves practicing techniques before labor begins that you can use to help trigger deep relaxation when the contractions start. You can practice these on your own or with a partner. Specialized classes now teach HypnoBirthing (see page 36). While research on the effectiveness of hypnosis

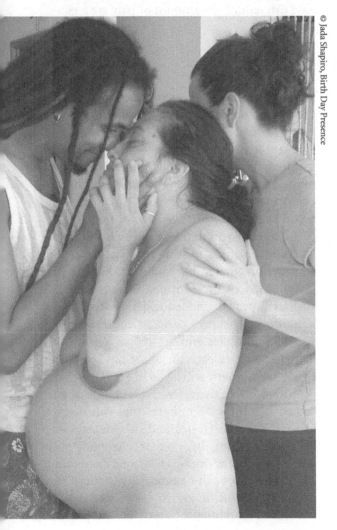

© Jada Shapiro, Birth Day Presence

is limited, several studies have found women using hypnosis in labor used less pain medication and reported greater satisfaction with their birth experiences.[11] A high hypnotic susceptibility may be required for a greater reduction in pain; however, relaxation and reduction of suffering were found to be a benefit regardless of how easily a woman responds to suggestions.[12]

Visualization

Visualization involves imagining different scenes or images to aid you with, distract you from, or help you integrate the experience of labor. The images—as in visualizing a hike to the top of a mountain or ocean waves coming and going—can reflect the rhythm of your labor. They can be peaceful and relaxing scenes, such as being on a warm beach or in a familiar place that evokes calm and relaxation. Women can use visualizations of flower buds opening as a symbol of the cervix opening and yielding to this process and the baby. Visualization can be done on your own, with the guidance of a tape or CD, or with a support person guiding you.

Stillness

Sometimes simply being very still, being quiet and focusing inward, or sleeping between contractions leads to deep relaxation. You may want to draw upon skills learned in yoga, meditation practice, spiritual work, or mindfulness-based childbirth preparation classes. Whatever resources you use to center yourself in your everyday life may work in labor as well.

TECHNIQUES THAT USE THE SENSES

These techniques work primarily by sending alternative or competing sensations into the nervous system and brain at the same time that the contractions are occurring. This can diminish the amount of pain you feel as your brain focuses on the competing stimuli instead of on just the pain signals from the labor process. For this effect to keep working, it will be important to change the stimuli throughout labor, trying new ones from time to time, because the body gets used to one sensation and then the technique becomes less effective.

Touch

The human touch in labor is a powerful way to relieve pain and reduce anxiety.[13] Touch may range from a supportive hand placed for reassurance in one spot, like on your arm, to a light stroking on your back and arms as you have a contraction, to a firm massage on your neck and shoulders between contractions. Foot massages can be helpful when you are resting, as can head and scalp massage.

Often, once you are in labor, you may not know exactly what would feel good and what wouldn't. A common error that friends and family make is to constantly ask you what you want. Doulas and those with more experience know that it is better to just say, "Is it okay if I rub your shoulder?" and then do so with your permission. If it doesn't feel right, you will let them know. You may find that for some or even all of your labor, you prefer not to be touched.

Counterpressure

Counterpressure is using a special kind of touch to help relieve back pain in labor. In one of the many methods for applying counterpressure, someone may place the palms of her or his hands over your lower back where the sacrum (the triangular bone at the base of the spine) is and then gently but firmly press in and support your back during a contraction, holding it until the contraction is over. Another technique is squeezing in on both hips, which places pressure on the outside of your pelvic bones. This in turn creates more space around your sacrum, where the nerves involved in back labor are located.

Heat and Cold

At times during labor, a warm compress on your lower back or abdomen may be just the right thing. At other times, a cold washcloth on your forehead or on the back of your neck may feel perfect. Someone may fan you between contractions and the cool breeze may soothe you and let you relax. At another time, a warm blanket wrapped around your feet may help you to sleep between the contractions. Using heat and cold during labor is a marvelous way to both nurture you and provide your body with lots of new stimuli and changing sensations. (This competes with your perception of the pain and can help to lessen it.)

The Comfort of Water

Being in water during labor can be wonderfully soothing and can help you relax. Many studies have shown water immersion during labor to be safe for both mother and baby while also reducing the mother's pain and her need for pain medication. Laboring in water can help you relax during early labor and may help babies rotate and get into a better position for birth.[14]

When using a tub, work with your midwife or physician to determine when and for how long you can be in the bath, so that you can avoid any negative effects. If a woman enters the bath before she is in active labor or stays in for more than one or two hours, labor progress can be slowed.[15] Laboring in water can make you dehydrated or raise your temperature if you are not drinking enough, or if the water is too hot.

Being immersed in water for pain relief is called "hydrotherapy." This is different from having a "water birth," which refers to actually birthing your baby under the water. Many hospitals offer hydrotherapy, but few offer water birth as an option. The combination of hydrotherapy and water birth is more commonly offered in birth centers and homes. In some settings, you will need to rent your own tub if you want to use a deeper tub that allows you to be more fully immersed in the water, so check with your planned birth site.

If a tub is not available, showers are also a good option during labor. Standing and swaying under the water or holding an extended showerhead and letting the water run over your belly can be very helpful. Some women stay in the shower for hours. The flow of hot water on your back can make a huge difference, especially if you experience contractions mostly in your lower back.

Focal Points

Some of us find it useful to focus our gaze on a particular object. You can use "focal points" such as a picture, flowers, or anything that has special meaning for you. In a hospital setting, some families bring a colored cloth for the over-the-bed table (the one with wheels) and set up a small "altar" of items for the laboring mother to focus on. Focusing into the eyes of someone you love is a powerful way to feel strength and support along your journey.

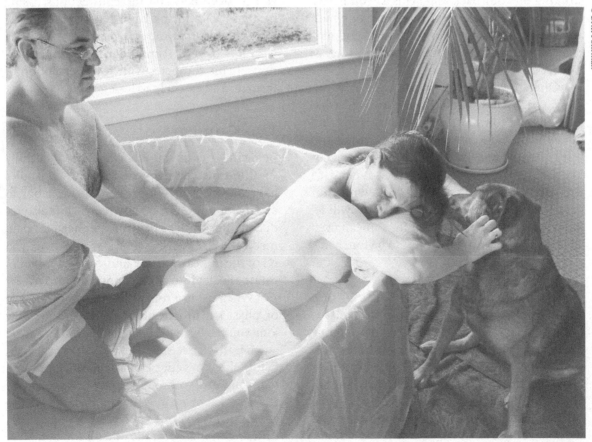

Music

Music and sounds have tremendous power to evoke emotions. Music can improve pain tolerance, increase energy, and elevate mood. It can also be used to help you maintain your chosen movements or breathing patterns. You may want to listen to music during some or all of your labor and birth. Choose whatever appeals to you. Those who walk into your labor room from another, possibly more hectic, space will instantly get the message that this is the tempo and mood of your space. If you are birthing somewhere other than your home, bring your own music player. (Also bring plenty of batteries, unless you know that power outlets will be available to you.)

Using Your Voice

Our voices are a powerful aspect of our laboring bodies. For many of us, the use of our voice in conjunction with our breath helps us through contractions. Often the sounds we make are almost like low moaning or a kind of low singing. As labor progresses, the sounds tend to get deeper and louder. Near the time of birth, in most cultures around the world, women give a "birth yell" that signifies that the baby is coming.

During labor, you may find comfort in singing, laughing, giggling, or making low, open sounds, "ohhhhs" and "ahhhhs" and "oms." You may fear that making sounds means that you are losing control or being undignified. In fact, it means that you are present and aware, working with the descending, opening process of giving birth. Feel the vibrations in your body and feel free to express them.

Aromatherapy

The sense of smell is heightened in pregnancy and labor. Aromatherapy is the practice of intentionally using certain scents to evoke physical or emotional responses such as relaxation, heightening energy, or a sense of peace. In one large study, more than half of the women who used aromatherapy (the scents of clary sage, lavender, rose, or chamomile) during labor found it helpful in relieving pain and reducing anxiety and fear. The aromatherapy also may have reduced their need for additional pain relief.[16]

Many books and practitioners can provide information about the use of aromatherapy. It can vary from simply picking an oil whose scent you like to using certain ones to try to achieve certain effects. (For example, lavender is commonly used for relaxation.) In a hospital setting, you may not be allowed to burn candles or use an oil diffuser, but perhaps you can put a drop of oil on a lightbulb, or a cotton ball inside a pillow, or use a mister to spray the scent into the air.

However, many women cannot tolerate strong smells of any kind in labor. Scents should be used in small amounts at first, guided strictly by your preferences.

TECHNIQUES THAT REQUIRE SPECIAL SKILLS

Acupuncture and Acupressure

Acupuncture has long been used to help induce women's labors. Some research has shown that it can be helpful for reducing labor pain and enhancing relaxation.[17] Licensed acupuncturists in most communities work with pregnant and laboring women. Acupressure, a simple alternative to acupuncture that doesn't involve needles, can be administered by a labor companion or care provider with minimal training. Some research has shown that acupressure can reduce labor pain.[18]

Sterile Water Injections

Women who experience back labor may benefit from a technique that involves using a tiny needle to inject a small amount of sterile water into four spots around the sacrum, the triangular bone at the base of the spine. These injections create an intense stinging sensation that dissipates quickly. Some women find that the pain of back labor is relieved within minutes of the injection and relief lasts up to two hours.[19] Although this is a simple, safe procedure, not all midwives or physicians offer it, so you may want to ask in advance, in case you experience back labor.

TENS Units

Transcutaneous electrical nerve stimulation (TENS) involves placing on your skin small pads with electrodes that emit very low-voltage pulses. The pulses feel like vibrations in rhythmic patterns against your skin. TENS units have been employed by mothers in labor in Europe for years. Although research has shown that TENS has little effect on reducing labor pain, some women say it helps.

Physical therapists and some massage therapists have TENS units, but you can also buy or rent one and learn to use it yourself. TENS is safe when used as directed.[20]

MEDICATIONS FOR PAIN RELIEF

Pain medications can be extremely helpful at certain times and in certain situations in labor. They can dramatically ease the pain of labor, and can be vital in managing long, complicated, or difficult labors. Yet, like many medical interventions, they carry risks for mothers and babies and should be used only with full knowledge of all options and alternatives as well as of the risks and benefits. Medications do not take the place of emotional support and encouragement, which is essential regardless of whether you are using medication or not. These medications are not available at outside-of-hospital births; if you are giving birth at home or in a freestanding birth clinic, you will have to transfer to a hospital if at some point you need or want them.

I have three children and have had three very different labor experiences, all in a hospital setting, and all wonderful and challenging in different ways. My first daughter was ten days late and I was ultimately induced. I was on Pitocin and the contractions came on suddenly, strong from the outset. I labored for ten hours and my cervix was slow to dilate, going from 1 centimeter dilated to 3 centimeters dilated over that time period. At that point I was exhausted and finally agreed to an epidural, which I had been trying to avoid. I tell you, it was bliss. I finally stopped fighting against the contractions and relaxed into them. As a result, I went from 3 centimeters to 10 centimeters (fully) dilated over only 45 minutes, and then pushed for only 30 minutes and Isabel was born. The more common belief is that epidurals can slow down the birth process, but I found the opposite was true, because I could be a more active participant when I wasn't in so much pain.

I went into my second delivery with an open mind, clear that I would happily take pain medication if I felt the need, but wanting to try to do it without medication if possible. As it turned out, I did not have a choice. My son Jamie was born very quickly, literally 3 minutes after I stepped foot into the hospital. No pain medication for me! It was too late! Well, I thought I had a high pain tolerance but that was something. Unbelievable, really. At least it was over quickly! Some have said to me, "Aren't you glad you did it without pain medication and know you can do it?" Well, sure I can do it, but I wouldn't say "glad."

For my third and final delivery I was sure I wanted pain medication. I felt no need to prove to myself that I could do it pain free, and, having done it both ways, I felt I had been able to be more present for the birth of my child when the pain was controlled. Bring it on! I was very clear on this from the minute I entered the hospital. As it turned out, my third delivery was my hardest. My daughter was what is called "face presentation" and was very difficult to move through the birth canal as a result. She was stuck behind my pubic bone for a long while, and even the epidural did not control this bone pain, though I am sure it substantially helped. The labor was long, and I was so tired. I am very thankful that I was able to get some pain relief. In the end, I was able to deliver Hannah vaginally and all went well.

There are two basic ways that pain medications are used during labor: *systemically,* that is, affecting the entire body, and *regionally,* affecting a targeted area. The systemic medications are usually narcotics (but they also include nitrous oxide; see box below). Epidurals use medications regionally, generally as a mixture of local anesthesia (numbing medicine) and narcotics.

SYSTEMIC MEDICINE

Opioids (also called narcotics) are the most commonly used systemic medicines given to

---

NITROUS OXIDE

Nitrous oxide is an odorless, tasteless gas that you breathe in through a mask. Exactly how nitrous oxide works is not well understood, but many women who use it during labor find it beneficial. Although women who use nitrous oxide don't necessarily report less pain, they report feeling that while they still have some pain they are not as bothered by it. Nitrous oxide can be administered by an anesthesiologist, a midwife, or an obstetrician. It is the most commonly used form of analgesia in the United Kingdom, where midwives use it in hospitals and carry it with them to home births, and three of every five women use it at some time during labor.[21]

Nitrous oxide has not been used much in the United States. Yet it provides better analgesia than morphine, meperidine (Demerol), or fentanyl.[22] In a 2002 national survey, 52 percent of the women who used nitrous oxide found it to be very or somewhat helpful.[23] It is safer than the narcotics/opioids and doesn't have any of the adverse side effects for mothers or babies that can occur after using narcotics/opioids or epidurals.[24] Another advantage is that it takes effect in about a minute and the effect stops quickly once you stop breathing the gas through the mask.

Some women find it difficult to synchronize use of the gas with the timing of their contractions in order to achieve maximally effective pain relief. In the UK, mid-

(continued)

wives teach women how to do this during prenatal care. Some women find that a mask makes them feel claustrophobic or don't like the way the gas makes them feel. Some women experience dizziness or nausea.

Nitrous oxide for relief of labor pain is mixed half-and-half with oxygen and delivered through a mask or tube that the laboring woman holds. The gases are delivered either from a hospital pipeline through the walls into the labor rooms or from two separate portable cylinders. Women must begin breathing the mixture through the mask at least 1 minute before the onset of a contraction and continue until the contraction begins to ease.

Self-administration is an essential safety measure. You must hold the mask or tube yourself and not let another person hold it for you. If you breathe too much of the gas, you will become drowsy, your hand will relax, and the mask or tube will fall away from your face, so that you breathe normal room air. Self-administration also allows the woman to control management of her pain.

Nitrous oxide is not widely available for use in labor in the United States. Laboring women in the United States have fewer options for pain relief than women in most other countries in the industrialized world. It is unclear why nitrous oxide is not used often in obstetrics in this country. Ether and chloroform, the other anesthetic gases that were used by women in labor in the early 1900s, were associated with complications and therefore most gas anesthetics went out of favor as other medications became available. Used with current equipment and procedures, nitrous oxide is safe, is effective enough for many women, and has important advantages compared to other, much more commonly used methods of labor analgesia. More women should have access to this method.[25] (For more information on nitrous oxide, see www.ourbodiesourselves.org/childbirth.)

relieve pain during labor. They include morphine (usually used only in early labor to help women get some sleep when this stage of labor is long), meperidine (Demerol or Pethidine), nalbuphine (Nubain), butorphanol (Stadol), and fentanyl (Sublimaze). Specific medicines used vary by provider and location.

When used systemically, opioids are given to you through an intravenous line (an IV) or by an injection into your arm, leg, or buttock. They work by being absorbed into the bloodstream and going to the receptors in your body that diminish pain perception. In general, they make you feel relaxed, sleepy, and possibly a little dizzy, and you tend to feel your contractions less. They may make it easier for you to rest for longer periods of time between the contractions.

Each opioid works for only a limited length of time and can be safely given only at certain times during labor. After a peak of effectiveness, the medicine begins to wear off. The length of time varies from one medicine to another. One to two hours is common, with the peak often being less than half an hour after the medicine is given.

Advantages and Disadvantages of Systemic Medicines

One advantage of systemic medicines is that they are short-acting. They therefore can be used at a time in the labor when you just need some help to make it through a challenge. The use of morphine for women who are exhausted in early labor is one example. Another common example is a one-time dose of systemic medicine if you are in the middle of labor and feel exhausted or like giving up; it may be what you need to get through this short but tough time. Mothers who try this may get a "second wind" and do fine without further medication. Others may have an even harder time coping with labor because of the way the narcotic makes them feel ("high" or disoriented). Another advantage to choosing to use systemic medicine over regional medicine like an epidural is that you either can avoid the possible adverse effects of the epidural altogether, or you can delay getting the epidural until later in the labor, which may diminish the impact of some of the epidural's negative effects.

But the main disadvantage of systemic opioids (narcotics) is that their use in labor has generally been found to have limited effect on controlling women's pain. When women rate the effectiveness of all the techniques used to minimize pain during labor, systemic opioids are less effective than immersion in water.[26] They are also much less effective for pain relief than epidurals. They will not take the pain away completely. The medicine may "knock you out" between contractions, or it may "take the edge off" by not allowing you to feel the buildup and the letdown of the contractions, thus making the contractions seem farther apart and allowing you to rest more between them. Some women experience a welcome feeling of relaxation; others feel a bit out of control.

Other disadvantages of systemic medicines are:

• The use of these medicines may prevent the production of your own endorphins (self-made hormones that naturally reduce your perception of pain).
• They are short-acting, and there is a time limit for when you can get another dose. So, after you have been given one dose, there is usually a waiting period before you can have more if the first dose doesn't work as well as you want. Some women find this waiting period very difficult.
• Just as they circulate throughout your body, systemic medicines get into the baby's circulation as well. There, they will have the same effect on the baby that they do on you. If a baby is born too soon after this type of drug is given to the mother, the baby may need help to breathe or may be given special drugs to wake her or him up. For this reason, many care providers will not give systemic pain medication to mothers if birth is likely to occur soon.
• Babies of mothers who receive these medicines can also have trouble initiating breastfeeding successfully and may not be able to suck correctly during the first few hours or days of life.[27]

REGIONAL MEDICINE

This type of medicine affects a certain region of the body, rather than the whole body. It may involve use of local anesthesia, which works by taking away sensation through a numbing effect on nerves. Or it may involve narcotic medications, or a combination of local anesthesia and narcotic medications. The region of the body that feels less pain depends on where the medicine is placed, how many nerves are involved, and how large an area they affect. There are two main categories of regional medicine for pain relief in labor: (1) the epidurals and spinals, and (2) the targeted regional anesthetics (such as paracervical or pudendal blocks), which are used much less frequently.

Epidurals and Spinals

"Epidural" and "spinal" refer to the areas where pain medicine is placed. In an *epidural,* medicine is infused into the area right outside the spinal canal (the epidural space); in a *spinal,* medicine is placed inside the spinal canal, where the spinal fluid is. Today there are epidurals, spinals, and combined spinal-epidurals.

Different medicines may be delivered by spinal injection or epidural catheter. How you will feel depends in part on the characteristics of your labor and the dose of local anesthetic (numbing) medicine and/or narcotic that is used. If narcotics are used in an epidural or spinal, they affect the nerves directly (unlike when they are used for systemic medication). You generally won't feel the dizziness or other negative systemic effects you might get with an IV or injection, just less pain.

Some anesthesiologists say it is normal to feel about 80 percent relief if the medicine is working correctly. You will still feel your contractions, but for the most part they will feel like pressure, not pain.

The type and amount of medicine—narcotics, local anesthetics (numbing medicine), or a combination—affect your mobility. When relatively low concentrations of local anesthetics and/or narcotics are used, as is now common practice, you will be able to move your legs. You may even be able to walk, although you may need continuous assistance to do this and some hospitals will not allow you to walk because of safety and legal liability concerns.

To place an epidural or spinal, an anesthesiologist or nurse-anesthetist first numbs a small area of skin on your back. For an epidural, she or he uses a needle to place a catheter (a tiny, flexible plastic tube) into the epidural space. With the catheter in place, medicine can be infused through a pump that controls the dose and the rate throughout your labor. In "patient-controlled" epidural anesthesia, you have a button that activates the pump when you push it. (It has controls that won't allow you to overdose yourself.)

A spinal is usually used for short-term pain relief. Spinals are often used for cesarean sections, and sometime for forceps or vacuum extractor births. A lower dose of medicine is put into the spinal for women in labor. In a spinal, the medicine is injected in a single dose, instead of being given continuously. In order to get the medicine into the spinal space, a very thin needle is used.

In some hospitals, a one-time dose of medicine is injected into the woman's spinal fluid and then a catheter is left in place in the epidural space for use when the spinal medicine wears off. This is known as a *combined spinal-epidural.* The advantage of the combined spinal-epidural is that if relief from the spinal wears off before the birth, the anesthesia staff can add anesthetics to the epidural catheter instead of having to give you another shot.

An epidural or a spinal will be accompanied by continuous electronic fetal monitoring of the baby. In addition, women who have an epidural will have an IV. Most women will need a temporary urinary catheter to empty the bladder, as well as equipment to monitor blood pressure.

Your ability to move and change positions in labor may help the baby to descend and assume a good birth position. Because epidurals and spinals can limit this, and have other potential adverse effects (listed on facing page), you may wish to avoid the medication unless and until you feel you can't go on without it. This is what author Penny Simkin calls "late and light" medication.

If you are having your first baby and want an epidural, it would be unusual to wait so long that you would not have the time to have one. If you are having your second or third baby, labor can be fast; depending on where you are in your labor, a combined spinal-epidural might be appropriate because the spinal part would give you more immediate relief.

I thought that I was going to die—literally DIE—before I got my epidurals. I would have killed my husband and my midwife if they had tried visualization, aromatherapy, or something similar on me while I was waiting the hour for my epidural. I was too busy concentrating on not dying. The good experiences I had in my two labors were after the epidurals. Before just totally sucked because of the pain. I believe in using the safest pain medication available if you want it. As my stepmother put it, "They don't give out prizes for suffering." My mother had me naturally and said it was a mistake that she did not repeat with my younger sister. I planned on having epidurals with both my children, but I was not prepared for how badly labor hurt up until the point I got the epidurals.

Advantages and Disadvantages of Regional Medicines

The greatest advantage of epidurals (and spinals) is that they can take away the greater part of the pain women feel in labor and while giving birth. An epidural can provide much-needed rest for an exhausted mother, especially when other approaches to getting that rest have

failed. An epidural can be helpful in the case of a very long labor. Psychological issues or individual circumstances may make experiencing the physical sensations of labor too difficult for some mothers at some point. Finally, some women choose epidurals simply in order to eliminate most labor pain.

The disadvantages of regional medications used for labor pain are:

- Sometimes the insertion of the epidural is ineffective and the process has to be repeated. Because of differences in the anatomy of the epidural space and the positioning of individual catheters, you may not get any relief in a small area of your abdomen or back (an "epidural window"). Sometimes such areas can be anesthetized with higher doses of medication.
- You are more likely to have problems during your labor with low blood pressure,[28] which may be associated with a drop in the baby's heart rate. This may necessitate changing positions, administration of medicine to raise your blood pressure, the placement of oxygen, and perhaps placement of an internal monitor to better track the baby's response to these actions. Your blood pressure generally comes back up without any lasting effect on you or the baby.
- This type of medication can increase the amount of time that you are in labor.[29]
- You may be more likely to need Pitocin, a synthetic form of the hormone oxytocin, to make your contractions stronger.[30]
- If you have an epidural, you may be more likely to get a fever during labor than women who don't have epidurals. Because your providers cannot know if a fever is from an infection or from the epidural, if you get a significant fever in labor, your providers will start antibiotics and your baby may be sub-

jected to more tests in the first hours after birth.

- You may be more likely to have forceps or vacuum delivery.[31] If you have a forceps birth, you are more likely to have a serious tear (a third- or fourth-degree tear) in your vagina.[32]
- One or two of every one hundred women who get an epidural, and fewer than one of every one hundred women who receive a labor spinal, get a bad headache called a "spinal headache." The headache usually doesn't start until the next day; if it occurs, effective treatment is available.

Evidence is mixed on whether there is an association between epidurals and problems in establishing breast-feeding; such problems seem more likely to be linked to high-dose opioid epidurals than to other epidurals.[33]

Paracervical Block

A paracervical block involves injecting a local anesthetic into the area next to the cervix. The medicine blocks pain signals from the nerves that come from the cervix. It is an effective and relatively simple way to provide pain relief for an hour or two, before the pushing stage of labor. Paracervical blocks are not commonly performed because they can cause a decrease in the baby's heart rate, although such a decrease almost always lasts for only a very short time and rarely causes problems for the baby.

Pudendal Block

A pudendal block involves injecting an anesthetic into nerves that will numb the perineal area around the opening of the vagina. This type of anesthesia is now rarely used during labor because of the advent of epidurals, but it is sometimes used for the pushing stage of labor, for forceps delivery, or for episiotomy repair. It provides temporary relief.

CONCLUSION

Learning about our options for coping with pain and working with a support team that is knowledgeable about them can help us feel less anxious as we anticipate labor and birth. We can arrive at informed decisions about the approaches we prefer, recognizing that we may need to make changes based on how our labor unfolds.

I was scared of the pain. I wanted to avoid interventions if possible, but I also wanted my limits to be respected. I wanted to see a midwife because I believed that her philosophy of birth, practical techniques, and continuous support would help me have the kind of birth I wanted. But I needed to know that if my labor was really hard or lasting forever or if I was totally exhausted, she would support me in getting an epidural.

The first midwife I interviewed when I was pregnant didn't seem to hear my fears; she just said that women's bodies were designed to give birth, and that my body would do so also. The second midwife, the one I chose, was more reassuring: she said she knew lots of nondrug techniques to help me cope and manage with the pain, but that she was committed to helping me have a good birth, whatever that meant to me. She said that there were times when epidurals were extremely helpful. In the end, I didn't have an epidural, but knowing that it was an option—and knowing that my midwife wouldn't see me as a failure if I had one—may have been part of what helped me avoid one!

When I was pregnant with my son, I was determined to have a natural birth. I prepared myself for this event by doing prenatal yoga, taking HypnoBirthing, hiring a doula, and learning about coping techniques from childbirth classes and books. During labor, I did things that comforted me. In early labor, I found it soothing to walk in my garden in the summer sunshine. I found the car ride to the hospital was extremely uncomfortable because the lack of mobility made the pain seem so much more intense. When I got into my hospital room, I was able to get into the tub. Bliss! The nurses discovered that my baby's head was crooked and if we couldn't get him to change positions, I wouldn't be able to push him out vaginally like I'd hoped. I was thankful I was still able to move and my doula suggested position changes [for me] to help get his head straightened out. The pain was intense but I used breathing and visualization to cope and it was only a half hour later that I was ready to push!

After five hours of pushing, the doctor told me that maybe [my baby's] head just wouldn't fit and that I should get a cesarean. I asked her if the situation was urgent and if there was anything else I could do. She said if I could push his head low enough, it was still possible to push him out. I'd been up for two nights and didn't have much energy left, so I agreed to get Pitocin knowing that it would strengthen my contractions. Because of the slow progress, they really had to pump up the Pitocin and they recommended I get an epidural so I could handle the pain. At this point I had exercised every coping technique and comfort measure I knew and I was determined to have my baby vaginally, so I agreed. Edmund was born healthy with the aid of forceps, weighed nine pounds, one ounce, and had a very large head. In retrospect, I am so grateful for learning all I did about coping techniques and pain medication because I know that I made the best choices I could for me and my baby.

NOTES

1. D. C. Wertz, "What Birth Has Done for Doctors: A Historical View," *Women & Health* 8, no. 1 (1983): 7–24.
2. "Cruelty in the Maternity Ward," *Ladies' Home Journal,* May 1958, 45.
3. Penny Simkin and April Bolding, "Update on Nonpharmacologic Approaches to Relieve Labor Pain and Prevent Suffering," *Journal of Midwifery & Women's Health* 49, no. 6 (November–December 2004): 489–504.
4. Ibid.
5. E. D. Hodnett, "Pain and Women's Satisfaction with the Experience of Childbirth: A Systematic Review," *American Journal of Obstetrics and Gynecology* 186, no. 5 (2002) S160–172.
6. Childbirth Connection, "Labor Pain: What Is Labor Pain Like?" accessed at www.childbirthconnection .org/article.asp?ClickedLink=262&ck=10191&area= 27#laborpain on September 29, 2006.
7. E. D. Hodnett, S. Downe, N. Edwards, et al., "Homelike Versus Conventional Institutional Settings for Birth," *Cochrane Database of Systematic Reviews* 2005, Issue 1. Art. No.: CD000012. D01: 10.1002/14651858. CD000012.pub2.
8. Penny Simkin and April Bolding, "Update on Nonpharmacologic Approaches to Relieve Labor Pain and Prevent Suffering," *Journal of Midwifery & Women's Health* 49, no. 6 (November–December 2004): 489–504.
9. S. Michel, A. Rake, K. Treiber, B. Seifert, R. Chaoui, R. Huch, et al., "MR Obstetric Pelvimetry: Effect of Birthing Position on Pelvic Bony Dimensions," *American Journal of Roentgenology* 179 (2002): 1,063–1,067.
10. In her book *Pregnancy, Childbirth, and the Newborn,* Penny Simkin describes these labor strategies as the three R's: Relaxation, Rhythm, and Ritual.
11. A. M. Cyna, G. L. McAuliffe, and M. I. Andrew, "Hypnosis for Pain Relief in Labour and Childbirth: A Systematic Review," *British Journal of Anaesthesia* 93, no. 4 (2004): 505–511. See also C. A. Smith, C. T. Collins, A. M. Cyna, et al., "Complementary and Alternative Therapies for Pain Management in Labour," *Cochrane Database of Systematic Reviews* 2006, Issue 4. Art. No.: CD003521. DO1: 10.1002/14651858.CD003521. pub2.
12. P. R. Appel and J. Bleiberg, "Pain Reduction Is Related to Hypnotizability but Not to Relaxation or to Re-

duction in Suffering: A Preliminary Investigation," *American Journal of Clinical Hypnosis* 48, nos. 2–3 (2005): 153–161.

13. Simkin and Bolding, "Update on Nonpharmacologic Approaches."

14. P. P. Simkin and M. O'Hara, "Nonpharmacologic Relief of Pain During Labor: Systematic Reviews of Five Methods," *American Journal of Obstetrics and Gynecology* (May 2002): S131–159

15. Ibid.

16. E. E. Burns, C. Blamey, S. J. Ersser, et al., "An Investigation into the Use of Aromatherapy in Intrapartum Midwifery Practice," *Journal of Alternative and Complementary Medicine* 6, no. 2 (2000): 141–147.

17. E. Skilnand, D. Fossen, and E. Heiburg, "Acupuncture in the Management of Pain in Labor," *Acta Obstetrica Gynecolica Scandinavia* 81 (2002): 943–948. See also A. Ramnero, U. Hanson, and M. Kihlgren, "Acupuncture Treatment During Labour—A Randomised Controlled Trial," *BJOG* 109 (2002): 637–644; B. I. Nesheim and R. Kinge, "Performance of Acupuncture as Labor Analgesia in the Clinical Setting," *Acta Obstetrica Gynecolica Scandinavia* 85, no. 4 (2006): 441–443; and Simkin and Bolding, "Update on Nonpharmacologic Approaches."

18. S. T. Brown, C. Douglas, and L. P. Flood, "Women's Evaluation of Intrapartum Nonpharmacological Pain Relief Methods Used During Labor," *Journal of Perinatal Education* 10, no. 3 (2001): 1–8. See also U. L. Chung, L. C. Hung, S. C. Kuo, and C. L. Huang, "Effects of LI4 and BL 67 Acupressure on Labor Pain and Uterine Contractions in the First Stage of Labor," *Journal of Nursing Research* 11, no. 4 (2003): 251–260; M. K. Lee, S. B. Chang, and D. H. Kang, "Effects of SP6 Acupressure on Labor Pain and Length of Delivery Time in Women During Labor," *Journal of Alternative and Complementary Medicine* 10, no. 6 (2004): 959–965.

19. Simkin and Bolding, "Update on Nonpharmacologic Approaches."

20. D. Carroll, M. Tramer, H. McQuay, et al., "Trancutaneous Electrical Nerve Stimulation in Labour Pain: A Systematic Review," *BJOG* 104 (1997): 169–175.

21. M. A. Rosen, "Nitrous Oxide for Relief of Labor Pain: A Systematic Review," *American Journal of Obstetrics and Gynecology* 186 (2002): S110–126.

22. Ibid.

23. Eugene R. Declercq, Carol Sakala, Maureen P. Corry, Sandra Applebaum, and Peter Risher, *Listening to Mothers: Report of the First National U.S. Survey of Women's Childbearing Experiences* (New York: Maternity Center Association [now Childbirth Connection], 2002.

24. Rosen, "Nitrous Oxide."

25. Adapted with permission from Judith Bishop, "Administration of Nitrous Oxide in Labor: Expanding the Options," *Journal of Midwifery & Women's Health* 52 (2007): 308–09; Judith Rooks, "Use of Nitrous Oxide in Midwifery Practice—Complementary, Synergistic, and Needed in the United States," *Journal of Midwifery & Women's Health* 52 (2007): 186–89.

26. Declercq et al., *Listening to Mothers.*

27. S. Jordan, S. Emery, C. Bradshaw, et al., "The Impact of Intrapartum Analgesia on Infant Feeding," *BJOG* 112, no. 7 (2005): 927–934. See also A. B. Ransjo-Arvidson, A. S. Matthiesen, G. Lilja, et al., "Maternal Analgesia During Labor Disturbs Newborn Behavior: Effects on Breastfeeding, Temperature, and Crying," *Birth* 28, no. 1 (2001): 5–12.

28. M. Anim-Somuah, R. Smyth, and C. Howell, "Epidural Versus Non-epidural or no Analgesia in Labour," *Cochrane Database of Systematic Reviews* 2005, Issue 4. Art. No.: CD000331. DO1: 10.1002/14651858. CD000331.pub2.

29. Ibid. A meta-analysis of trials involving nearly 2,400 women found that epidural analgesia prolonged labor by an average of 42 minutes in the first stage and an average of 14 minutes in the second stage, when compared with systemic opioid analgesia. See Holger Eltzschig, Ellice Lieberman, and William Camann, "Regional Anesthesia and Analgesia for Labor and Delivery," *New England Journal of Medicine* 348, no. 4 (January 23, 2003): 322; Stephen H. Halpern, Barbara L. Leighton, Arne Ohlsson, Jon F. R. Barrett, and Amy Rice, "Effect of Epidural Versus Parenteral Opioid Analgesia on the Progress of Labor: A Meta-analysis," *JAMA* 280 (December 23, 1998): 2105–2110.

30. Anim-Somuah et al., "Epidural Versus Non-epidural or No Analgesia."

31. Ibid.

32. Ibid.

33. Siranda Torvaldsen, Christine Roberts, Judy Simpson, Jane Thompson, and David Ellwood, "Intrapartum Epidural Analgesia and Breastfeeding: A Prospective Cohort Study," *International Breastfeeding Journal* 1, no. 24 (December 11, 2006). See also Sue Jordan, "Infant Feeding and Analgesia in Labour:

The Evidence Is Accumulating," *International Breast-feeding Journal* 1, no. 25 (December 11, 2006); J. Riordan, A. Gross, J. Angeron, et al., "The Effect of Labor Pain Relief Medication on Neonatal Suckling and Breastfeeding Duration," *Journal of Human Lactation* 16, no. 1 (2000); A. B. Ransjo-Arvidson, A. S. Matthiesen, G. Lilja, et al., "Maternal Analgesia During Labor Disturbs Newborn Behavior: Effects on Breastfeeding, Temperature, and Crying," *Birth* 28, no. 1 (2001): 5–12.

CHAPTER 12

Special Concerns During Labor and Birth

When anything out of the ordinary happens while we are in labor or giving birth, we may feel scared, confused, or both. We need our medical providers and support people to explain what is happening and help us make informed choices about how to deal with any complications that may arise. While this may seem to be a difficult time to ask questions and insist on what you need for yourself and your baby, it is important to do so. In most circumstances, you will have at least a few minutes, and sometimes more time than that, to get information and consider your options.

This chapter looks at a range of complications that can occur during labor and childbirth. It explains what can be done about them and how safe and effective various treatments and interventions are, on the basis of available research.

PROLONGED OR STALLED LABOR

Once you're in labor, how long is too long to keep going? Prolonged labor can be tiring for the mother, the baby, and the mother's support team. Usually, unless these are other complications, there is no reason to hurry the natural process of labor.

Infection (see page 218) is more common if labor lasts a long time. Avoiding frequent vaginal exams can decrease that risk. If you have regular contractions in the active phase of labor but your cervix does not dilate after two to four hours, it may be that the contractions are not strong enough. In this case you may be offered some intervention to help make the contractions stronger and more effective. Occasionally, a small catheter will be carefully inserted through the cervix into the uterus so that the intensity of each contraction can be measured more accurately.

Nonmedical methods to stimulate or speed up labor include acupressure, acupuncture, certain herbal treatments, nipple stimulation, and possibly walking. It's difficult to know how effective these methods are or what risks they may involve, as very little research has been done, but they have been used in many cultures for generations. Your older relatives and their friends may have used them or may know about them. You can talk with your support team about the possibility of using them.

Both physicians and midwives use synthetic oxytocin (Pitocin) and/or artificial rupture of membranes to speed up labor. (For more information on Pitocin, see page 180. For more on rupture of membranes, see page 180.)

My son was born after forty hours of labor. My labor started at 10 P.M. with contractions at regular intervals about 10 minutes apart. The length [of time] between contractions and the intensity remained relatively constant, so I labored at home for the first nine hours. In the morning we called our midwife and doula and arranged to meet them at the freestanding birth center where we planned to have a natural, drug-free water birth. After I labored at the birth center for six hours, the midwife suggested we go back home, as I was only dilated a few centimeters. At home I spent the next several hours walking around the block with my doula and [my] husband in an attempt to speed up labor.

After about twenty-one hours of labor, my contractions sped up to about 4 minutes apart, so we went back to the birth center. I labored in the tub for several more hours, at which point the midwife wanted to see how dilated I was. I was 7 centimeters dilated, and she noticed that my cervix was swollen. At that point the midwife decided that I needed to go to the hospital. At the hospital they started Pitocin and I made the decision to get an epidural. It was a tough decision, but after twenty-eight hours of labor I was ex-

hausted and needed to rest. The epidural allowed me to sleep for three hours—the best three hours of sleep I've ever had! After waking up I was dilated to 10 centimeters and started to push. I pushed for four hours, during which time a C-section was discussed. Because the baby's heart rate was fine, I asked them to continue to let me push, which they did. After I had been pushing for four hours, the doctor decided that he needed to use forceps because the baby was coming out at an angle. The doctor positioned the forceps and with two more pushes our little boy was born!

"BACK LABOR" / "POSTERIOR" BABY

If the back of your baby's head is positioned toward your back, in what is called a "posterior" presentation, you may feel the strength of your labor contractions mainly in your back ("back labor"). Many babies are in this position at the start of labor. Most babies will rotate as labor progresses, so that the back of the baby's head is toward the front of the mother's body. Only about five of every one hundred babies are still in that position at birth.[1] In most cases, the baby's head fits more easily through the birth canal when the back of the head is toward the front of the mother's body. A mother may need to push longer for a baby who remains in the posterior position. There's also a greater chance that the mother may need either a vacuum or forceps delivery or a cesarean section to give birth. (For more information about vacuum and forceps deliveries, see page 185.)

It is unclear why some babies don't rotate—the shape of the mother's pelvis may have something to do with it—but epidurals may also increase the chance that a posterior baby will not rotate to the opposite (anterior) position.[2] Some health care providers try to get the baby to rotate by gently pushing on the head and rotating it manually through the vagina. This can be very effective in speeding labor if the rotation is successful.

Sometimes changing your position can help your baby rotate. A woman who gave birth at home in her late twenties describes an approach her midwife used:

*I had been at 7 centimeters for about five hours, and was feeling kind of stuck. My midwife checked me and found that the baby was posterior, . . . which can make labor much harder. Contractions had slowed down and I was tired but wanted to get things going again, so she made me a vile concoction of black cohosh (*Cimicifuga*) & partridgeberry (*Mitchella repens*) herbs with lots of honey, which I drank, and then she spread the Sunday paper on the floor beside my bed, where I got into a deep squat to see if we could bring the baby down on the cervix and encourage rotation. . . . In 20 minutes, I was completely dilated and pushing my big ten-pound son out. I remember it as an ecstatic, sexual feeling, breathing the baby out so slowly.*

Sometimes the baby rotates back to posterior or won't rotate at all. In that case, the pushing stage often lasts longer, and, depending on the size of the baby, she or he may have to be delivered by cesarean.

VARIATIONS IN FETAL HEARTBEAT

Fetal heart rate monitoring is used to assess whether the baby is getting enough oxygen. If you are healthy, your pregnancy is not complicated, and you are not taking pain medication during labor (no epidural or Pitocin), the baby's heartbeat should be listened to periodically. (For more information, see page 175.) Continuous fetal heart rate monitoring is ap-

propriate if an epidural is in place, Pitocin is being used, or there is some concern about whether the baby is getting enough oxygen.

Continuous fetal monitoring is very good at reassuring providers that the baby is doing well, but it is rather poor at predicting whether a baby is having problems. Providers need to take the whole pattern that the monitor shows into consideration, not just the small area that may look problematic. It is not unusual for babies' heart rates to vary during the course of labor. Some of the changes are normal and are related to pressure on the baby's head as the cervix opens, or to pressure on the umbilical cord, often seen after the bag of waters has broken. Research has shown that most variant fetal heart patterns are false positives—that is, the baby is fine despite the unusual pattern.

If your provider is concerned about your baby's fetal heart rate pattern, she or he may give you oxygen through a mask, increase your fluids if an IV is in place, or ask you to change your position (move from one side to the other). These changes can often result in a more reassuring heart rate pattern.

Your provider may also choose to insert an internal fetal monitor to assess the heart rate more accurately. To do this, she or he will insert a small wire (fetal scalp electrode) through your vagina and cervix and attach it to the baby's head.

If the fetal heart rate pattern is irregular, your provider will use different techniques to determine whether the heart rate pattern is likely to compromise your baby's well-being. If she or he determines that your baby is at risk, interventions can be used to try to increase the amount of oxygen the baby receives. If problems persist, a cesarean section may be necessary.

HEMORRHAGE

Hemorrhage (heavy bleeding from the vagina) during labor may be caused by a low-lying placenta, placental abruption (see page 222), rupture of the uterus, or tearing of the cervix or vagina (see "Lacerations [Tearing]," page 218). If the placenta is implanted in the uterus with one edge very close to the cervix, bleeding may occur during labor as the cervix thins and dilates. Bleeding can also be caused by a condition known as *placenta previa,* in which the placenta completely covers the cervix. Since most women today have at least one sonogram during pregnancy, placenta previa is usually discovered before labor starts, and delivery options and plans can be put in place before labor begins. (For more information about placenta previa, see "Bleeding in the Second and Third Trimesters," page 133.)

Lacerations (tears) of the cervix are not common if labor progresses normally and the baby comes out without assistance. Your provider should check for tears after the birth if bleeding continues and there seems to be no other cause. Lacerations of the vagina, however, are very common. They occur as the baby passes through the vagina, but they rarely cause true hemorrhage unless the birth happens very quickly or instruments (forceps or vacuum cup) are used to help with the birth.

Sometimes the bleeding will stop as the baby descends through the birth canal, and labor can continue. Usually, if the bleeding is heavy during labor, the mother will need a cesarean section.

RETAINED PLACENTA

Sometimes there is a delay in the delivery of the placenta after the baby has been born. In other instances the placenta is delivered, but it is clear that some fragments remain in the uterus. It is extremely important that these fragments be removed, as they may allow blood vessels to remain open, causing hemorrhage either shortly after delivery or several days to weeks after delivery. You are also at risk for infection in the uterus if the fragments are not removed.

If your placenta does not come out spontaneously within about thirty minutes after you give birth, your provider may gently massage your abdomen, ask you to push, and/or attempt to stimulate uterine contractions by giving you Pitocin or asking you to breast-feed. If these techniques are not successful, she or he may attempt a manual extraction of the placenta (removing it by hand). Your provider may also use suction or a scraping instrument to remove small fragments, under ultrasound guidance if it is available.

Sometimes the placenta seems to have been expelled completely, but days or weeks later a woman may have a sudden episode of heavy bleeding that continues or comes and goes, often accompanied by moderate to severe cramping. If this happens to you, call your health care provider immediately.

POSTPARTUM HEMORRHAGE

After about one in twenty births, the woman experiences heavy bleeding (postpartum hemorrhage). This happens most commonly in the first twenty-four hours after birth, but occasionally a few days or even many weeks later.

By far the most common cause of postpartum hemorrhage is that the muscles of the uterus do not contract well enough, a condition known as *uterine atony.* This condition is most common in the first day after birth. If you experience heavy bleeding, your provider may vigorously massage your abdomen to empty the uterus of any blood clots. Your provider may also manually remove blood clots from inside the uterus, through the vagina. If these approaches are not successful, the condition can be treated with various medications, ranging from those that have been available for many years, such as synthetic oxytocin (sold under the brand name Pitocin) and methylergonovine (Methergine), to newer medications, such as misoprostol (Cytotec) and carboprost tromethamine (Hemabate). The other causes of hemorrhage right after birth are retained placenta (see page 217) and unrecognized lacerations of the vagina and cervix (see "Lacerations [Tearing]," below).

Delayed postpartum hemorrhage, occurring up to twelve weeks after birth, is often due to retained fragments of the placenta or to infection (for more information about these conditions, see sections above and below this one). If your bleeding is heavier than the heaviest day of your period, you are soaking a pad every hour, or you have a fever, call your health care provider right away.

INFECTION

Usually the cervical mucus plug, amniotic membranes, and amniotic fluid protect your baby from the bacteria that normally live in your vagina. Occasionally, when the membranes have been ruptured for a long time or with long labor, an infection can develop. An infection of the amniotic membranes, or bag of waters, is known as *chorioamnionitis* (*KOR-e-o-am-ne-on-I-tis*).

Fever is one sign of an infection. (Fevers can also be caused by dehydration and are associated with the use of epidurals.) If your providers think it's very likely that you have chorioamnionitis, you will probably be given IV antibiotics until you no longer have a fever and your labor will be induced if you are not already in labor.

If your waters break a long time before labor starts, and if you have sex or vaginal exams that introduce bacteria from the vagina into the cervix and uterus, there's a greater chance of developing chorioamnionitis. Some women develop an infection without having had any vaginal exams, just because the protective barrier between the fetus and the outside world has ruptured and let bacteria get in. Chorioamnionitis may spread from the membranes to the uterus and cause a uterine infection, known as *endomyometritis*, after the baby is born.

The usual treatment for chorioamnionitis is inducing labor, usually with oxytocin (for more information, see page 146), and giving you intravenous antibiotics. Your baby will also need blood tests and intravenous antibiotics for forty-eight hours after birth. Endomyometritis is also treated with intravenous antibiotics. If you develop a uterine infection, you may have to stay in the hospital for at least forty-eight hours after the birth.

LACERATIONS (TEARING)

The process of giving birth can lead to lacerations, or tearing, of the cervix, the vagina, and most often the perineum (the area between the vagina and rectum). Waiting until your cervix has fully opened prior to pushing virtually eliminates the risk of a tear in the cervix (unless instruments are used). The slow, steady progress of your baby down the birth canal allows your tissues to stretch and minimizes tearing of the perineum. Certain birth attendants are more skilled at coaching you during the pushing so that you can avoid severe tears. Vacuum- and especially forceps-assisted vaginal births are more likely to cause severe lacerations of the perineum and vagina, and doctors are more likely to perform an episiotomy when these instruments are used.

An episiotomy is a cut made to enlarge the vaginal opening so that the baby can get out more easily. This procedure was routinely used in the past to avoid tearing of the perineum. Today, routine use of episiotomy is no longer recommended because it has been found that a woman is more likely to suffer a tear into the anus or rectum with an episiotomy than without.[3] (For more information about episiotomy, see page 185.)

I had some tearing during the birth of my daughter. I pushed for about two hours and my tissue wasn't stretching enough for the baby to come out, so they cut a tiny episiotomy, which then tore some more. I was told it was not a very bad tear, but I was so uncomfortable with the stitches afterwards. My entire vaginal area was so swollen and it was a bit numb; it didn't feel like my own tissue and I was afraid it wasn't healing well. Soaking in the bathtub helped a lot. . . . After about three or four weeks I started feeling normal again "down there" and eventually everything healed great, no problems with sex or anything.

Massaging the perineum during pregnancy can reduce the chances of tearing while giving birth.[4] This technique involves applying gentle pressure with fingertips just inside the vaginal opening, using a lubricating oil. (For more information, see page 38.)

MECONIUM-STAINED AMNIOTIC FLUID

Usually, a baby has her or his first bowel movement (meconium) after birth. Sometimes, however, a baby has a bowel movement before or during birth. If this happens, the amniotic fluid released when the mother's bag of water breaks will have a greenish tint. Up to one in every five babies born after 34 weeks' gestation has meconium in the amniotic fluid.

Most of the time, this is not a problem. However, if the baby is not getting enough oxygen before or duing birth, she or he may take a breath and inhale some meconium. The meconium can irritate the baby's lungs and cause lung problems that are usually temporary and mild, but can be severe. If the meconium is thick, your provider will ask you to wait (pant, not push) after the baby's head is out, so that the baby's mouth and breathing passages can be cleared by suction before the rest of the baby is birthed. In most hospitals, a pediatrician, anesthesiologist, nurse, or other attendant will be present at the birth of a baby who has passed meconium, to attend to the baby if needed. Most babies who pass meconium before or during labor are healthy and do not need any special attention, but it is safer to have qualified personnel available in case their expertise is needed.

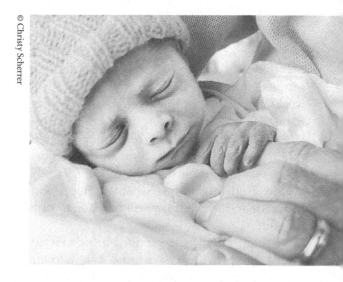
© Chrisy Scherrer

PREMATURE BIRTH

About eight out of every one hundred women go into premature labor, defined as labor before 37 weeks (see page 134). If this progresses to premature birth, the baby may need special care. The closer the baby's birth is to "full term," or 37 weeks, the lower its risk of medical complications. Babies who are born before 28 weeks have a greater risk of dying, and those who survive may have lasting medical problems. Fortunately, the care in neonatal intensive care units has greatly improved the healthy survival of very premature infants.

"Preemie" babies are vulnerable to many complications, such as breathing, neurological, and intestinal problems. Depending on how early the baby is born, she or he will be evaluated by a pediatrician immediately after birth and may need to be cared for in the neonatal intensive care unit (NICU). For more information see "Preterm Labor," page 134.

PRETERM LABOR IN THE SECOND TRIMESTER

Babies born at 22 weeks or less almost never survive more than a few hours after birth. Between 22 and 24 weeks of gestation, most babies don't survive, and almost all who do have serious, crippling health conditions. At 24 weeks, about half of the preemies survive, but many will have severe, long-term health problems. It is rare that babies are born in the sixth month of pregnancy, but if you are in this situation, it is important that you and your family are involved in planning what will happen at the birth and what efforts will be made to care for your baby.

Sometimes there is a conflict between what health care providers advise and what parents want. For example, you may not want a breathing tube and CPR (cardiopulmonary resuscitation) for a baby who has a minimal chance of surviving—you may prefer just to keep the baby comfortable. Because doctors are trained to do everything they can to save the baby, you may need to speak up about your preference. Or, you may want all efforts made to save the baby, even when the pediatricians think your newborn has no chance of survival. Health care providers and hospitals are constrained by local laws and standards of care. State and federal laws are not all the same regarding parents' and doctors' rights to decide whether or not to revive extremely premature infants.[5] If you experience preterm labor at between 22 and 24 weeks, ask to speak about your options with the pediatrician on call as soon as possible. If there is time, you can also ask for an ethics consultation, at which the hospital team of nurses, doctors, and social workers who help parents and physicians with difficult decisions will be made available to you.

If your baby does not survive, your grief may feel overwhelming. You can get help—you don't have to deal with it alone. In addition to getting support from family and friends, you may find it helpful to talk with other women who are going through the same painful loss, through bereavement groups and other resources. The neonatal intensive care unit (NICU) can help put you in touch with a chaplain, a social worker, and a support group. (For more about coping with losing a baby, see Chapter 9, "Childbearing Loss.")

PREVIOUSLY UNRECOGNIZED PRE-ECLAMPSIA

Sometimes pre-eclampsia (a condition characterized by high blood pressure and kidney problems) is not diagnosed during pregnancy, because the woman has not developed signs of the condition. The symptoms can develop during labor or after a woman has given birth. If you have a terrible headache or vision problems during labor and delivery or right after the baby's birth and your blood pressure is elevated, your provider should test your blood for liver or kidney abnormalities and your urine for protein.

If you have pre-eclampsia, you should be treated with an intravenous solution of magnesium sulfate, to prevent convulsions (eclampsia) from developing.[6] After you give birth, the hospital may keep you under close observation for a while, just to make sure you don't have convulsions. (For more on pre-eclampsia, see page 140).

UNCOMMON PROBLEMS DURING LABOR AND BIRTH

SHOULDER DYSTOCIA

In a small number of births (fewer than one in every one hundred), the baby's head is delivered but the shoulder gets stuck and the body does not come out quickly. This is called *shoulder dystocia*. It is an emergency situation because the baby can be deprived of oxygen, which, if the deprivation lasts for several minutes or more, can cause brain damage. Shoulder dystocia is more common when the baby is very big at birth (around ten pounds or more), but it can happen to smaller babies as well. It is also more common when the mother has diabetes during pregnancy. Babies born to women who have diabetes can be larger than average, and they tend to have bigger shoulders that are more likely to get stuck in the birth canal.

A health care provider will try to get the shoulder free through various maneuvers, including flexing the mother's thighs up against her abdomen, pressing on her abdomen just above the pubic bone, asking her to get into all-fours position, delivering a posterior arm befoe the stuck shoulder, or trying to rotate the shoulder manually so it slips under the pubic bone. In some cases, shoulder dystocia is associated with broken bones and nerve damage in the arm. Most of the time, the arm will heal well and the baby will not have any problem. In rare instances, the baby can suffer long-term damage to the nerves in the arm. This injury can also occur in babies born by cesarean section, with and without labor. Shoulder dystocia is unpredictable, and there is no good strategy for preventing the associated complications.

BREECH PRESENTATION

Sometimes the baby's feet or buttocks come out first, instead of the head. That happens to about three or four of every one hundred full-term babies, mostly for no apparent reason. In most cases, the baby is discovered to be in the breech presentation before labor begins. Occasionally, it is not discovered until labor starts or is well established. Sometimes the baby may have turned just prior to labor. An ultrasound can be used to determine the baby's position.

Even very experienced providers occasionally fail to spot a breech baby until labor begins, and thus miss the opportunity to try to turn the baby. (For more about turning a breech baby in the womb, see "Breech Baby," page 145.) Studies have shown very low rates of success of turning the baby once the waters have broken, so most providers won't try to do it at that point.

The midwife checked me from behind—I could see some poop on the pad below me and was a bit embarrassed—but she informed me that my baby was breech and it was his poop coming out! I asked her what that meant—were we supposed to go to the hospital? I'd never had an ultrasound and the baby had never been head up in any of our exams—who knew when he flipped? The midwife said that normally, that was the protocol, but we didn't have time, as he was clearly almost here. I turned and looked her in the eye and said I felt like it would be all right—I didn't want to go to the hospital. She felt the same way and got out her birth stool. I sat down and my son basically shot out in one push.

Some breech babies can be safely delivered vaginally; for others, a cesarean birth is safer. (For more information, see "Breech Baby," page 145.)

PLACENTAL ABRUPTION

Placental abruption, a rare complication of birth, occurs in about one in one hundred pregnancies. Abruption occurs when the placenta or part of the placenta separates from the uterine wall, causing bleeding in both mother and baby. In rare cases this bleeding can be life-threatening. Giving birth quickly, often by cesarean section, helps to minimize complications.

The symptoms of abruption may include abdominal pain between contractions, extremely strong and/or frequent contractions, and bleeding from the vagina. Occasionally there are no symptoms until late in the process. Abruption can be associated with the use of drugs such as amphetamines and cocaine, severe trauma to the abdomen (such as that caused by a motor vehicle accident or physical violence), smoking, and high blood pressure in the mother.

PROBLEMS WITH IMPLANTATION OF THE PLACENTA

In rare instances, the placenta implants abnormally, often in a scar from a previous cesarean section or other surgery on the uterus. The placenta can then grow into this scar and occasionally even through the wall of the uterus into other organs, such as the bladder. These abnormalities in attachment of the placenta are called *placenta accreta*, *placenta increta*, and *placenta percreta*, depending on the depth of invasion of the uterine wall. Placenta accreta, the most common of these serious complications, is becoming more common and now is discovered in about one in every twenty-five hundred births. The increase is thought to be related to the increase in the rate of cesarean sections. Abnormal attachments of the placenta are also seen more commonly with placenta previa.

The diagnosis of these conditions can now often be made by ultrasound or magnetic resonance imaging (MRI) during pregnancy. The abnormal attachment makes the placenta very adherent to the uterine wall so that it is difficult to remove after birth. If implantation problems are not diagnosed before birth, severe hemorrhaging can occur during and after birth. Your provider will attempt to stop the bleeding with a variety of interventions such as blood transfusions and exploratory surgery with the goal of avoiding a hysterectomy.

CONCLUSION

Most births are uncomplicated. However, if either you or your baby experiences complications, labor and birth can be frightening, especially if you don't understand what is happening and what can be done about it. Good support from your family or others close to you will help you if you are faced with unexpected complications. It's also important to have providers you trust caring for you. If you do not feel comfortable with the advice your doctor, midwife, or nurse is giving, it may help to have your partner or somebody else you trust speak to your provider. Sometimes, you may want to ask for an opinion from another provider. When you, your loved ones, and your health care team are cooperating with one another, even unexpected events can usually be managed in a way that is safe and satisfying for both you and your baby.

When I broke my bag of waters at 33 weeks and realized I wasn't going to have the home birth I'd wanted, I felt sad and scared at the same time. I wanted the best care for my baby but I wasn't sure I could ask for what I wanted and I wasn't sure I knew what to ask. Once we were in the hospital, our midwife introduced us to nurses, the obstetrician, and a pediatrician from the intensive care nursery. We talked to everyone and learned as much as we could about premature babies. That helped a lot. We kept learning about how to take care of her after she was born as we visited her in the intensive care unit and learned more about her heart defect. The first few months were an intense focus on feeding and caring for this baby who had a heart that was working too hard and on getting well from surgery myself. Now, many years later, we look back on her first years with pride for how we came together as a family to love her and care for her and deal with difficult health issues all at the same time.

NOTES

1. A. J. Satin, "Abnormal Labor: Protraction and Arrest Disorders," *UpToDate* 14.3 (August 2006), accessed at www.uptodate.com/physicians/index.asp.
2. Ellise Lieberman, Karen Davidson, Aviva Lee-Parritz, and Elizabeth Shearer, "Changes in Fetal Position During Labor and Their Association with Epidural Analgesia," *Obstetrics & Gynecology* 105, no. 5 (May 2005): 974–982.
3. "Episiotomy," *ACOG Practice Bulletin* no. 71 (April 2006). See also V. Myers and J. Goldberg, "Episiotomy: An Evidence-Based Approach," *Obstetrical & Gynecological Survey* 61, no. 8 (2006): 491–492.
4. K. Hartmann, M. Viswanathan, R. Palmieri, G. Gartlehner, J. Thorp Jr., and K. N. Lohr, "Outcomes of Routine Episiotomy: A Systematic Review," *JAMA* 293 (2005): 2,141–2,148. See also M. M. Beckmann and A. J. Garrett, "Antenatal Perineal Massage for Reducing Perineal Trauma," *Birth* 33, no. 2 (June 2006): 159.
5. Sadath A. Sayeed, "Baby Doe Redux? The Department of Health and Human Services and the Born-Alive Infants Protection Act of 2002: A Cautionary Note on Normative Neonatal Practice," *Pediatrics* 116, no. 4 (October 2005): e576–585. See also E. F. Krug III, "Law and Ethics at the Border of Viability," *Journal of Perinatology* 26 (June 2006): 321–324.
6. L. Duley, A. M. Gulmezoglu, and D. J. Henderson-Smart, "Magnesium Sulphate and Other Anticonvulsants for Women with Pre-eclampsia," *Cochrane Database of Systematic Reviews* 2003, Issue 2. Art. No.: CD000025. DO1:10.1002/14651858.CD000025.

CHAPTER 13

Cesarean Births

My first baby was a face presentation, mentum posterior, and there was no way he would have made it out alive, vaginally; that position wedges the baby's face between the sacrum and the pubic bone, with no room to descend. I had a C-section in a small local hospital. The OR [operating room] was actually warm. . . . My midwife and my partner were with me, right in the OR! It was a good way for this skeptic to learn that yes, a surgical birth can be a positive event. I had minimal anesthesia, and had the baby back with me within an hour or so of his birth.

In certain circumstances, cesarean sections are clearly needed for the safety of the mother and/or the baby. In other circumstances, it can be difficult to determine whether or not the surgery is medically necessary. Providers may not be able to say that the surgery is absolutely necessary but may recommend it for safety. The risks and benefits of a cesarean vary according to your specific situation. Ideally, you will discuss during prenatal visits the possibility of having a cesarean section, although many of the circumstances that require birth by cesarean section emerge only during labor.

If your provider recommends that you have a cesarean and you are not in an emergency situation, ask about the benefits and risks—both short-term and long-term—to you and your baby. If a cesarean is recommended to you during prenatal care, consider seeking a second opinion and find out as much as you can about your options.

REASONS FOR RECOMMENDING A CESAREAN

The most common reasons a cesarean is recommended include the following.

BEFORE LABOR BEGINS

Prior Cesarean Section or Other Uterine Surgery

If you have given birth by cesarean before, or have had previous uterine surgery, giving birth by cesarean section may be recommended. However, in certain circumstances, you may be able to give birth vaginally (a process called "VBAC," for "vaginal birth after cesarean"). (For more information, see "VBAC or Repeat Cesarean Section?" page 233.)

Abnormal Location of the Placenta

Occasionally, at the end of a pregnancy, the placenta lies over the opening of the cervix (a condition known as *placenta previa*). About one in five hundred women experiences placenta previa at the end of pregnancy; when this happens, a cesarean section is the safest way to give birth.

Usually placenta previa is seen during an ultrasound in the first half of pregnancy. Most of the time, the placenta moves up off the cervix as the uterus grows during pregnancy, so that the placenta no longer covers the cervix by the beginning of the third trimester. (For more information, see "Bleeding in the Second and Third Trimesters," page 133.)

Early Separation of the Placenta

In rare cases, a normally placed placenta may separate prematurely from the uterus (a condition known as *placental abruption*). If the amount of blood loss is life-threatening or if the baby's condition reflects lack of oxygen or nutrition because of the lost placental function, a cesarean section is warranted. (For more information, see "Placental Abruption," page 222.)

Multiple Babies

No high-quality research currently supports giving birth to all twins by cesarean section. It is usually safe to give birth to twins vaginally if the first twin is positioned well, with her or his head down. In addition to the position of the babies in the uterus and in relation to each other, their size and how far along you are in your pregnancy, as well as the skill and experience level of your health care provider, are factors in deciding whether vaginal birth may be appropriate.

With three or more babies, a cesarean section is generally recommended. Vaginal birth can be dangerous for the triplets who come second and third.

Have a careful discussion of your birth plans with your provider if you are carrying more than one baby.

Breech Position of Baby

About 4 percent of babies are in a feet-first ("footling breech"), buttocks-first ("frank breech"), or legs-crossed ("complete breech") position at the end of gestation. If your baby is in a breech position, your provider may be able to use a process called *external cephalic version* to manually turn your baby to a head-down position about three or four weeks before your due date. In some circumstances, a cesarean section may be the safest way for your baby to be born. In other circumstances, you may be able to give birth vaginally. (For more information, see "Breech Baby," page 145.)

Pre-eclampsia

Pre-eclampsia is a condition characterized by maternal high blood pressure and protein in the urine (see page 55.)

Once the diagnosis of pre-eclampsia is

made, your provider may recommend that you give birth right away rather than wait for labor to start spontaneously. She or he will most likely suggest induction of labor (see page 146), as it is safest for you to give birth vaginally. However, you may require a cesarean section if your blood pressure is uncontrolled or if there is evidence that the condition is harming your baby. (For more information, see "Pre-eclampsia / Hypertension," page 140.)

Maternal Infection

Active maternal infections such as active genital herpes can be transmitted from mother to infant during a vaginal birth, because the baby is in contact with open sores in the birth canal. If a woman has active genital herpes sores at the beginning of labor or when the bag of waters breaks, there is a small but serious risk that the baby will be infected during vaginal delivery. This risk can be reduced by giving birth by cesarean section. Women with a history of genital herpes can consider using a medicine such as acyclovir in the last month of pregnancy to reduce the risk of developing an active lesion at the time of delivery. If no lessons are present when you go into labor it is safe to proceed with a vaginal birth.

For some pregnant women who are HIV-positive, having a cesarean greatly reduces the risk of transmitting the virus to the baby. In the past, it was recommended that all HIV-positive pregnant women give birth by cesarean section. Now the recommendations depend upon your viral load. If your HIV is untreated, or if you are taking antiretrovirals but your viral load is more than 1,000 copies per milliliter, having a planned cesarean will reduce the chances of your baby becoming infected. (For more information, see page 141.)

Large Baby

The main reason to consider a cesarean section for a large baby is concern about shoulder dystocia. *Shoulder dystocia* refers to difficulty in delivering a baby's shoulders (and, therefore, the rest of the baby) after the head has emerged from the birth canal. (For more information about shoulder dystocia, see page 221.)

Estimates of the baby's size are not consistently accurate at full term, whether they are arrived at through ultrasound or through examination by a midwife or doctor. Additionally, there is no accurate and safe way to measure the mother's pelvis to determine whether a particular baby will fit through. Therefore, routine delivery of a "large baby" by cesarean section is not justified. The American College of Obstetricians and Gynecologists advises physicians to consider a cesarean if they estimate the baby's weight at more than eleven pounds in a woman who does not have diabetes or more than about ten pounds in a woman who has diabetes.[1] However, the evidence to support this position is inconclusive.

Other Reasons to Plan a Cesarean

For women who have certain medical conditions—including heart, kidney, or neurological diseases; fibroids (noncancerous tumors of the uterus) that obstruct the birth canal; or specific pregnancy-related illnesses—it may be safer to give birth by cesarean. Similarly, if there is evidence that a baby is ill or is unable to tolerate labor, birth by cesarean section may be recommended. In all of these cases, it is important to work with health care providers who understand your views and preferences.

DURING LABOR

Lack of Progress in Labor

Occasionally, a woman may be in labor for longer than is usual. In such cases, the provider may recommend a cesarean section. Determining whether a cesarean is medically necessary in this situation can be difficult.

Generally, labor should be allowed to continue on its own as long as progress is being made and no other complications are present. (For more information, see "Prolonged or Stalled Labor," page 214.)

Changes in Fetal Heart Rate

Continuous electronic fetal heart rate monitoring sometimes raises concerns about fetal well-being, but this does not always mean a cesarean is necessary. Changes in the fetal heart rate are most often transient and not a sign that the baby is in trouble. (For more information, see "Variations in Fetal Heartbeat," page 216.) However, changes in fetal heart rate occasionally can suggest infection, problems with the umbilical cord, or problems with the placenta delivering oxygen to the baby. If these changes are not preceded and followed by reassuring patterns in the baby's heart rate, a cesarean section may be warranted.

Prolapsed Umbilical Cord

In rare instances, when the bag of waters breaks, the baby's umbilical cord comes into the vagina in front of the baby's head. This is called a "prolapsed" cord. The pressure of the baby's head on the umbilical cord interferes with the delivery of oxygen to the baby. This is more likely to happen if the baby is a footling breech (in a feet-down rather than a head-down position).

This is an emergency that almost always requires a cesarean section.

HOW CESAREAN BIRTH WORKS

If you are giving birth by cesarean section, whether planned or not, the process will start in an operating room, where you will usually receive spinal or epidural anesthesia to make you completely numb below the level of your ribs. Your partner or support person may be asked to wait outside the operating room while the spinal or epidural is being set up, but in most instances he or she can return to the room to support you during the surgery. If an epidural catheter (tube) is already in place when the decision for surgery is made, the level of anesthesia will be increased so that you are completely numb.

In the rare instance when a cesarean section needs to be performed very quickly, you may be given general anesthesia (which makes you unconscious), because it is faster than making you numb with a spinal or epidural. General anesthesia is also used in the rare instances when an adequate level of anesthesia is not obtained with a spinal or epidural.

For most cesarean sections, your belly will be scrubbed and your pubic hair clipped, and often you will be given a dose of antibiotics during the procedure to reduce the risk of infection. In addition, a small tube (catheter) will be placed in your bladder to keep it empty during the procedure. A drape will be placed between your chest and the lower part of your body to create a sterile area for the operation. The drape also prevents you from seeing the surgery as it happens. Sometimes the drape is close to your neck, but you can turn your head to the side if it makes you feel claustrophobic. Your arms are likely to be taped down at your sides. You will have an IV inserted and devices

COMPARING THE RISKS OF CESAREAN BIRTHS VERSUS VAGINAL BIRTHS*

While most mothers and babies who have cesarean births do fine, cesarean sections involve more risks than "spontaneous" vaginal births (births that do not involve the use of forceps, vacuum extraction, or a cesarean). Women who have cesarean sections have more infections after the birth (usually in the uterus, bladder, or incision, and including infections resistant to antibiotics), more pain, longer recovery periods, and a greater chance of being rehospitalized. Women who have cesareans are also at a slightly increased risk of rare complications such as blood clots and bowel obstructions.

A woman who has had a cesarean section is more likely to have a cesarean section in future pregnancies. As the number of C-sections increases for a woman, the risk of complications in future pregnancies also increases. Potential complications include ectopic pregnancy (pregnancy that develops outside the uterus), placenta previa (when the placenta attaches near or over the opening of the cervix) and other placental problems, and, during birth, rupture of the uterus. With each cesarean section, it is common to encounter more scar tissue in the area of the previous incision. This can lead to greater blood loss and a longer operating time for the next cesarean. A rare complication of repeat cesarean sections that is being seen more often because more cesareans are being performed in the United States is an abnormal attachment of the placenta, in which the placenta grows deeply into or through the wall of the uterus in the area of the previous scar. The placenta may even grow into the wall of the bladder. It then becomes difficult to remove, resulting in blood loss that is difficult to control and possible injury to the bladder. In cases such as this, a hysterectomy may be needed at birth to prevent severe hemorrhage.

In addition, babies born via cesarean section are more likely to have mild respiratory problems in the newborn period than babies born vaginally, and they are more likely to experience asthma in childhood and adulthood. Babies born via cesarean section are less likely to establish breast-feeding, although plenty of such babies do breast-feed.[2]

Unless there is a clear, compelling medical reason for you to have a cesarean section, having a vaginal birth is likely to be the safest option for both you and your baby.

* The information in this box is adapted from the Childbirth Connection booklet "What Every Pregnant Woman Needs to Know About Cesarean Section." The booklet provides an extensive review of the best available research on cesarean sections and is available for free download at www.childbirthconnection.org.

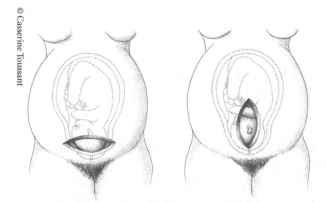

A horizontal ("bikini cut") incision for a cesarean operation is more common than a vertical incision.

will be attached to your skin to monitor your vital signs. In most hospitals, if you do not have general anesthesia a support person or partner can be present during the surgery, staying at the head of the bed, next to your head, behind the drape.

After the anesthesia has taken effect, the surgeon will usually make a horizontal incision in your skin, low down near the pubic bone—the "bikini cut." (Vertical cuts are now reserved for special situations.) The surgeon will then cut through the uterine muscle and ease your baby out. The incision on the skin is not always in the same direction (horizontal or vertical) as the incision on the uterus. The type of incision that goes through the uterine muscle will determine whether you should consider a vaginal delivery if you give birth again. (For more information, see "What You Need to Know About VBAC," page 234.)

I looked up at my husband. There he was, looking quite ridiculous in his blue scrubs and hairnet. He was standing slightly, just enough to see over the draped curtain. His eyes [were] intently staring. I can't even be certain he blinked. When the doctor announced the birth of our daughter, there was no need for him to say it. I saw it on my husband's *face, the birth of his daughter. His eyes widened at first, almost as if someone had stomped on his toe, then he began to cry. The look on his face was amazement, pride, love. I saw the birth of our daughter that day, too . . . through the eyes of my husband. It was beautiful.*

The surgeon will clamp and cut the umbilical cord and hand your baby to a nurse or other attendant who will suction your baby's nose and mouth if needed and assess the baby's breathing. Once the baby is breathing normally and has been bundled into a warm blanket, your partner can hold your baby and you can welcome your child even as the doctor removes the placenta, sews up the incision, and closes the skin with sutures or staples. Your provider can save the baby's cord blood and the placenta if you like. (For more information about storing cord blood, see page 41.) The entire procedure usually takes about an hour.

RECOVERY

Following your surgery, you will be cleaned up in the operating room and taken to a recovery room, where you can focus on getting to know your baby. This is an important time to start breast-feeding if you have chosen to do so. The baby is usually alert for the first hour or two after birth. Ask for help if you feel that you cannot start breast-feeding on your own. During this time, if you have had a spinal or epidural, the anesthesia will gradually wear off. If you received an opioid medicine in the spinal catheter, you shouldn't have much pain the first twenty-four hours. If you did not have the opioid medicine in the spinal catheter, you will be given IV pain medication as needed. Usually, after a few hours you are ready to go to your postpartum room.

During the first few days after a cesarean

PREPARING FOR A CESAREAN SECTION*

If you know you are going to give birth by cesarean, the following suggestions can help make your experience safer and more comfortable. Discuss them with your provider as you plan for the surgery.

- **Schedule a planned cesarean after week 38 of your pregnancy if possible.** Babies born before the thirty-ninth week of pregnancy are more likely to have breathing problems. (Some doctors require that an amniocentesis be done to ensure the baby's lung maturity for any nonemergency cesarean done before 39 weeks. Establishing an accurate due date in early pregnancy eliminates this worry.)
- **Use epidural or spinal anesthesia.** These are forms of regional anesthesia, which numbs you from your ribs down. Regional anesthesia is safer for you and your baby than general anesthesia (which makes you unconscious). It also allows you to be awake to greet your baby and start breast-feeding.
- **Have the bladder catheter inserted after you are numb.** Otherwise, the procedure may cause discomfort.
- **Confirm that your doctor administers one dose of antibiotics at the time of the cesarean.** Antibiotics reduce the chance of infection. You do not need them afterward unless you develop an infection.
- **Have a narcotic (opioid) medication injected into the epidural catheter at the end of the operation.** This increases the chance that you will feel comfortable enough to hold and breast-feed your baby in the first hours after the surgery.
- **Talk with your provider and anesthesiologist about keeping your arms free, rather than taped down.** A woman's arms are sometimes taped down during a cesarean so that she will not move her hands into the area of the surgery, but this precaution is not required in all settings. If having both arms free for the whole surgery isn't allowed, you may be able to have at least one arm free to help hold the baby during the second half of the surgery.
- **Keep your support team with you throughout.** Your partner and/or other labor companions can help you through the surgery, share the moment of birth, and greet your baby with you. Most hospitals allow only one support person in the operating room. You may want to ask to have a doctor or nurse explain what is happening throughout the process, or ask if you can have music of your choice (generally through your own headphones and music player) during the procedure. If you want to witness the moment that your baby leaves your body, ask that the drape be lowered enough for you to see the baby. (Some obstetricians may

* The content in this box is adapted from Childbirth Connection's "Tips and Tools: C-Section," available at www.childbirthconnection.org/article.asp?ck=10170.

be unwilling to comply with this request if they believe that lowering the drape could increase your risk of developing an infection.)

- **Take steps to reduce the risk of developing blood clots.** For most women, this will mean getting up and walking soon after the operation and staying well hydrated. Moving your feet and legs at least hourly while you are in bed also helps. If you are considered at greater risk of developing blood clots, you may also wear elastic support stockings or take blood-thinning medication.
- **Keep your baby with you after the birth.** Ask that the baby be held against you "cheek to cheek" while the surgical repair is being done. Ask to hold the baby after the surgery is completed. Skin-to-skin contact can foster breast-feeding success and your early relationship. If your baby has to be separated from you for care in a nursery, your partner or another support person can go along and then bring back word of your baby's condition.
- **Ask for "multimodal" pain medication on a fixed schedule after the surgery.** When you are given a combination of pain medicines that work in different ways (opioids/narcotics and nonsteroidal anti-inflammatory drugs, or NSAIDs) you will have better pain control and you will need a lot less of the opioid/narcotic.

section, most women can breast-feed and care for our babies. Some women have difficulty due to the pain from the healing incision. It may be challenging to hold your baby, since the incision will limit your movements. Your pain can be controlled with a narcotic and other medications such as ibuprofen. These medications are considered to be safe during breast-feeding. Narcotic pain relievers may cause constipation (see page 242). It is important to take enough pain medication so that you can move around comfortably, with very little pain.

If you are finding breast-feeding to be a challenge, ask your nurse for help. Many postpartum nurses have had special training in breast-feeding. Many hospitals also have certified lactation consultants on staff who can help you with more difficult problems. Your partner or others can help with moving the baby from one breast to the other, burping, and diaper changing. Certain ways of holding your baby while breast-feeding can minimize the pressure on your abdomen. (For more information, see Chapter 14, "Your Physical Recovery and Your Newborn," and Chapter 15, "Feeding Your Baby.")

It is important that you move around and walk as soon as you comfortably can after your cesarean. Walking will reduce your risk of developing blood clots in your legs, encourage you to take deep breaths (doing so helps with recovery), and generally help you feel better. The catheter draining your bladder will generally be removed one day after your operation, and this will give you greater freedom to move around.

You can start eating foods and drinking liquids again as soon as you feel ready. If you develop nausea, it may indicate a slowing down of bowel function or be a side effect of the narcotics used to relieve pain. In general, your own appetite will usually let you know what you can safely eat, but you will probably want to start out slowly.

With my planned C-section, they wanted me not to have eaten for twelve hours before. After the section, I felt great and brazenly ate two grilled cheeses. Approximately 15 minutes later I violently threw them back up. That was one feeling I would not like to repeat. Ouch!

Digestion and bowel movements usually return to normal within a few days, although some women experience gas and constipation or diarrhea for a few days. Take a shower as soon as you can. It can make you feel better after the stress and effort of your surgery (and labor, if you had it).

During the first few days after a cesarean section, some women experience worsening in leg swelling that was present during pregnancy. As long as the swelling involves both legs, it is a natural process related to the surgery and the fluids you were given. This swelling generally resolves within a few days, although it can take up to a few weeks. If you have swelling that is painful and involves only one leg, it may indicate that there is a blood clot in the leg. This should be addressed immediately to prevent any clot from traveling to the lungs and causing serious problems.

If your incision was closed with staples, they will likely be removed while you are in the hospital. However, if your wound does not appear to be healing well, you will need to arrange an office visit or have a visiting nurse remove your staples seven to ten days after surgery. (If you had sutures, they will likely dissolve over a few weeks and will not need to be removed.) You will experience some vaginal bleeding, which may last six to eight weeks and will become lighter toward the end (see "Lochia," page 240). Foul-smelling discharge from your vagina, worsening cramping in your belly, redness around your incision, and fever are all good reasons to call your provider immediately, as you may have developed an infection. You should plan to see your provider about six weeks after your surgery to make sure you are healing well. (Some providers may want to see you in two weeks as well.)

A cesarean section is major abdominal surgery. It will take time for your abdominal muscles to regain their strength and flexibility, and for you to regain your overall strength. Six weeks after a cesarean, most women are able to resume all normal activities, including exercise, driving, and sex with vaginal penetration. It is important to have the six-week postpartum visit to be sure that you can resume these activities. Remember to start any exercise program slowly, since you have had at least six weeks of limited activity. (For more information on recovery and the postpartum period, see the chapters in "Becoming a Mother," the next part of this book.)

I was told that after the C-section I shouldn't walk up or down stairs for several weeks. I had to laugh. We call our place "the treehouse." There's two flights of stairs up to our son's room, three to our bedroom, four to my office, one down to the kitchen. Even if I'd wanted to, I couldn't have heeded the recommendation. But I healed quickly. It was September and I was able to walk outside to the hospital's garden the day after [the baby] was born. I think it's all very individual. I didn't force myself to do anything, and was gentle with myself, and I think because I kept moving, but moved slowly, I healed more easily.

The hardest part about my C-section was when the morphine wore off and I tried to stand up. I thought my guts would spill out. I held a pillow to my belly for most of the next few weeks with a heat pad to ease the throbbing pain.

As you are limited in what you can lift or carry for a few weeks, including not being able to drive a car, make sure that you have enlisted a lot of help for the first four weeks. I needed basically twenty-four-hour care for two weeks, as I had a toddler I could not lift.

VBAC OR REPEAT CESAREAN SECTION?

A substantial proportion of cesarean sections (more than one in three) are repeat procedures.[3] If you are pregnant and have had a cesarean section in a previous birth, you will need to decide whether to attempt a vaginal birth after cesarean (VBAC) or have a planned cesarean section. Because both VBACs and cesarean deliveries involve some risks to both mothers and babies, making this decision can be a challenge. There is not a single answer that is right for everyone.

Often the condition that makes a cesarean necessary in one birth will not exist in the next, and many women who have had a cesarean section can go on to have a safe vaginal birth. The majority of women (at least three out of every four) who plan a VBAC with supportive caregivers will go on to have one, instead of needing a cesarean section, although it has become increasingly difficult to find a setting that supports VBACs.[4] Women who give birth vaginally avoid the known risks of cesarean section. (See "Comparing the Risks of Cesarean Births Versus Vaginal Births," page 228.)

My first child was delivered via C-section due to breech presentation and advancing PIH [pregnancy-induced hypertension] within me. I had a long recovery and wanted so much to try for a VBAC with my second child. We talked to my OB about all possible aspects of the hospital experience. One thing we discussed and I am glad I followed through on later was asking for a "hep lock" [heparin lock, a catheter that is inserted in your vein like an IV but is capped off instead of being constantly connected to a bag of fluid] instead of the full IV. I was more mobile with the hep lock.

We hired a wonderful doula—someone who knew what we wanted from the birth and would be with us at all times during the labor and birth watching for any signs of uterine rupture (our doula was a retired birthing center nurse). With the help of my husband, our doula, and two very supportive delivery room nurses, I delivered my second child vaginally with no pain medication. The VBAC met my goals for a shorter recovery. It was a wonderful experience.

VBAC has its own set of risks. The most serious complication that can occur is a separation of a previous uterine scar (a *uterine rupture*) that, in rare instances, can result in excessive bleeding, the need for a hysterectomy, and even the death of the baby. However, a large proportion of what have been termed uterine ruptures are asymptomatic—that is, they have no medical consequences. The risk of uterine rupture during an attempt at vaginal birth after one prior cesarean section with a lower uterine horizontal incision is about one in one hundred, and the risk increases with the number of previous cesarean sections.[5] (Uterine rupture can occur in the absence of scars on the uterus from a previous cesarean. However, the single factor that increases the chance of uterine rupture dramatically is a prior cesarean.)[6]

Women who attempt VBACs and ultimately need cesarean sections may feel that the physical and emotional toll of laboring and then having cesarean surgery was worse than the toll of a planned repeat cesarean would have been.

As you consider whether you want to pursue a VBAC, learn about how different factors

WHAT YOU NEED TO KNOW ABOUT VBAC

If you had a cesarean and want a VBAC, it is essential to talk with your health care provider before you go into labor. As you consider whether you want to try to have a VBAC or schedule a repeat cesarean section, you will want to know two very important things: First, what is your individual chance of having a successful VBAC? And second, what is your individual chance of having a uterine rupture?

The following factors can affect your chance of having a successful VBAC:

1. The events that occurred during your previous labor and the reason you had the surgery. Was the reason for your previous cesarean a problem such as a breech presentation, which is not likely to happen again, or was it something such as arrest of dilation or fetal descent that is more likely to recur?
2. The previous number of cesareans or uterine surgeries that you have had.
3. Any history of previous vaginal births.
4. Your practitioner's philosophy regarding VBAC.
5. The birth center's or hospital's guidelines and practices regarding VBACs. A growing number of hospitals and providers are refusing to allow women to attempt VBACs, for multiple reasons, including concern about uterine rupture and its complications, fear of lawsuits, and lack of immediately available anesthesia. Hospitals that cannot provide twenty-four-hour in-house anesthesia and obstetrical coverage usually do not allow VBAC attempts.

Your chance of having a uterine rupture is increased if you:

1. Have a vertical scar on your uterus. Most of the time, the surgeon will make a horizontal cut into the uterus (*low transverse cesarean section*). Rarely, if this is not possible or the cesarean is performed in an emergency, a vertical incision will be made in the uterus (*low vertical* or *classical*). If you have a horizontal/transverse scar on your uterus, your chance of uterine rupture is lower and a VBAC is safe to try. If you have a vertical incision, the chance of the uterus rupturing is much higher and a VBAC is not recommended. The visible scar on your belly is not always in the same direction as the scar on the uterus beneath. If you don't know what kind of incision was made in your cesarean, you can find out by asking for your medical records. In rare cases, a surgeon may make both a horizontal and a vertical cut in the uterus, creating a scar in the shape of an upside-down T; if this happened in your previous cesarean, it is not safe to give birth vaginally.

2. Had your cesarean section within the past eighteen months. This makes your chance of having a uterine rupture a little higher than if your cesarean section was done more than eighteen months ago.
3. Had an infection in the uterus after the previous cesarean section. Your surgical scar may be slightly weaker and your chance of having a uterine rupture is a little higher.
4. Have your labor induced or augmented with oxytocin during this VBAC attempt.

in your previous cesarean experience may affect your likelihood of success in giving birth vaginally and your chances of uterine rupture. (For more information, see "What You Need to Know About VBAC," page 234.)

If you decide to attempt a VBAC, it's essential to choose a setting with available emergency care, in case you need to undergo a cesarean section. Also, find out the provider's and hospital's VBAC rates. To try to get a sense of how comfortable the nurses and physicians are with caring for women having VBACs, ask your provider about her or his feelings about trials of labor, about how the covering obstetricians feel, and about the support that you can expect in the hospital.

Many women as well as some obstetrical providers have become interested in trying to find ways to decrease the rate of cesarean births. In 1982, a large group of concerned parents and professionals founded the International Cesarean Awareness Network, Inc. (ICAN, first called the Cesarean Prevention Movement). It aims to prevent unnecessary cesareans, to provide support for cesarean recovery, and to promote VBAC.

In a practice guideline article published in 1988, the American College of Obstetricians and Gynecologists (ACOG) embraced the position that VBACs are a safe and reasonable alternative to repeat cesareans. They reaffirmed this position in 1991. In 1998 and again in 1999, ACOG added the caution that VBAC should be attempted only in institutions equipped to deal with uterine rupture. The rate of VBAC declined from more than one in four women in 1996 to fewer than one in ten in 2004.[7] The national *Listening to Mothers II* survey reported that a majority of women (57 percent) in 2005 who wanted the option of a VBAC were denied that choice, primarily because their provider or hospital was unwilling to do a VBAC.[8] If you are interested in a VBAC, try to find a hospital where VBACs are allowed and get a list of that hospital's providers. Childbirth educators, midwives, and doulas in the area may be able to help identify VBAC-friendly caregivers and hospitals.

None of the local hospitals would even let me do a VBAC except for the [hospital-based] birthing center where I had my first baby. They had many stipulations, such as, I couldn't get in the tub, or the shower, I had to have a hep lock put in my hand as soon as I went into labor should I need a C-section, I had to have constant fetal monitoring, and I couldn't use a midwife because a doctor had to be on the premises for a VBAC. These stipulations were a combination of the birthing center and my ob-gyn practice. I remember calling my doula and saying, "I feel like not telling them when I go into labor so I can get to the birthing center just in time for pushing to avoid all of these crazy interventions." My doula responded with the exact answer I needed. She said, "So, you are feeling like you have no power or control in your birthing process." I said, "Yes," and she told me that I needed to take back control. I immediately went to work researching VBAC statistics. . . . I wrote a letter to my practice saying that I wanted to be able to labor in the tub or the shower, [that] I did not want constant fetal monitoring unless something in my labor indicated that I needed it, and that I wanted to use the midwife or I was leaving the practice. It took many painful conversations, but they finally agreed to my terms. . . . I was so thrilled and felt so in control again. It was an amazing feeling.

AFTER A CESAREAN SECTION

Women who have complicated labors and obstetric emergencies appreciate the necessity of cesarean sections. Yet even when it is lifesaving, cesarean birth may raise complicated emotions. Some of us experience the surgery as intrusive, a violation of our bodies. Many of us fault ourselves, feeling guilty or defensive that we didn't do "everything possible" to have a vaginal birth. In fact, we do the best we can, given our physical circumstances and the information and support available.

We planned on the "perfect" birthing center natural birth. I saw midwives during my entire pregnancy, and even went to a birthing class focusing on a natural childbirth. . . . Yet birth is such an unpredictable thing. Anything can happen. For months I was depressed, think-

ing . . . that I had failed. I realize now that although meaningful, your birth experience is such a small part of the relationship with your child. I now know that bonding is so much more than the initial moments. I write this hoping that if someone else's birth doesn't go as "planned," she will know that she is not a failure and that she can still have a wonderful relationship with her child.

NOTES

1. American College of Obstetricians and Gynecologists, "Fetal Macrosomia," *ACOG Practice Bulletin* 22 (November 2000): 514.
2. Childbirth Connection, "Cesarean Section: Best Evidence: C-Section," accessed at www.childbirthconnection.org/article.asp?ck=10166 on July 25, 2006.
3. Physicians Committee for Responsible Medicine, "When Is Surgery Unnecessary?" accessed at www.pcrm.org/resources/education/society/society3.html on September 6, 2006.
4. Childbirth Connection, "Options: VBAC or Repeat C-Section," accessed at www.childbirthconnection.org/article.asp?ck=10211 on July 26, 2006.
5. Julie Welischar, MD, and Gerald Quirk, MD, PhD, "Vaginal Birth After Cesarean Delivery," UptoDate Online, updated August 29, 2006; accessed via www.utdol.com (a subscription-only service) on January 25, 2007.
6. M. Barger, E. Declercq, A. Nannini, J. Weiss, and L. Bartlett, "Uterine Rupture," American Public Health Association, October 2001.
7. Brady E. Hamilton, Joyce A. Martin, Stephanie J. Ventura, Paul D. Sutton, and Fay Menacker, "Births: Preliminary Data for 2004," *National Vital Statistics Report,* accessed at www.cdc.gov/nchs/data/nvsr/nvsr54/nvsr54_08.pdf on December 14, 2006.
8. Eugene R. Declercq, Carol Sakala, Maureen P. Corry, and S. Applebaum, *Listening to Mothers II: Report of the Second National U.S. Survey of Women's Childbearing Experiences* (New York: Childbirth Connection, 2006).

Becoming a Mother

CHAPTER 14

Your Physical Recovery and Your Newborn

In the first hours and days after giving birth, you will likely experience a range of feelings, from exhilaration to exhaustion, joy to sadness, and confidence to uncertainty. It's not unusual to feel multiple, contradictory emotions, all at the same time.

She was placed on my chest and I began to cry from the overwhelming sense of emotions I felt. I was feeling so many things simultaneously: relief, love, excitement, awe, astonishment, pride, and achievement. It was truly a momentous occasion, very surreal and very beautiful. When I looked deeply into my newborn daughter's eyes for the very first time, I kissed her softly and whispered: "Hi, Baby. Welcome to the world, we've been waiting for you."

YOUR PHYSICAL RECOVERY

The moments and hours after giving birth are a good time to rest and recover from the exertion of bringing your child into the world.

Immediately [after the birth] I felt surprisingly good—alert and pumped full of adrenaline, and finally hungry and thirsty. [But] when they tried to get me up to use the bathroom I nearly fainted. That caused quite a stir, and I had to be wheeled in a chair. I continued feeling light-headed for about a day. . . . We stayed in the hospital two nights, and I was grateful to have someone taking care of me and the baby.

Whether you have given birth in the hospital or in your own home, had an unmedicated birth or required numerous medical interventions, your body will go through many physical changes in the hours and days after giving birth.

SORENESS

Nearly all women experience some kind of body soreness after labor and birth. Back pain or other body aches can result from the physical exertion of labor, or from particular labor positions. These aches and pains during the first few days are completely normal.

Soaking in tubs, getting massages, and moving around can help alleviate general soreness. (For information about specific cramps and pains, see "Cramping" below, and facing page.) If the pain is severe, is not controlled by self-help techniques or pain medicines, or gets worse, notify your midwife or doctor.

LOCHIA

Both women who have vaginal deliveries and women who have cesarean sections will experience vaginal discharge after childbirth. This discharge, called *lochia,* is blood mixed with material from the uterine lining that supported the baby in the womb. It is initially red, then will lighten to pink, then brown, before becoming clear or yellowish and finally stopping two to eight weeks after the birth. Women who have C-sections may have lochia for a shorter period of time, because much of this material is removed during surgery.

The lochial discharge is a normal, healthy process. Although it is common to see some small, coin-sized clots at first, the amount of bleeding should steadily decrease over the first few weeks. Most hospitals and pharmacies have large maternity pads (oversized maxi pads) you can use. Do not use tampons, which are not absorbent enough and are a potential source of infection (in addition to being very uncomfortable after a vaginal birth). If you have large clots or unusually heavy bleeding (a large maxi pad soaked in under an hour), the blood has a bad odor, or you have fever and chills, you should call your health care provider. These may be signs of an infection or of a retained piece of placenta. Do not be surprised if your bleeding becomes slightly heavier for a day or two when you become more active. If this happens, you may be doing too much; try resting for a day. If your bleeding continues to be heavy, do not hesitate to call your health care provider.

No one ever talks about it, but a postpartum woman's best friend is a box of high-quality overnight maxi pads—with wings! A friend told me to bring my own before I went into the hospital—and double up on them, front and back—so that I wouldn't have to rely on the hospital's awful ones that move and don't absorb anything anyway. It was great advice. I even wore them while laboring because I had already broken my water and didn't like the feeling of sitting in a pool of wet all night.

CRAMPING

Like lochia, uterine cramping is a normal part of recovery from childbirth. This cramping is a sign that the uterus is contracting and returning to prepregnancy size. Uterine cramping is often more intense for women who have had previous pregnancies. Breast-feeding can make the cramps occur during the first few days. These "afterpains" generally stop being painful by the third day after giving birth.

To relieve the cramping, hold a pillow or a heating pad over your abdomen, lie on your stomach if this is comfortable, or lie on your side with a pillow between your legs and over your stomach. Over-the-counter pain medicines such as ibuprofen (sold under brand names like Motrin or Advil) can be taken if you have afterpains that are very intense and if you do not have other medical conditions that can be made worse by taking ibuprofen. The usual recommendation is to take ibuprofen about fifteen minutes before breast-feeding.

I hardly remember the cramping after the birth of my first child. . . . Not so with my second. The pain was like extraordinarily intense menstrual cramping. It shocked me. My breasts would fill painfully with milk, and I would happily put the baby to nurse, but the moment she started to suck, the cramping would begin. It made me dizzy, it was so intense. I got used to propping the baby on a pillow on my aching stomach— nursing pillow and cramping pillow in one. . . . Gazing at my new baby hungrily nursing away helped distract me from the pain.

PERINEAL PAIN

Perineal pain due to episiotomy, tears, stitches, or just the stretching of vaginal birth is also very common. Perineal pain may make it uncomfortable to walk or sit.

During the initial period of recovery (the first twenty-four hours), most women find it helpful to apply ice packs, which not only assist with pain relief, but can help reduce the swelling in the area. After twenty-four hours, women may find comfort in warm compresses or sitz baths, soaking the vulvar/perineal area in tepid water in the bathtub or in a special insert—a sitz bath—that can be placed on the toilet. You may also use pain medication for perineal pain. If your pain is not relieved by these strategies or if it worsens, contact your health care provider.

To relieve the stinging that can occur as urine comes in contact with sutures or small tears, you can keep a squirt bottle with warm water in the bathroom and use it to spray water on your vulvar area when you urinate. It is important to avoid constipation in the postpartum period as straining during bowel movements may be painful to the perineum.

SPINAL HEADACHE

In rare cases, women who have had epidural or spinal anesthesia experience anesthesia-related headaches after giving birth. These headaches are worse when sitting or standing, and are usually relieved by lying down. A spinal headache is initially treated with fluids and over-the-counter or prescription pain medication, and should resolve in two to four days. If it does not go away or is particularly severe and includes symptoms such as double vision or neck pain, notify your health care provider as soon as possible. The spinal headache can often be treated with an injection into the epidural space, which will make the headache go away more quickly.

PAIN AFTER CESAREAN SECTION

If you have had a cesarean section, you will need stronger pain relief medication than women who have had vaginal births. Talk with your health care providers about post-surgical pain relief, both for the first few days and then for the first two to three weeks after going home. During the first day in the hospital, you

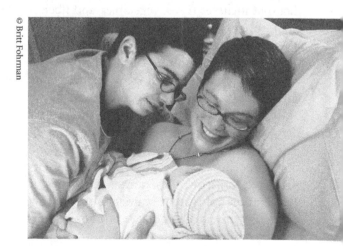
© Britt Fohrman

may require intravenous medication, followed by a gradual change to pain medication you can take by mouth. You may be given a liquid diet initially, and then solid foods should be added slowly. Eat what you feel you can tolerate. When you go home, usually four to five days after surgery, you likely will need to continue to take prescription medicines for pain relief. It is best to take opioid pain medication only when it is really needed, because such medicines can cause constipation. Your provider will probably give you a strong dose of ibuprofen, which often works better for post-surgical pain than opioids do. Be sure that you get enough pain relief to be able to comfortably care for yourself and your baby. (For more information about medications and nursing, see page 263. For more information on recovering from a C-section, see page 229.)

CONSTIPATION

You may not move your bowels for a day or two after birth. This is normal.

To make the first bowel movement easier and prevent future constipation, drink plenty of water, move around as soon as possible after delivery (it will probably take a day to begin walking again after a C-section), and eat a balanced diet that includes fruits, vegetables, and fiber. A stool softener can help with constipation. If needed, laxatives in the form of either pills taken by mouth or suppositories can also help ease severe constipation. Before using suppositories, check with your health care provider.

Bowel movements may be uncomfortable if you have developed hemorrhoids during either pregnancy or birth. Witch hazel pads and sitz baths can ease the discomfort of hemorrhoids, as can over-the-counter medicines. If your hemorrhoids are very uncomfortable, talk with your provider about prescription creams and suppositories that can help.

ABDOMINAL AND PELVIC FLOOR WEAKNESS

You may experience some abdominal muscle weakness after birth, as well as pelvic floor weakness, which can lead to urinary incontinence (leaking urine). Women can also have bowel incontinence due to weakened pelvic floor muscles. Kegel exercises can help you recover pelvic muscle tone. (For more information on Kegels, see page 38.)

If you have had a vaginal birth, light abdominal exercises can help recover abdominal muscle tone. If you have had a cesarean section, your abdominal muscle tone will take longer to recover. During the first few days, you can press a folded towel or a pillow over your abdomen when sitting up or you can turn onto your side to sit up. The towel or pillow and your arm will help you move without having to use your abdominal muscles as much. In the days and weeks immediately following delivery, do not pick up anything heavier than your baby.

FATIGUE

Fatigue is a major factor in the days immediately after you give birth. You are recovering from the physical demands of labor and birth and, at the same time, your sleep is being interrupted by your baby. If possible, have your partner or a support person sleep in the room with you—even if you are in a hospital or birthing center—to help support you in your recovery and facilitate your bonding with the baby.

In the first days either at home or in the hospital, be choosy about the visitors you see. Their job is to help you, not the other way around. A visit that interferes with a much-needed chance to rest should be avoided. Ask friends and relatives to stay for a few minutes only or to delay their visits. Many will be happy to share their concern and generosity in another way, like volunteering to care for your other children, do simple errands, or drop off meals for your family. If phone calls are feeling intrusive, consider turning off the ringer or screening your calls, particularly during those precious times when the baby is sleeping.

If at all possible, limit your activities during the immediate post-recovery period to initiating breast-feeding (if you are nursing), bonding with your baby, and resting, which will help you recover physically. Ask for help from your partner, a family member, or another support person. When possible, sleep when the baby sleeps, and postpone or delegate the demands of your household and everyday life for at least a few weeks.

Excessive fatigue can also be a sign of anemia, or low iron in your blood. You may need to increase your intake of high-iron foods, including meat, eggs, leafy greens, and legumes. Another way to prevent anemia is to continue taking your prenatal multivitamin supplement, which contains iron.

The first week after the birth I wasn't good for much of anything—I was really weak, and it was especially frustrating at the hospital because I was barely strong enough to hold the baby, much less do anything else for her besides feed her. After that first week, though, things started to improve. I really took seriously the injunction to do nothing for the first two weeks, and that really helped me start feeling better.

TEMPERATURE INSTABILITY

You may experience hot and cold flashes as your body adjusts its levels of hormones and shifts fluids. If you are nursing, you may feel a rush of warmth when your breasts engorge with milk.

MOOD CHANGES

Many new mothers experience "baby blues" after delivery and some experience more serious depression. (For more information, see page 281.)

SORE BREASTS

Your milk will come in on the second to fifth day after your baby is born. After your milk comes in, your breasts may feel uncomfortable, hard, and engorged. If you are breast-feeding, this engorgement will go away within a few days. (For more information, see Chapter 15, "Feeding Your Baby.") If you are not breast-feeding, the milk will stay in your breasts, and your breasts may feel hard and uncomfortable a bit longer. Wearing a tight-fitting bra, binding your chest, using ice packs, and/or taking over-the-counter pain medicines can help with the discomfort. After several days, your body will stop making milk and your breasts will gradually soften and become smaller.

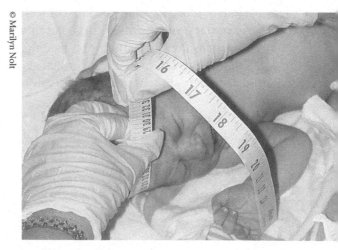

© Marilyn Nolt

Soon after being born, your baby will probably be measured to provide a baseline to chart her or his growth. The average baby is about 20 inches in length.

YOUR NEW BABY

EARLY SIGNS OF HEALTH

In the first few minutes after birth, your health care provider will judge how your newborn initially adapts to being outside the womb. This evaluation, called the Apgar score, is based on five signs: heart rate, breathing, muscle tone, reflexes, and color. Your baby will be evaluated at one and five minutes of life and given a score of 0, 1, or 2 for each sign. Although a score of 10 is perfect, very few babies get a score of 10 because most have some bluish color in their hands or feet for several minutes after birth. A score of 7 or more at 5 minutes is normal, and is seen in healthy babies. A score of less than 7 at 10 minutes will lead health care providers to observe the baby carefully.

THE INITIAL ALERT PERIOD

Most babies are quite alert during the first hour or two after birth. During this time period, your baby has good muscle control and a heightened ability to learn how to nurse. This alert period is ideal for skin-to-skin contact, lots of eye contact, verbalizations from parents and caregivers to the baby, and breast-feeding. You and your baby can look at each other, get to know each other's touch, and start to develop a bond.

After the initial alert period, most babies experience a sleepy period that usually lasts for three to five hours. Take advantage of this opportunity to rest, bathe, and recover from your birth.

DRESSING

Many babies enjoy being swaddled, or wrapped tightly in a receiving blanket, and can be dressed easily in kimono-style shirts or other clothes that do not have to be put over the head. Some prefer to have their arms and hands free. Newborns aren't able to control their temperature well during the first twenty-four hours or so. A hat will protect your newborn from losing a large amount of heat through her or his head.

SLEEPING

Some hospitals have a central nursery where babies are watched by nurses assigned to that room. Other hospitals have a policy of "rooming in," whereby mothers and babies stay together and both are cared for by nurses who staff the postpartum floor. Most hospitals keep babies who are born by cesarean section in a central nursery until the mother is alert enough to call for assistance if needed. Some hospitals also take babies to a central nursery right after birth for a short observation period. However, if you and/or your support people are able to take care of the baby, you can request that your baby stay in the room with you.

Rooming in will help you and the baby get to know each other. Often, for instance, a mother rooming in with her baby will quickly become familiar with the signs that her baby is hungry, wet, or otherwise in need of attention well before the infant begins to cry. Rooming in can also facilitate more frequent nursing. (For more information, see "Baby-Friendly Hospitals," page 254, or "Mother-Friendly Care," page 23.) Whether you are at home or in a hospital or birthing center, you can keep the baby with you in bed, particularly when you are awake.

To reduce the risk of sudden infant death syndrome (SIDS), always have the baby sleep on her or his back. The American Academy of Pediatrics recommends that infants sleep on their backs during the first twelve months of life, in a crib, preferably in the same room as their parents. Wherever your baby sleeps, create a safe space, where the baby is secure from falling and from suffocation hazards, including comforters or pillows.

Some research indicates that bed sharing may increase the incidence of SIDS, particularly if the baby is sleeping on soft bedding or on her or his stomach.[1] This is a controversial issue. A recent review of the research suggests that the increase in SIDS that has been associated with bed sharing is likely related to other factors, such as an adult in the bed drinking alcohol or smoking or being extremely tired; overcrowded housing conditions; and/or when sleeping takes place on a water bed or soft sofa or the infant is placed under a heavy comforter.[2] Many health care providers and researchers suggest that when bed sharing is practiced safely, it has benefits for infants and parents, including better sleep and easier nighttime feedings.[3]

While bed sharing may be controversial, room sharing is not. Having your baby in close proximity to you, either in a crib in the same room or in a co-sleeper (a three-walled, crib-like baby bed that attaches to your bed), allows you and your baby to respond to each other more easily than if you are in separate rooms. It also may reduce the risk of SIDS.[4]

TESTS AND TREATMENTS FOR YOUR NEWBORN

Most providers in all settings collect blood from the umbilical cord after the cord is cut. This blood is used to test for the baby's blood type. (For information on saving cord blood, see page 41.) Health care providers in the United States are required by law to administer an eye ointment that protects newborns against blindness from gonorrhea or chlamydia to all newborns in the first few hours after birth. Most babies get a shot of vitamin K at the same time that this eye ointment is given. Health care providers are also required by law to draw some blood from your baby's heel for tests that can detect certain harmful or potentially fatal disorders. This blood is usually obtained just before you go home. Finally, hospitals offer a few other tests and treatments that are part of the "routine" assessment of newborns. If your baby is premature or has special health needs, she or he may need additional medical attention. (For more information about premature birth, see page 219.)

EYE ANTIBIOTICS

Every state in the United States requires health care providers to place a small amount of antibiotic ointment under babies' eyelids within the first four hours after birth. This treatment, as mentioned above, is to prevent eye infections and blindness that can occur if the baby is infected with gonorrhea or chlamydia. The ointment does not hurt the baby. For an hour or so, it may give your baby's eyes a goopy appearance, but this will pass as the antibiotic gets absorbed.

If this eye treatment is done immediately after birth, it can interfere with you and your baby making good eye contact during the initial alert phase. You can request that the treatment be postponed for an hour or two. Although the practice is rare today, some hospitals may still use silver nitrate instead of antibiotic ointment for the eye treatment. Silver nitrate can be irritating and slightly painful. You can check with your hospital in advance and request antibiotic ointment if the hospital is still using silver nitrate.

VITAMIN K

In most settings in the United States, babies are given an injection of vitamin K after birth to protect against a severe and sometimes fatal bleeding disorder caused by vitamin K deficiency. Although the disorder is very rare, vitamin K is offered to all babies, since their livers, where vitamin K is made, are immature and may not make enough of the vitamin.

Some parents object to the vitamin K injection because a report in the 1990s from the United Kingdom suggested that infants who get a shot of vitamin K have a higher rate of cancer in childhood. More recent studies from the United States have not found any relationship between the shot of vitamin K and cancer that occurs several years later. Another possible concern is that the vitamin K shot, like all injections, is a little painful. Vitamin K can be given by mouth in two different doses, but oral doses do not prevent vitamin K deficiency disease as well as the shot does. Although the standard policy in the United States is to give vitamin K as one shot in the first several hours after birth, you can request the oral form if you want.

NEWBORN SCREEN

When your baby is about one to three days old, her or his blood will be tested for a number of genetic and congenital conditions. This test is usually performed by drawing blood from the baby's heel and sending it to a state testing facility. The results are available in one to two weeks. Your newborn can be tested for many disorders with this one sample of blood.

Every state in the United States requires health professionals who care for newborns to perform newborn screening. However, the number of tests that are done varies a great deal between the different states. All states require newborn screening for phenylketonuria (PKU), benign hyperphenylalaninemia, sickle-cell disease, thalassemia, transferase-deficient galactosemia, and congenital hypothyroidism. A few states require HIV testing for newborns. Speak to your health care provider to learn exactly which diseases are tested for in your state.

You have the right to refuse newborn testing, or to request additional tests, particularly if you are aware of certain metabolic diseases in your family or if you have given birth to a previous child with an inherited condition. If the hospital is unable to provide the particular test you request, you can discuss with your health care provider how to get your baby tested.

HEPATITIS B VACCINE

If you give birth in a hospital, you may be asked if your newborn can be given the first of three injections to protect against hepatitis B. Hepatitis B is a disease of the liver that is transmitted from person to person though blood and body fluids. Hepatitis B immunity is required for most school-age children. Some care providers may put this initial injection off until a later pediatric visit. However, if you are already diagnosed as a hepatitis B carrier, your baby will need a hepatitis B vaccine and an injection of hepatitis B immunoglobulin immediately after birth. If your hepatitis B status is unknown at the time of birth, it is recommended that your baby be given the vaccine immediately after birth.

HEARING TEST

If your baby is born in a hospital or birthing center, she or he will likely be given a hearing test prior to going home. If your baby is born at home, your pediatrician or nurse will schedule this test shortly after birth.

JAUNDICE

Your baby will also be given a full head-to-toe examination by a nurse-practitioner, family care practitioner, or pediatrician within the first day or two of life. This will include checking for jaundice, a condition that causes a yellow coloring of the skin and the whites of the eyes due to a buildup of bilirubin, a breakdown product of red blood cells. Many babies get a little jaundice in the first week after birth because the fetal blood cells are breaking down to make room for regular blood cells. This sort of jaundice will go away without treatment after one or two weeks. Your health care provider can determine if your baby has a more harmful level of jaundice. Sometimes, the provider may need to check blood bilirubin levels a few days in a row. If the levels are high, your baby may be treated with a special light or blanket to help break down the bilirubin.

CORD CARE

Your newborn baby won't have that adorable baby's belly button until the remnant of the umbilical cord, the umbilical stump, falls off in five to ten days. Until then, keep the stump clean and dry and fold diapers down so that they do not to rub against it. In the past, parents were advised to clean off the umbilical stump with alcohol, but recent research shows that alcohol treatments are no better than keeping the umbilical stump clean and dry. Many health care providers will rub the cord with a one-time antibiotic treatment that protects this area from infection.

Do not rub any cosmetic clay on the stump, use a belly band, place a coin on it, or do anything to constrict it. Although these practices may be traditional in some communities, they can lead to infection. You should also refrain from tugging or pulling at the cord, which in its last days often looks like it's "hanging by a thread."

After the cord is completely off, there may be some minor yellow or clear discharge from the site for a day or two until it dries completely.

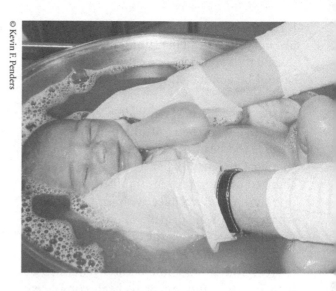

Any prolonged discharge, bleeding, redness, or irritation at the site may be a sign of infection; if this occurs, seek medical care.

CIRCUMCISION

Circumcision is a surgical procedure that removes the fold of skin that covers the tip of a boy's penis (the foreskin). While the practice is rooted in historical and cultural tradition, medical organizations and health agencies around the world do not recommend routine circumcision of baby boys.[5]

Some scientific studies have suggested that circumcision may provide some protection against urinary tract infections and some sexually transmitted infections, including HIV infection. But the procedure also carries some small risks, including bleeding, infection, injury to the head of the penis, and possibly diminished sensation.[6]

If you choose to have your son circumcised and he was born in the hospital, the procedure will usually be done before you go home. Some families choose to have their newborn circumcised in a religious ritual outside of the hospital. In either case, speak to the person performing the circumcision about her or his plan to provide anesthetic (numbing) pain relief during the surgery. Circumcision is painful and should be conducted only with pain relief for the baby.

In the first few days after circumcision, apply plenty of petrolatum (petroleum jelly) around the head of the penis every time you change your son's diaper. The diaper should be changed often to prevent the site from coming into too much contact with urine or feces, which could lead to pain or infection. There may be some blood in the diaper, mild swelling of the head of the penis, or a yellowish discharge. You should not bathe a circumcised baby in a tub until his penis heals completely. Fever, redness, or swelling may be a sign of postoperative infection and should be brought to the attention of your care provider.

If you decide not to circumcise, do not expect your son's foreskin to be retractable immediately. Indeed, in many uncircumcised boys, the foreskin cannot be fully pulled back for a number of years; this is completely normal. The penises of uncircumcised boys don't need any special care, just routine cleaning.

ARE YOU READY TO GO HOME?

If you have given birth somewhere other than in your home, you and your health care provider will discuss when you should go home. The standard hospital practice is for women to go home two days after vaginal births and three to four days after cesarean births. These numbers are often just guidelines; your stay may depend upon how you and your baby are doing as well as upon your insurance coverage.

I was scared to go home. I was hoping [the providers at the hospital] would keep me through the weekend, because—I think it was just more nervousness than anything. This baby girl, it's just gonna be me and her when I [go] home. And I knew I had the support of family and friends who would stop by and make sure I ate but . . . it was just, I didn't want to be left alone. [I wondered:] "Am I doing everything right? Why is she crying? I just changed her, fed her!" . . . Half of me was ready to go home, and the other half was like, "Maybe I should stay a little bit longer, just in case anything happens."

Particularly in places like birthing centers, women who desire to do so may be able to go home within hours after a normal vaginal birth. This is true if you have adequate support at

PAPERWORK

During the few days after delivery, the hospital staff will help you fill out your baby's birth certificate. If you had your baby at home, your midwife or doctor will complete the birth certificate, file it with the appropriate office, and give you information about how to get an official copy for yourself. You may also get information about how to apply for a Social Security number for your baby.

home and plan close follow-up with your health care provider. If your medical condition is stable, your pain control adequate with oral medications, your support team in place, and your baby robust and healthy, you can discuss with your care provider the possibility of being discharged early.

You will need diapers, a place for the baby to sleep, some clean blankets and washcloths, baby clothing appropriate to the season, bottles and formula if you are not breast-feeding, and a car seat to bring the baby home. Consider how you will welcome your new baby home, and who will be there to greet her or him. Will this be an important occasion for family and friends, or a quiet time of adjustment and rest? Are there siblings and will your new baby bring any older brothers or sisters "gifts" to help smooth the arrival?

We were so excited to introduce her to everything that would be hers. We were tired but exhilarated on the ride home. Then as we stood in front of the house, time sort of stood still and we heard every small background noise like a song. We started up the steps slowly, talking to this baby in my arms, and we told her, "This is your apple tree," "This is the porch you can play on," "These are the flowers we will teach you the names of." We opened the door with tears of welcome and excitement.

NOTES

1. Peter S. Blair, Peter J. Fleming, Iain J. Smith, Martin Ward Platt, Jeanine Young, et al., "Babies Sleeping with Parents: Case-Control Study of Factors Influencing the Risk of the Sudden Infant Death Syndrome," *BMJ* 319 (December 1999): 1457–1462, accessed at http://bmj.bmjjournals.com/cgi/reprint/319/7223/1457 on August 21, 2006.
2. J. J. McKenna and T. McDade, "Why Babies Should Never Sleep Alone: A Review of the Co-sleeping Controversy in Relation to SIDS, Bedsharing, and Breastfeeding," *Pediatric Respiratory Reviews* 6 (2005): 134–152.
3. For more information, see policy statement, American Academy of Pediatrics, Task Force on Sudden Infant Death Syndrome, "The Changing Concept of Sudden Infant Death Syndrome: Diagnostic Coding Shifts, Controversies Regarding the Sleeping Environment, and New Variables to Consider in Reducing Risk," *Pediatrics* 116, no. 5 (2005): 1,245–1,255. For co-sleeping and crib sleeping guidelines, see www.askdrsears.com/html/7/T070600.asp.
4. McKenna and McDade, "Why Babies Should Never Sleep Alone."
5. For more information, see American Academy of Pediatrics, Task Force on Circumcision, "Circumcision Policy Statement," *Pediatrics* 103, no. 3 (March 1999): 686–693, available online at http://aappolicy.aappublications.org/cgi/content/full/pediatrics;103/3/686. See also the Circumcision Information and Resource Pages, "Circumcision: Medical Organization Official Policy Statements," accessible online at www.cirp.org/library/statements.
6. For more information, see the Circumcision Information and Resource Pages, "Frequently Asked Questions About Infant Circumcision, at www.cirp.org/pages/parents/FAQ.

CHAPTER 15

Feeding Your Baby

I had read all the books about how good breast milk is for babies, and I wanted to nurse my child, but before he was born I still felt a little strange about it. I never had any experience like that before, so I didn't know what it would be like to have this little person sucking on my breast almost twenty-four hours a day. I was almost wishing deep down that formula was better for babies. Then, after the birth and when we were in the hospital and started trying to breast-feed, I had this total change in attitude. I was like, "This isn't as weird as I thought it would be. This is a bonding thing."

I thought I would like breast-feeding, but I was surprised by how lovely it turned out to be. I felt awkward at first—was I holding him correctly? was any milk coming out?—and my nipples were a little sore, but both the baby and I quickly found our rhythm.

I'd had a cesarean section, and it hurt to hold my son in my lap. So I'd sit on the couch, scoop him up like a football, and place him on a fat cushion by my side. I'd tuck his feet behind me and lift his head to my breast, and he would latch right on. Those first moments of sucking brought such a physical and emotional release. I'd sigh and stare into his eyes or close my eyes and drift. Eventually he'd pop off my nipple, give a contented "ah," and fall asleep. Days and nights passed in that drifting, dreamy, milky state.

Many of us find great pleasure and pride in our body's ability to nourish new life. In addition, breast-feeding offers many benefits to both mothers and our babies.

Breast milk is the best food for babies. It provides exactly the right balance of nutrients, adapting to your baby's changing requirements as she or he grows in the first months of life. Breast milk has unique nutritional properties that benefit infants' health and that are not available in formula.

Babies who are formula-fed are more likely than babies who are breast-fed to develop ear infections, gastrointestinal problems, asthma, diabetes, lower respiratory tract infections, and eczema. Both sudden infant death syndrome (SIDS) and childhood leukemia, while rare, are more common in babies who are formula-fed.[1]

Mothers' health is also affected by breast-feeding. Women who do not breast-feed are more likely to develop breast cancer, ovarian cancer, and type 2 diabetes. Women who do not breast-feed or breast-feed for only a short period of time are also more likely to experience postpartum depression.[2]

In addition to being good for our babies' health and our own health, breast-feeding has practical advantages: When you breast-feed, you don't have to spend money on formula or deal with bottles (except when you're separated from your baby).

The American Academy of Pediatrics recommends that children be exclusively breast-fed for six months, and then, after solid foods are introduced, given breast milk on a continuing basis to a minimum age of twelve months, "and thereafter for as long as mutually desired."[3] The World Health Organization recommends that breast-feeding continue up to two years.[4]

In several specific situations, such as when a mother is HIV-positive, breast-feeding is not recommended (see "Reasons Not to Breast-Feed," page 252). In addition, some of us are unable to breast-feed. In these rare circumstances, formula is a vital alternative. (For more information, see "Formula Feeding," page 272.)

DECIDING TO BREAST-FEED

I remember at age five watching my mother breast-feed my youngest brother. He was born by forceps and he had a scrape on his cheek by his

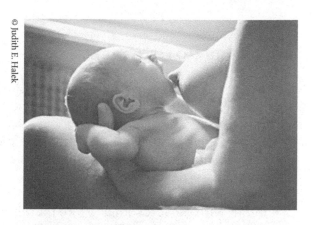

ear from the forceps blade. My mom told me that she would take extra vitamin C that would go through her breast milk to help Scott heal and grow. I remember her saying, "Even though a lot of women don't breast-feed, in this family, we breast-feed all our babies!" Every time she nursed him, I would climb on the sofa next to her and watch his cheek heal. And years later, when I was handed my own newborn, I felt my mother and my grandmother's love through that memory of "in this family, we breast-feed all our babies!"

The attitudes and assistance of the people who surround you play a significant role in supporting breast-feeding. Many of us make the decision to breast-feed before our babies are born. This can be helpful, because it allows us to plan in advance. We may sign up for a breast-feeding class, purchase nursing bras and nursing pillows, and choose birth settings and pain relief options that will maximize our chances of breast-feeding success. (For more information, see "How Birth Practices Affect Breast-Feeding," page 252, and "Planning Ahead," page 253.) Of course, many women don't plan in advance and are still able to breast-feed just fine.

Some of us hesitate to breast-feed, for a variety of reasons. We may not know women who nurse; we may feel concerned about exposing our breasts in public. If you are pregnant and trying to decide whether you will breast-feed

REASONS NOT TO BREAST-FEED

In a few specific situations, breast-feeding is not safe for the baby. The American Academy of Pediatrics cites the following reasons not to breast-feed:

- HIV-positive status in the mother (see page 141)
- active, untreated maternal tuberculosis
- some maternal medications
- illegal drug use by the mother
- infant with galactosemia (a rare metabolic deficiency)
- mother positive for HTLV (human T-cell lymphotropic virus type I or II)
- maternal exposure to radioactive materials (breast-feeding is not recommended for as long as there is radioactivity in the milk)
- herpes simplex lesions on mother's breast (infant may feed from other breast if that breast is clear of lesions)[5]

your baby, ask nursing mothers, female friends, or relatives to share their stories, and learn more about the process of breast-feeding.

If your hospital doesn't provide sufficient breast-feeding support or if you have to go back to work in a matter of weeks, you may feel as if the decision not to breast-feed—or not to continue for long—has been made for you. But any breast-feeding is better than none, because of the health benefits it provides to both you and your baby. You also may be able to overcome obstacles that initially seem daunting.

HOW BIRTH PRACTICES AFFECT BREAST-FEEDING

If you plan to give birth in a hospital, be sure to check out the facility's breast-feeding policies. For example, you can ask if the hospital helps each mother to hold her baby skin-to-skin right after giving birth and to begin breast-feeding within an hour; practices "rooming in," which allows mothers to keep our babies with us twenty-four hours a day; and does not give for-

mula to breast-fed newborns except in urgent medical situations. (For more guidelines, see "Baby-Friendly Hospitals," page 254.)

If your hospital doesn't offer these services, try to find another hospital that does. If you can't or don't want to switch hospitals, make it clear before your birth that you want to breast-feed your baby and that she or he should not be given any formula or pacifiers. Write a note stating this fact and ask that it be placed in your file and above the baby's bassinet. Ask that your baby not be cleaned up and given tests until you have had a chance to nurse, unless there is a medical necessity for separating you from your baby in the first hour after birth.

Learn about how medications and pain relief measures administered to you during labor and birth may affect your baby's ability to breast-feed. Studies show that babies who do not have medication in their system at birth and who are left undisturbed on their mothers' bellies for at least an hour are much more likely to begin nursing without a problem.[6] Still, even if you have pain medication such as an epidural

A BRIEF HISTORY OF BREAST-FEEDING RATES

Before 1900, most infants were breast-fed by their mothers. Some were breast-fed by relatives, neighbors, or hired or enslaved "wet nurses." The majority of babies who were not able to receive breast milk died, as there was no safe alternative to human milk. In the mid-twentieth century, scientists learned how to alter cow's milk to create a replacement for human milk. Commercial formulas soon became affordable and readily available in many parts of the world. Breast-feeding rates in North America and Europe began to decline rapidly. In the United States, the decline continued until 1971, when just one in four babies (25 percent) was breast-fed while in the hospital, according to the Ross Mothers Survey, a study conducted annually by the formula maker Abbott Laboratories.[7]

After hitting bottom in 1971, breast-feeding rates began to climb. The efforts of breast-feeding advocacy organizations such as La Leche League helped raise in-hospital breast-feeding rates in the United States to as high as 70 percent in 2002, according to the Ross survey. One in three babies that year was still breast-feeding at six months, and one in five was breastfeeding at twelve months. The Centers for Disease Control reports that almost 73 percent of new mothers started breast-feeding in 2005, with almost two in five still breast-feeding at six months and one in five at 12 months.[8]

Studies show that most women in the United States want to breast-feed but that practical barriers, early difficulties, and misinformation often jeopardize success. In countries such as Sweden and Norway—where about 98 percent of mothers begin breast-feeding and 70 percent are still breast-feeding after six months—social acceptance, supportive hospital practices, and extended maternity leave all contribute to helping women achieve their breast-feeding goals. Unfortunately, in the United States, society's influences are different, and at six months after giving birth, less than 40 percent of mothers are breast-feeding. Breast-feeding rates are particularly low among poor women and African-American women.[9]

during labor and/or if your baby is separated from you immediately after birth, your baby is likely to nurse well, although it may take more time to get breast-feeding well established in the first few days. Holding your newborn skin-to-skin as soon as possible will help the baby to feed well when she or he is ready.

You may also want to ask your provider whether a lactation consultant or other breast-feeding assistance is available in your planned birth setting.

PLANNING AHEAD

While you are pregnant, you don't need to do anything specific to prepare your body for breast-feeding. Your breasts will prepare themselves. As a pregnancy progresses, breasts develop milk-making structures and the flow of blood to the breasts increases. Your breasts will get bigger and heavier, and often nipple color will darken. By the fifth or sixth month of pregnancy, your breasts are fully capable of producing milk for your baby. You may even notice drops of *colostrum,* a milky substance, on your nipples. Some of us find that using soap to wash our nipples has a drying effect, and therefore avoid this during the last months of pregnancy.

You may want to purchase one or two nursing bras before your baby is born, within the last two months of pregnancy. It is best to try on a nursing bra before buying one, but you can also order bras online. Avoid nursing bras that are too tight or have underwires. Both cause compression of breast tissue and can contribute to plugged milk ducts or mastitis. Also, buy a bra that has plenty of room to stretch, because your breasts will get even bigger when your milk comes in. Be sure to wash new bras before wearing them.

Although many new-mom books talk about the importance of supportive bras, nursing bras, and certified bra fitters, women all over the world happily breast-feed without any of these. Do what is comfortable and practical for you. It's better to avoid wearing a bra if you don't have one that fits comfortably.

If your nipples are inverted or flat, you do not need to do anything special during pregnancy to prepare them for breast-feeding. (For information about breast-feeding with flat or inverted nipples, see illustration page 265.)

BABY-FRIENDLY HOSPITALS

Not so long ago, it didn't seem likely that Boston Medical Center (BMC) would ever become an internationally recognized site for breast-feeding excellence. At the cash-strapped inner-city hospital with a maternity ward that treats mostly poor women of color, it seemed that time and money would be better spent on things other than increasing breast-feeding initiation rates.

"Everyone said BMC was an unlikely place for this to happen," says Bobbi Philipp, MD, a BMC pediatrician and one of three cochairs for the hospital's breast-feeding task force. "It was outside attitudes that made us want to prove to the world that our mothers and babies deserved to breast-feed just as much as anyone else."

Convinced of nursing's health benefits, BMC's breast-feeding task force began the process of becoming an internationally recognized "Baby-Friendly" hospital, a designation created by the World Health Organization and the United Nations' International Children's Emergency Fund to acknowledge hospitals that take the Ten Steps to Successful Breastfeeding. The steps are:

1. Maintain a written breastfeeding policy that is routinely communicated to all health care staff.
2. Train all health care staff in skills necessary to implement this policy.

3. Inform all pregnant women about the benefits and management of breast-feeding.
4. Help mothers initiate breastfeeding within one hour of birth.
5. Show mothers how to breastfeed and how to maintain lactation, even if they are separated from their infants.
6. Give infants no food or drink other than breast milk, unless medically indicated.
7. Practice "rooming in"—allow mothers and infants to remain together 24 hours a day.
8. Encourage unrestricted breastfeeding.
9. Give no pacifiers or artificial nipples to breastfeeding infants.
10. Foster the establishment of breastfeeding support groups and refer mothers to them on discharge from the hospital or clinic.[10]

In December 1999, BMC earned a Baby-Friendly designation, making it just the twenty-second hospital in the United States with such an accreditation. In the years since, the number of Baby-Friendly hospitals in the United States has grown, but not much. As of December 2006, only 55 hospitals in the United States were considered officially Baby-Friendly, though the designation has been awarded to more than 19,000 hospitals in other parts of the world—including 6,500 in China alone.

The campaign at BMC has paid off in hospital-wide breast-feeding initiation rates that range between 82 and 88 percent, according to Philipp, who adds that these numbers are remarkable because poor African-American mothers—who make up more than half of the women giving birth at the hospital—generally have very low breast-feeding rates.

"One of our proudest achievements is that we've been able to take what was once a formula-feeding culture and turn it into a breast-feeding culture," Philipp says. "Our moms are behind this change, too. We're busting stereotypes here; we're all proud of that."

ESTABLISHING BREAST-FEEDING

Right after your baby is born, hold her or him against your chest, skin-to-skin. Most babies can locate the nipple and initiate feeding on their own. Babies who have the opportunity to initiate feeding themselves are more likely to feed well later.[11] A healthy newborn will be ready to nurse within the first hour after birth. After the first hour or two, most babies will sleep, then awaken ready to feed again four or five hours later. Your colostrum (sometimes called the "first milk") is the best fuel for your baby during this learning phase. (For more information about colostrum, see "How Your Milk Comes In," page 260.)

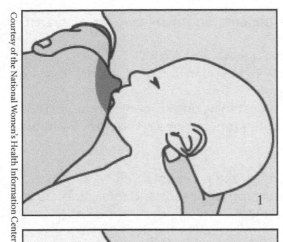

Courtesy of the National Women's Health Information Center

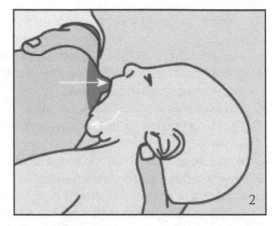

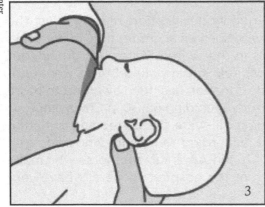

1. Tickle the baby's lips to encourage her or him to open wide.
2. Point your nipple to the roof of the baby's mouth and when she or he opens wide, pull her or him onto the breast, chin and lower jaw first.
3. Watch the lower lip and aim it as far from base of nipple as possible, so the baby's tongue draws lots of breast into the mouth.

LATCHING ON

I was lucky. My kids latched on right away after they were born. It's like they were showing me how to do it.

Establishing a good "latch" for breast-feeding is the single most important thing mothers can do to prevent sore nipples. A healthy latch is one that is not painful for the mother and allows the baby to draw an adequate amount of milk from the breast. For most mother-baby teams, *practice* is the key to establishing such a latch.

Watch your baby and follow her or his signals. Learn to respond to the more subtle signs of hunger before your baby becomes agitated and starts to cry. Among the newborn's first signs of interest in food are little movements of the body, especially the hands moving near the head, smacking the lips, mouthing movements, seeking with the lips, rooting (turning the head in response to anything that touches the cheek), and bobbing the head. Many of these movements, also called "feeding cues," happen when the baby's eyes are closed, although the baby is not asleep. This "quiet alert" state is the best time for newborns to learn to feed. Babies who are awake and somewhat hungry will respond to the smell of their mother's milk and the closeness of her nipple by opening their mouths widely and sealing onto the breast and nipple.

Babies draw both nipple and breast tissue into their mouths when breast-feeding. To help your baby do this, line the baby up so that her or his nose is opposite your nipple. Lean back a bit, or use a pillow under your baby's body or your arm, so that you do not tire of supporting the baby's weight in your arms. Use your hand to support your baby's upper back and neck so that the baby can extend her or his head back and open the mouth as wide as possible. When babies smell the nipple, most will open their mouths. When your baby's mouth is open wide, gently bring your baby to your breast, and insert your entire nipple and as much of the areola (the darker skin around the nipple) as possible into her or his mouth. (Do not lean over and try to push your breast toward the baby.) The baby's lower jaw should be on the breast as far as possible from the nipple, so that the lower jaw and the tongue can stroke milk from the breast. Think of having the baby's nose closer to the nipple and the lower jaw farther away, rather than centering your nipple in the baby's mouth.

Once the baby is latched, pause to look and listen. Your baby's cheeks should touch your breast, hiding the baby's mouth. Your baby's lips, if you can see them, should be rolled slightly outward, away from your breast. If your baby's lips are curled in or under, gently break the suction by putting your pinkie between the nipple and the baby's mouth, and then try again. Your baby's chin should be firmly planted on the breast. A good latch position will allow you to have good eye-to-eye contact with your baby. Listen for the sounds of swallowing and a shift in breathing between sucks. Watch to see if the baby's ears move—a sign that she or he is swallowing. If your baby is correctly positioned, you should not feel any pain. If feeding is painful, ask a nurse or lactation specialist for help.

She took right to the breast. Ahhhh, such a glorious feeling! Nothing in the world can match it. Such relief physically and mentally.

Another important part of establishing a healthy latch is getting comfortable with a few

basic ways to cradle your baby while breast-feeding. Nurses and lactation consultants often encourage mothers to start newborns out with the "crossover" and "football" holds; both of these nursing positions are relatively easy to master and provide a mother with good control of her baby's delicate head and neck. In any position, it is important to keep the baby's head in alignment with her or his body and keep the baby horizontal, with her or his head, chest, navel, and knees all facing you. (See illustrations of the different holds, page 258.)

If detailed instructions about latch and positioning make your head spin, it's important to remember that breast-feeding is, at heart, a human instinct. While it may take time and effort to get a healthy nursing relationship started, within a matter of days or weeks, you and your baby learn about each other and the relationship is established. Rather than worrying about picture-perfect holds, listen to and look for your baby's cues. Trust yourself. Filter out unhelpful, unsolicited opinions. Respond to your baby's—and your body's—needs. And don't hesitate to seek help if you need it, as many women do.

Hannah was put to my breast almost immediately after being born and she nursed with great gusto. It was amazing to see her nurse, because she seemed like an old pro, whereas I had no clue what to do! I simply followed her lead and tried to respond to any cues she gave indicating her need to nurse, which was often and for long periods of time.

Problems with Latching

He had trouble nursing right off the bat, and was grunting for air a bit. He would latch on, but he had a weak suck. I had him latched on wrong for the first day or two, and wound up with sore nipples and spoon-feeding him the colostrum be-

FEEDING POSITIONS

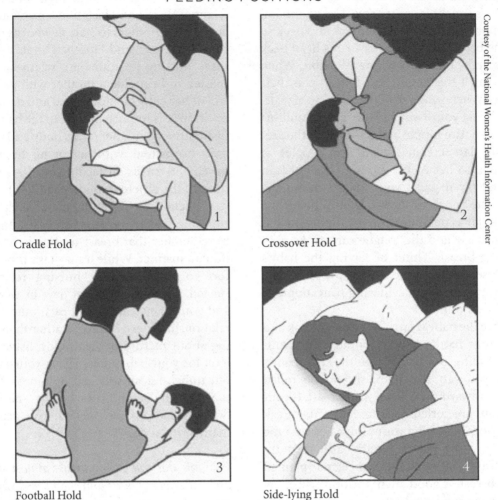

Cradle Hold

Crossover Hold

Football Hold

Side-lying Hold

Courtesy of the National Women's Health Information Center

Try different breast-feeding positions, such as these, to find what works best for you and your baby.

1. *Cradle hold:* Hold your baby's head in the crook of your elbow, cuddled up to the breast.

2. *Crossover hold:* Hold your baby's head and body with the hand and arm opposite to the breast she or he will nurse from (that is, use your right hand if you will be nursing from your left breast). This is a good position for small babies.

3. *Football hold:* Hold your baby's head in one hand with your wrist and forearm supporting the baby's neck and upper back. Pull the baby to a semi-sitting position and then down and toward your breast on the same side of your body. The baby's legs will be tucked between your arm and your side. This is a good position if you've had a cesarean birth, if your breasts are especially large, or if your baby is small.

4. *Side-lying hold:* Lie on your side, tummy to tummy with your baby. Use a couple of pillows to support your head, and to help incline the baby. This is a good hold for mothers who find it painful to sit, or who have large breasts. It's also a helpful position for co-sleeping because both mother and baby can drift off to sleep after a feeding. (For more information on co-sleeping, see page 245.)

258   OUR BODIES, OURSELVES: *Pregnancy and Birth*

cause it hurt so badly. The nurse / lactation consultant came out on the second day to check up on us. . . . It took me a couple weeks to fully adjust to nursing him; it was still uncomfortable, but not painful. After that, I was able to nurse him for nearly two years without problems. I am so glad I did.

Getting a baby started at the breast seems like it should be easy—and for many mothers it is. But some mothers and babies have a harder time establishing an effective latch.

Some babies, especially those born prematurely, may not have a strong enough suck to draw the nipple fully into the back of the mouth, which is necessary in order to draw milk from the breast and start the suck-breathe-swallow cycle. They may also tire more easily than full-term infants. Sleepy or jaundiced babies may prefer napping to nursing during the first few days of life and may need to be woken frequently to nurse. In rare cases, babies have anatomical conditions that can interfere with the establishment of a healthy latch. These can include a markedly recessed chin (the baby is born with an underdeveloped chin and an overbite that can make latching difficult) and tongue-tie (the baby's *lingual frenulum,* the strip of tissue that connects the tongue to the floor of the mouth, extends so close to the tip of the tongue that the tongue cannot move freely during feeding and the baby may have difficulty getting enough milk). A minor medical procedure can correct the problem of tongue-tie. A lactation specialist can help identify effective positions for feeding babies with receding chins or other problems.

FEEDING TWINS

Many mothers of twins prefer nursing our babies at the same time, simply because it cuts breast-feeding time in half, while others find it

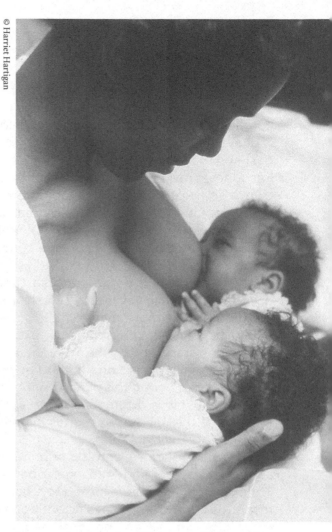

Some mothers of twins find it more efficient to breast-feed both at once.

difficult to nurse simultaneously or prefer to nurse one at a time. You may want to master feeding on one breast before attempting to feed on both. If you do decide to nurse both babies at once, it is often easiest to hold both babies in the football hold, one twin in each arm. Other mothers prefer holding both babies in the "cuddle" hold, with their legs crossed over each other. At the beginning, mothers may need assistance to feed two babies at once. This can be provided in the hospital by a nurse, and later at

HOW YOUR MILK COMES IN

From the earliest moments of your child's life, your breasts create and secrete *colostrum,* a yellowish, milky substance that's tailor-made for a newborn. Colostrum contains the proteins, minerals, and calories a newborn needs before breast milk is available. Colostrum also has antibodies to help fight infection. It is easy to digest and the temperature is just right. Colostrum helps "seal" the inside of the baby's intestines, preventing the invasion of bacteria. If ingested in frequent doses, colostrum also helps to remove bilirubin from a baby's body, reducing the risk—and severity—of jaundice. (Bilirubin is a breakdown product of the extra red blood cells a baby no longer needs after birth.) There is no artificial equivalent of colostrum, no formula that provides its unique combination of benefits for newborn development.

After the baby is born, your breasts start to make mature milk. For the first few days, the baby receives mostly colostrum, and after that, a mixture of colostrum and mature milk. As more mature milk is made, your breasts will get bigger and feel fuller. The fullness is caused by the extra blood supply that is in the breasts as milk production starts and by the milk that is now being produced and is filling the ducts. Fullness usually occurs on the third or fourth day after giving birth, and resolves a few days later. During this period your breasts may feel quite hard and often warmer than usual. This is a temporary phase. Feelings of hardness and pressure will go away once the milk production is initiated, but the breasts will remain larger now that they are fully lactating.

The milk you make consists of hundreds of nutrients and micronutrients, as well as growth factors and immune properties that are specific for your environment. For example, if you are exposed to a germ at home or in your workplace, your body responds by creating a specific antibody to fight that germ. That antibody will also enter into your milk and be consumed by your baby, who will become better able to respond to the same germ. In this way, every feeding is an immunization against microbes in the environment. A baby's own immune system isn't fully functional for months, so breast-feeding helps protect the baby during this time.

home by a partner or other support person. A lactation specialist who has experience working with mothers of multiples can also be a great help, as can mothers who have breast-fed multiples. The National Organization of Mothers of Twins Clubs (NOMOTC) can give you referrals to women in your area who can help you (248-231-4480; www.nomotc.org). In time, you will develop a feeding pattern that works for you.

EARLY BREAST-FEEDING PATTERNS

At the very beginning, most babies seem to want to do three things: eat, poop, and sleep.

They also enjoy gazing into their caretakers' eyes, and being held and rocked.

Breast-fed newborns need to nurse at least eight to twelve times each day. All that suckling, while providing nourishment for your baby, is also stimulating your breasts to ramp up their milk production, so as your baby grows, your supply will grow, too.

Frequent nursing is important for your baby's health and development as well as for building your milk supply, but this does not mean that you need to stick to a regimen. Not so long ago, doctors used to insist that babies be kept on a strict nursing schedule, feeding for as little as 15 minutes a breast for as few as six times a day. This recommendation was based on bottle-feeding routines and on erroneous beliefs that length of time (rather than positioning) was what caused sore nipples. The current advice is to breast-feed whenever your infant shows hunger cues, which will usually be at least eight to twelve times every twenty-four hours.

All babies are different and have different nursing styles. Some babies are very efficient and may get on and off the breast quickly. Others like to linger. Sometimes babies cluster-feed (nursing every thirty to forty-five minutes right after or before sleeping) and then take long naps in between. As long as the baby is nursing, and milk transfer is occurring, the occasional nap that lasts longer than four hours is not a concern. If your newborn baby takes several naps longer than four to five hours in a row, it may be necessary to wake the baby and encourage her or him to suckle and eat. Premature infants tend to be sleepier and may need to be woken up to eat more often. You may find that your baby seems to have "hungry days," when she or he nurses more than usual. This may signify a growth spurt.

The first few weeks after she was born she would get on the breast, nurse for about 5 minutes, and then fall asleep. I was so worried she wouldn't get enough milk to grow. At first we both got frustrated because she would wake up again 45 minutes later and be hungry, and then get on the breast, nurse for 5 minutes, and then fall asleep. After two or three days, my milk came in and I just settled in and learned her signs that she was getting tired. I started switching breasts just before she would get tired and that way she got more milk. We kept at it. Finally I noticed that she would fall asleep after 7 minutes, then 10 minutes, and finally, by the time she was three weeks old, she was taking both breasts and could last two to three hours between feedings.

When babies are finished nursing from one breast, they usually remove themselves from the breast. When your baby does this, offer her or him your other breast. Don't worry if the baby doesn't take the other breast. (Small babies in particular may want to nurse only on one breast at each feeding.) If this happens, offer the other breast first when the baby shows an interest in feeding again.

In general, your baby will show you when to end a feeding. Babies who have had enough milk show signs of fullness by releasing the breast; appearing relaxed, with the hands open and arms and legs curled in; closing or relaxing the eyes; and softening the facial muscles.

You may wonder if your baby is getting enough milk. Usually, you do not have to worry about this. Your baby will drink what she or he needs, and your body will make whatever your baby needs. Breast-feeding works on the principle that the more your baby sucks, the more milk you will make. If your baby is nursing and looking good, she or he is doing fine. Still, in the first few days it makes sense to watch for other signs that the baby is getting enough.

The common guide for many years was "at least six wet diapers a day." However, some babies urinate and pass stool at the same time and it can be difficult to tell how many times your baby has urinated. Diapers holding only urine should be well saturated every couple of hours. Some babies can't tolerate wet diapers and cry as soon as they are wet. For these babies, it is easier to count.

Urine is normally a very light yellow and smells like ammonia. If your baby's diaper is a dark yellow or if it looks as if it has a "brick dust" coating, the baby is not getting enough fluids; speak to your pediatric care provider immediately.

Feces should be soft and easily passed. Breast-fed babies may at first have very watery stool, which progresses to a soft, semi-formed consistency. The color will progress from greenish black in the first day or two to mustard color for several weeks and eventually to the typical brownish color. The frequency of babies' stools in the early days is a better indicator of how much milk the babies are consuming than how much they urinate. During the first two weeks after birth, your baby should have four or more stools every day; if not, contact your pediatric care provider.

Infants who are well hydrated will sleep after feeding, in most cases. The baby's lips, tongue, and mouth should be moist. Dehydrated babies can be lethargic, and they don't give the normal cues of hunger such as fretting and crying.

Many breast-feeding mothers find this early round-the-clock stage exhausting.

At the beginning, nursing felt like an unpleasant chore. It was really uncomfortable, even painful. My nipples were amazingly sore. To put it lightly, it wasn't something that I looked forward to. Plus, at first the baby nursed for a really long time. I would sit there for 45 minutes to an hour, and then I'd have to change his diaper, and before you knew it, I had to start over again. It felt like I was always nursing him.

My daughter ate daintily every two or three hours. She seemed to like to sleep more than she liked to eat and be held. Although I loved nursing her, I felt that I was doing all the work. I was really surprised by my second baby, her brother. He wanted to nurse all the time, he got on the breast very easily, and he was comforted most by being on my breast as much as he could. He was easier to nurse, but I got a lot less sleep when he was a newborn. There was only one thing that was the same. When they were full, they would fall asleep and fall off my breast with a little drop of milk on their smiling lips. I, too, felt peaceful and happy at the end of each breast-feeding experience. It was a several-times-a-day gift to me for a total of three years.

Some women find that sleeping in the same room or even the same bed with our babies makes nighttime breast-feeding far less challenging. (For more information about co-sleeping, its benefits, and safety precautions, see page 245.)

UTERINE CRAMPS AND OXYTOCIN

First-time nursing mothers are often surprised that early breast-feeding is accompanied by several distinct sensations. In the first days—and sometimes even weeks—after birth, nipple stimulation created by a breast-feeding baby causes the mother's uterus to contract. These contractions, which feel like menstrual cramps or even the beginning contractions that signal labor, are stimulated by the release of oxytocin, the powerful hormone that's also released in labor and during orgasm.

This cramping is healthy. It is a sign that your uterus is returning to its prepregnancy size. It is also a great illustration of the complex, interconnected way our bodies work. Breast-feeding stimulates the release of oxytocin, which leads to "let-down," when the breast contracts and a rush of milk flows out of the nipple. Let-down may be accompanied by a tingling sensation in the breasts that some of us start to feel a few weeks after we start breast-feeding regularly. Sometimes the nursing baby may pause or even choke momentarily before adapting to the fast flow of milk.

At the beginning, I had contractions every time he nursed, and I kept having them a bit longer than I expected. . . . They were really strong. He would suck, and I'd get this crampy contraction. Once I got used to it, I kind of liked it. It was like our bodies were working together like they did when he was growing inside me. It felt satisfying, like things were working the way they're supposed to.

The hormone oxytocin contributes to the feelings of intense closeness and bonding that mothers who breast-feed often describe experiencing after nursing.

FEEDING YOURSELF WHILE FEEDING YOUR BABY

While adjusting to breast-feeding, be good to yourself. Try to get as much rest as possible, sleeping or resting when the baby sleeps. Drink plenty of water. Eat lots of healthy food. Don't worry about picking up around the house or making elaborate meals. Ask friends and family to help out. Many mothers need to return to work not long after our babies are born, but if your job offers any maternity leave at all, take as much as you can.

Just as when you were pregnant, when you are nursing, you are not the only one who is "eating" what you put in your body. Many of the nutrients—and, unfortunately, the chemicals—contained in a mother's food, drink, and medicine can be passed on to her infant during breast-feeding.

There are no specific foods to avoid while nursing. Smoking while breast-feeding is not

---

RESOURCES ON MEDICATIONS AND BREAST-FEEDING

If a doctor suggests that you take medication while you are breast-feeding, learn as much as you can about the effects of the medication on breast-feeding mothers and babies. Talk with your maternity care provider, a lactation specialist, or your local La Leche League leader. Read the drug package insert, available from your pharmacy or on the Internet at www.fda.gov/cder. (The insert will tell you about rare adverse effects that some people have experienced.)

The best source of information is the book *Medications and Mothers' Milk* by Dr. Thomas Hale. Ask your provider if she or he has a copy, or look in your local library. The book is also available online for a fee at www.ibreastfeeding.com. Another excellent resource is LactMed (http://toxnet.nlm.nih.gov/lactmed), a free online database of research on the effects of different drugs on breast-feeding.

advised, but if you are a smoker, breast-feeding is still more beneficial for your baby than formula feeding. (If possible, avoid smoking inside your home, so that your baby will be exposed to less secondhand smoke.) Alcohol and many illegal drugs pass through a mother's milk and affect the baby. The risks of this vary by the type of drug and are not always fully understood. It is best to be cautious and not use illegal drugs or drink alcohol to the point of intoxication.

Although many over-the-counter and prescribed medicines and medicinal herbs are compatible with breast-feeding, they do pass into the breast milk in small amounts. Some prescription drugs have been proven to be unsafe for use while breast-feeding; for many others, the safety is unknown.

When I was nursing him I was ravenous. I could not get enough food in my body from the moment he arrived until probably six months into nursing, and I nursed for thirteen months. It was insane, it was just constant, it was wanting good healthy food, which is really unusual for me. I wanted apples and pears and water and good sandwiches and things like that, not the typical junk.

If it is difficult for you to afford nutritious food, WIC, the Special Supplemental Program for Women, Infants, and Children, can help. This federal program provides milk, fruit, cereal, juice, cheese, beans, peanut butter, and eggs to low- and moderate-income women and our children up to age five. WIC also provides education and support for breast-feeding women. The program may be housed in your local health department, school, or free clinic. For more information, see www.fns.usda.gov/wic. This website lists each state agency's 800 phone number. If you do not have Internet access, you can look in your phone book.

CHALLENGES TO BREAST-FEEDING

SORE NIPPLES

It started well for me—the baby latched on right away and sucked well—but then I got a cracked nipple and it was incredibly painful every time he nursed. And then the milk got stuck in some of the ducts in that same breast. So I needed him to nurse more on that side to get the milk moving, but every time he latched on it felt as if someone had set fire to my nipple. It took six weeks to get through all that. I didn't think I'd make it, but luckily I had a lot of support from my husband, my family, the midwives, and the lactation nurse at the clinic.

Some mothers complain of sore nipples for the first days or weeks—and some *limited* discomfort or tenderness is normal. But if you experience severe pain, or cracked or bleeding nipples, consult with a health care professional or lactation specialist immediately. These can be signs of an incorrect latch or of something more serious, such as an infection, that should be treated promptly.

The most common cause of nipple soreness is a poor latch. Your baby may be getting milk by "chewing" on the tip of the nipple, rather than opening wide and compressing as much of the areola as possible. If you have pain in the nipple with every suck, take the baby off the breast and reposition so that your nipple gets farther back in your baby's mouth.

Another cause of nipple soreness is a yeast infection commonly known as "thrush." Thrush is caused when an infection in the baby's mouth spreads to the mother's nipples. A newborn can get thrush if the mother had a vaginal yeast infection when giving birth, or if the mother was treated with antibiotics after the birth. A thrush infection can make a woman's nipples itchy, red, swollen, tender, and sometimes cracked. Many mothers with thrush complain of a severe burning or "cut-glass" sensation while nursing. If your baby has thrush, you may see white, cheesy patches on the inside of the baby's mouth that do not come off if you wipe them with a soft cloth or your finger. Yeast overgrowth can be easily treated with the prescription antibiotic nystatin. If nystatin treatment is not effective, other oral antifungal treatments are used. Check with your pediatric and obstetric care providers for diagnosis and treatment of this problem. It is important that both you and your baby receive treatment; otherwise you can pass the yeast infection back and forth between you.

Using plastic-backed nursing pads can also cause sore or infected nipples. When you are not nursing, your nipples should be kept as dry as possible, and these pads, which are used to keep breast milk from leaking onto your clothes, can also keep your nipples too damp and warm, and thereby encourage infection. Leaky nipples are common during the first few months of nursing. If you want to keep your clothes dry while keeping your nipples healthy, make a point of purchasing nursing pads without plastic liners or backing. If possible, let your nipples air-dry after nursing and then use a cotton breast pad inside of an appropriately fitted nursing bra. Avoid using a drying agent— such as soap or alcohol or some other antibacterial product—on the nipples.

Another cause of sore nipples, after the first month, may be some other infection (see "Mastitis," page 266).

ENGORGEMENT

Engorgement is a state of overfullness in the breast that is accompanied by extreme swelling, redness or shininess of the skin, increased temperature of the breast, and marked discomfort when the breast is moved or touched. Engorge-

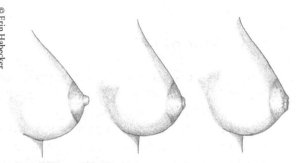

© Erin Habecker

The shape of your nipples may affect breast-feeding, but should not prevent it. If you have flat or inverted nipples (middle and right illustrations, respectively), you may need expert assistance in the early days to help your baby to latch and to make sure that the baby is receiving an adequate amount of milk. You may want to consult with a lactation specialist.

ment may occur in the first few days when your milk comes in, when extra fluid, blood, and lymph flow to the breast to provide raw material for milk making. Normally, this initial engorgement goes away after two to three days. Your breasts will continue to produce milk and may feel fuller as you get farther from your last feeding, but they will be soft and not painful.

Engorgement can also occur after nursing is established. Engorgement can happen when the baby is not removing enough milk. In addition, it can happen whenever feedings are regularly missed, including after mothers return to work or school or at holiday times or other events when schedules are disrupted. When breasts become *extremely* engorged, a woman's nipples can flatten out, making it hard for the baby to latch successfully for a day or two. The baby may suck just on the end of the nipple, causing nipple soreness.

If your areola is very hard and firm, you may want to express milk manually until your areola softens so that it is easier for your baby to latch on. Soaking your breasts in a basin of warm water may help your milk to flow. Cool compresses or cool packs (wrapped in a dish-

WHO CAN HELP?

If you face breast-feeding challenges such as latch difficulties, breast infections, or low milk supply, your health care provider (midwife, pediatrician, or ob-gyn) may be able to answer your questions.

For more specialized assistance, La Leche League is another resource, with more than three thousand groups in at least sixty countries. It holds local meetings that are free, providing information and support for all women who want to breast-feed. For more information, visit www.lalecheleague.org or call 1-800-LALECHE (1-800-525-3243) or 847-519-7730. The last phone number provides access to an automated system for finding leaders in the United States by entering a local zip code.

Another option is to ask your hospital or provider to connect you with a certified lactation consultant or counselor. The most experienced lactation consultants will likely have the credential IBCLC (Internationally Board Certified Lactation Consultant). To find a qualified lactation consultant on your own, visit www.ilca.org or call 919-861-5577.

For advice by phone, you can call the National Women's Health Information Center, which has breast-feeding peer counselors who are trained by La Leche League International and fluent in English and Spanish. These counselors can help you with common breast-feeding questions on issues ranging from nursing positions to pumping and storage. You can reach the Breastfeeding Helpline at 1-800-994-9662, Monday through Friday from 9 A.M. to 6 P.M. EST. If you call after hours, you can leave a message, and a peer counselor will return your call on the next business day.

cloth) may provide comfort before and after nursing. Having the baby nurse as often as she or he wants to is the best way to treat engorgement. Pumping your engorged breasts may overstimulate them and cause your body to make more milk than is needed. If you are engorged, keep your breasts comfortably supported, use cool packs for comfort, and let the baby breast-feed so that she or he determines how much milk your breasts need to make.

MASTITIS (BREAST INFLAMMATION)

Some nursing mothers develop mastitis, an inflammation in the breast. Inflammation is the body's response to infection, irritation, or trauma. Symptoms of inflammation include redness, heat, swelling, and pain in the affected area. Breast-feeding mothers may develop mastitis because of infection in the tissue of the breast, or just from the presence of milk in the tissue outside the milk-making cells. Noninfective mastitis may occur when milk is not being removed often enough from an area of the breast, increasing pressure in that area. Mastitis generally occurs in the first twelve weeks of breast-feeding, but may occur at any time. Anemia, a cracked nipple, or a plugged milk duct may be a contributing factor. Other factors that can increase the risk of mastitis include a too-tight bra, a skipped feeding or two, or infrequent changing of wet and/or plastic-backed breast pads.

It is important to distinguish between a plugged duct, mastitis, and an abscess (a local pocket of pus). A red, sore, or possibly even swollen spot on your breast may signify a plugged milk duct. To clear the blockage, try to gently massage the area while nursing, nurse frequently from that breast, and start each feeding from that breast. Apply moist heat to the area. Changing the infant's positions for feedings may also help drain the area more effectively.

If the blockage does not clear, you may develop mastitis. A full-blown case of mastitis feels like a bad case of the flu. You will be achy, feverish, and shivery. (Even if you don't feel hot, check your temperature; with mastitis, your temperature may be over 100 degrees Fahrenheit.) You may be tired and sore, and not feel the least bit like breastfeeding, but whatever you do, ***don't stop***. You've still got to keep your breasts draining or the mastitis could advance to a breast *abscess*, a rare but serious condition that can require surgical drainage.

If you think you have mastitis, contact your health care provider immediately. You will likely need antibiotics, which can be taken safely by nursing mothers. Your health care provider may also recommend a nonsteroidal anti-inflammatory medication, which is also considered safe when you are breast-feeding. While mastitis symptoms are present, try massaging your affected breast and changing nursing positions to more effectively drain your breasts. Also get plenty of rest and plenty to drink. You should start to feel better within twenty-four hours. If you are not starting to feel better, you still have a temperature, or you are feeling worse after three to four doses of an antibiotic, call your health care provider.

In rare cases, you may develop an abscess without having any symptoms of an infection.

If you have a hard, painful lump in your breast that doesn't go away during nursing, check with your health care provider. An ultrasound can diagnose a breast abscess.

LOW MILK SUPPLY

While the majority of mothers produce enough breast milk to feed our babies, a small percentage do not. For a mother who planned on nursing her child, finding that the milk she produces is insufficient can be distressing.

Concerns about possible low milk supply usually arise several days after birth, if a baby has lost a significant percentage of her or his birth weight and has soiled or wet only a few diapers. In many cases, the cause of this "failure to thrive" may actually be poor latch or some other common breast-feeding difficulty.

But in rare cases, low milk supply is caused by *polycystic ovary syndrome*, by *hypoplastic breasts* (breasts that show insufficient development of glandular, or "milk-producing," tissue), or by the effects of previous breast surgery (see below). In addition, certain kinds of birth control pills can affect milk production. Because they can reduce milk production, oral estrogens should be avoided in at least the first six months of a breast-feeding baby's life. Progestin-only birth control pills can be used by breast-feeding mothers, but it is recommended that they are started only after the milk supply is well established and adequate in volume (usually three to four weeks after the birth). (For more information about birth control, see pages 268 and 296.)

Breast Surgery

Women who have undergone surgery to decrease or increase the size of our breasts sometimes experience reduced milk supply. This is because surgical techniques commonly used to alter the appearance of the breast can sever nerves and milk ducts. If you have had either breast reduction or breast augmentation and an incision was made around the areola, the milk ducts and nerves may be affected. Although most women are able to breast-feed after such surgery, you may not be able to produce a full milk supply. Any incisions on the breast can reduce the chances of successful breast-feeding; incisions around or across the areola are believed to be most likely to cause these problems. Implants can press on the milk-making cells, and this can also reduce milk supply. One resource for women regarding breast-feeding after breast surgery can be found at www.breastimplantinfo.org/augment _4faq2.html.

A mother who has had a mastectomy can nurse from the unaffected breast, and with frequent feedings may be able to breast-feed exclusively. Direct radiation to the breast for treatment of cancer may decrease the amount of milk produced by that breast.

BREAST-FEEDING AS BIRTH CONTROL

Regular breast-feeding inhibits ovulation and will delay the return of your period. Most women who are breast-feeding will resume menstruation between three months and two years after giving birth.[12] However, the fact that you aren't menstruating doesn't mean you can't conceive. It's possible to get pregnant before your period resumes, as you may ovulate before menstruating.

In certain circumstances, breast-feeding can be an effective form of birth control. A method known as the *lactational amenorrhea method* (LAM) can reduce your likelihood of pregnancy to 2 percent or less. You can practice LAM if you meet the following three criteria:

1. Your period hasn't returned since childbirth. Any vaginal bleeding before the fifty-sixth day after birth is almost always *anovulatory* (meaning that no egg has been released) and can be ignored. After the fifty-sixth day, any two days of consecutive bleeding should be considered a sign of resumed ovulation.

2. You are fully breast-feeding day and night (with no pacifiers or bottles). "Fully breast-feeding" means that you are not giving your baby any supplemental feeding. (If you are supplementing only on rare occasions, LAM can also be effective.)* The frequency of the baby's feedings are also important: She or he needs to be feeding at least every four hours during the day and at least every six hours at night. The shorter the intervals between feedings, the more likely it is that you will not be able to conceive. It is not clear if pumping or manually expressing the milk provides as much protection as breast-feeding.

3. Your baby is under six months old.[13]

LAM is unreliable once your period returns, if your breast-feeding is not regular, or if your baby is six months old (or older). If you do not meet the LAM criteria, it is best to use another method of birth control. (For more information about birth control, see page 296.)

* LAM is effective if you are "nearly fully" or "almost exclusively" breast-feeding. This means that your baby is receiving no more than 1 ounce per week of vitamins, minerals, water, juice, or other supplement in month one; no more than 2 ounces per week in month two; and no more than 3 ounces per week in month three.

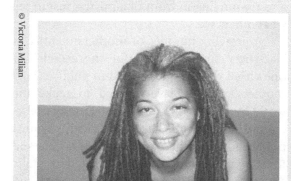

© Victoria Milian

"Any problems I had with nursing were all cultural."

Sharis Ingram

Choosing to breast-feed was the best decision I made for my family, but I didn't realize at the time how radical this was for a U.S.-born African-American woman.

I chose to do it because my mother and stepmother both breast-fed my much younger siblings. Most black women of my generation do not have experience with breast-feeding. We have not done it, and we have never seen it done. It is often stigmatized and associated with being "too poor to afford formula." Even when we're made aware of breast-feeding's benefits, our need to work outside of the home for extended hours prevents many of us from seeing it as a truly viable option.

I was fortunate that both my kids took to nursing immediately. It took a few minutes to work out how to get them to latch on properly and that was it. Any problems I had with nursing were all cultural. While I got a lot of support from my immediate family, from the surrounding culture I got very little. I can count on two hands the number of black women I know who breast-fed their kids, and still have a few fingers left over.

I found it very hard to be the one mother in my neighborhood who was nursing openly. When I did nurse in public, I got some strange looks and even the occasional negative comment. I once saw a woman in my neighborhood wearing a nursing shirt and was torn between wanting to go introduce myself as a fellow nursing mother and worrying that she'd think I was a stalker. Beyond my family, it was the men and women of my grandmother's generation who were the most kind and supportive of breast-feeding.

I found wearing nursing shirts helpful. The less skin that shows, the less likely people will figure out what you're doing, and if they do, the less likely you'll have a negative confrontation. I bought some nursing shirts, and also made some by cutting holes in stretchy undershirts, so that I could lift up my top layer and keep my belly covered.

With my second child, I no longer even think about it. I have nursed him everywhere, in the supermarket, on the subway or bus, at the playground, and I never think twice about it. Feeding babies should be unremarkable, no matter how it's done.

BREAST-FEEDING IN PUBLIC

Many mothers breast-feed our babies wherever we are. But in the United States and some other Western countries, cultural taboos and the sexualization of the female breast sometimes make women feel uncomfortable with nursing in public. Some of us nurse our babies at home or in seclusion, away from the prying or judgmental eyes of strangers. Others of us nurse in public but occasionally encounter resistance from people who see us.

In other parts of the world, it is not at all unusual to see a woman breast-feeding her child on the bus or in a park. If you nurse only in private, you may feel that breast-feeding limits your freedom. Because of this, you might wean earlier than mothers who nurse in public.

Part of becoming comfortable with public nursing is trying it out. Specially designed nursing clothes now make it easier to breast-feed discreetly, if discretion is your goal. You can also try nursing in front of a mirror, just to see what others see.

A growing number of mothers identify as "lactivists" and advocate for the exercise of one's legal right to breast-feed in public. Many mothers' groups have formed to make the world more accepting for breast-feeding mothers and babies. Some have filed lawsuits against public facilities where women have been asked to stop nursing and have participated in public "nurse-in" protests against coffee shops and restaurant chains with restrictive breast-feeding policies.

EXPRESSING AND STORING MILK

Many women express or pump breast milk sometimes, for a number of reasons. Pumping or expressing can make it possible for your

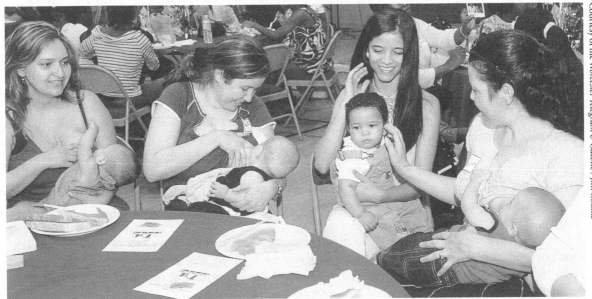

Courtesy of the Worcester Telegram & Gazette / Jim Collins

Several mothers and babies celebrate the sixth birthday of the Worcester (Massachusetts) Healthy Start Initiative. The Initiative receives federal funding to promote community-based programs for uninsured and low-income women and their babies.

HOW TO CHOOSE A BREAST PUMP

The two basic types of pumps are hand pumps and electric pumps. To decide which type of breast pump to use, it can be helpful to think about when and why you will be pumping. If you will mostly be with your baby and you just need to pump once or twice a week, hand-expressing your milk or using a hand pump will likely be sufficient. If you are regularly going to be apart from your baby for lengthy periods of time, you will likely want an electric pump.

Electric pumps vary by how portable they are, how much noise they make, how easy they are to use, and how efficient they are. They generally cost $200 to $300 and can sometimes be rented. Pumps that allow you to pump both breasts at the same time are the most efficient and the most expensive. If your baby is premature and unable to breast-feed yet, or if you are pumping to increase your milk supply, look for a rental-grade pump. Insurance often covers pump rental for mothers of sick or premature babies, although you may need a letter from the baby's physician to secure coverage. If you are on the WIC program, your nutritionist may be able to obtain a rental pump for you free of charge.

With the exception of rental-grade pumps, pumps are not meant to be loaned or shared between women, or purchased secondhand. It is possible for a pump to be contaminated with bacteria deep within the motor. For this reason, it is crucial to obtain a new pump, and to obtain and use your own breast-pump kit if you are using a rental-grade pump.

partner or another family member to take over nighttime or early morning feedings so that you can sleep, and is also a way for your baby to drink breast milk when you are at work or away.

While you are still in the hospital, a nurse or lactation specialist should coach you in how to express your milk by hand. Knowing this simple skill can help you remove milk whenever you need to, whether you have a pump or not. To hand-express milk, all you need is a clean bowl or other container and clean hands. You may want to begin by massaging your breasts gently, then stroking down the breast toward the nipple. Then, place your thumb on the areola an inch or so above your nipple and cup your breast with the remaining fingers under the nipple. Place the bowl on your lap, under your breast. Gently squeeze your thumb and fingers toward each other, while pulling back toward your chest wall. You may begin to see droplets of milk collecting on your nipple and dripping down your breast. When the droplets stop appearing, turn your hand so that you are compressing a different part of the breast. With practice, you will begin to collect streams of milk from the nipple. Many of us become adept at hand-expressing both breasts at the same time. For some of us, it is easiest to learn to express while taking a warm shower.

Hand-expression works very well for many women and not well for others. If hand-expressing does not work well for your circumstances, you might want to use a manual hand pump or an electric pump. (For more information see "How to Choose a Breast Pump," page 271.) Most women find it takes practice to collect milk quickly with any milk-expression technique.

Chill or refrigerate the milk as soon as you can after it is expressed. Human milk can be stored at room temperature for up to six hours (although it's best to keep it refrigerated as much as possible), in a refrigerator for up to three days, and in a freezer compartment with a separate door for up to three to four months. (If you have a separate freezer, where the temperature will not be too variable because the door will not be opened often, you can safely store breast milk in it for about six months.)

(For information on feeding breast milk to your baby from a bottle, see "How to Bottle-Feed," page 276.)

BREAST-FEEDING AND WORK

If you return to work after your baby is born, you can continue breast-feeding. Unless you work at home or have on-site day care in your workplace and can take breaks to breast-feed your baby, you will likely need to express your breast milk, store it, and then have your child's caregiver feed the child your milk from a bottle. Many mothers have continued producing breast milk for months—even years—after returning to paid employment.

It will be easier to continue breast-feeding if you have a breast pump as well as a workplace that provides you with a private, clean space and time for pumping. In some states, large employers are required to make these provisions for their workers. In others, it may be up to your employer's goodwill. If you want to pump breast milk after returning to work, it might be worthwhile to discuss your feeding plans with your employer prior to your mater-

nity leave. Many employers are eager to retain their employees, and may be able to help you work out a plan for breaks for pumping. When you return to work, breast-feed your child before leaving home each day and try to take two or three pumping breaks during an eight-hour workday. When you are reunited with your child after work, nurse frequently to maintain your milk supply.

About seven in every ten employed mothers with children younger than three years old work full-time. One-third of these mothers return to work within three months after childbirth and two-thirds return within six months.[14] Many workplaces and jobs are not amenable to pumping and continued breast-feeding. Mothers who are paid hourly to work in fast-food restaurants, in stores, or on assembly lines—disproportionately African-American and Hispanic—aren't often provided with lactation rooms or paid pumping breaks. Women who work in salaried positions are more likely to have such benefits. This division establishes a group of women who can afford to breast-feed beyond the first weeks and another group who cannot.

Our government needs to create more extensive family leave options and to encourage workplace support for breast-feeding mothers. In the United States, some states and municipalities have enacted legislation that requires large employers to establish breast-feeding-friendly work policies. Such polices should be enacted on a national level. (For more information, see Chapter 18, "Advocating for Mothers and Children.")

FORMULA FEEDING

I felt like I was cut loose from the system way before I was ready. I was discharged before my milk had even come in. Some of the people who

SUPPLEMENTING

Breast-feeding works on the principle that the more milk your baby (or a breast pump) effectively removes from your breast, the more milk you will make. If you give your baby formula as a supplement, your baby will typically nurse less, and as a result your body will produce less milk. If you stop producing enough for your baby, feeding with formula will become a necessity and your baby may be weaned prematurely. Therefore, caution is advised when considering supplementing your own breast milk with formula.

Supplementing temporarily may be advisable for an infant's health, if the baby is born very prematurely, experiences weight loss of over 10 percent, has low blood sugar, or has unusually high levels of bilirubin (a breakdown product of extra red blood cells that causes jaundice, a yellowing of the skin and the whites of the eyes).

You can supplement your own milk with banked human milk or with formula. The supplemental "milk" can be offered in bottles or at the breast with the aid of a supplemental nursing system, a device available through lactation consultants and health care professionals. If you feed supplementary formula in a bottle to an otherwise breast-fed baby, it is often easier to have someone other than you offer the bottle. The baby may prefer breast milk, and may want to nurse if she or he is with you. This can be a great opportunity for a partner, grandparent, or friend to feed the baby. (For more information on bottle-feeding, see page 276.)

Hospitals can acquire human milk for your baby by prescription. State-licensed and Human Milk Bank of North America–member milk banks follow a protocol that includes prescreening breast-feeding mothers who donate and ensuring the safety of donated milk by running bacteriologic tests and pasteurizing or otherwise heat-treating accepted milk. Pastuerized donor milk is expensive—as much as $4 an ounce—and it usually goes to premature infants but occasionally is also provided to adoptive parents and mothers with supply problems. It is not considered safe to acquire milk from other sources, including the Internet and friends and acquaintances, because the milk can contain infectious properties of which we are not aware. (The Human Milk Banking Association of North American provides more information on its website, www.hmbana.org.)

trained me at the hospital had not even nursed [their children] themselves. I felt like each individual tried her best, but it never came together for me. He never latched correctly. I never produced much milk. After a few days it felt like time was ticking away and my baby wasn't getting enough to eat. When I finally made the de-cision to say "I'm done with this. We're going to give you some formula," it was a huge relief. I felt like I could finally start trying to enjoy this new life.

For a number of reasons, not all mothers can breast-feed or choose to do so. If you will not be nursing your baby, you can use a variety of formulas. Formula is an acceptable alternative to human milk, although it does not have all the benefits. (For more information, see "Choosing a Formula," below.)

Infants cannot drink cow's milk or other animal milk as a replacement for human milk or formula because their digestive systems cannot process it in large amounts. Aside from the occasional taste of yogurt or cheese after four to six months, your baby should not be drinking animal milk until the age of at least twelve months.

In the not-so-distant past, many nursing mothers felt like they were singled out for choosing to breast-feed their children. Now that health care providers and government officials are touting the benefits of breast milk, many formula-feeding mothers feel that we are judged each time we feed our babies from a bottle.

There was always an assumption that I was going to breast-feed, and every time I pulled out the bottle, I always felt like I had to explain myself. People assume that everyone can nurse their babies. But not everyone can. I don't want to be judged for that.

CHOOSING A FORMULA

Infant formula is sold under different brand names and can be purchased in most large grocery stores and drugstores. Typically, there are only minor differences between standard formulas made by different companies. Unless your infant has a health problem, you may feed her or him any of the commercially available formulas.

All formula is made from either modified cow's milk or soy products, with additional nutrients added. (Because soy milk and cow's milk are not appropriate foods for human newborns, they are altered when used in formula to make them safer for babies.) Some formulas are modified to feed babies with special needs, such as premature babies or infants sensitive to cow's-milk protein.

Soy formula gained popularity in the 1990s because of concerns about allergies to cow's-milk protein. But babies can be intolerant of soy protein as well. If your family has a sensitivity to cow's milk or soy products, consult with your pediatric care provider to choose the formula that is best for your baby.

Some concerns have been raised about soy formula causing reproductive or thyroid problems because it contains isoflavones that are similar to female hormones. But no research has found short-term or long-term differences in growth or in frequency of illness in babies who are fed cow's-milk formula when compared with those who are fed soy formula.[15] There is no known advantage of soy formula over other formula, except for kosher and/or vegan families that want a formula without cow's milk.

Most formula is fortified with iron to prevent childhood anemia. Iron is an important nutrient for formula-fed babies. The added iron may make the baby's stool darker and also drier, leading to difficult bowel movements. If you think your baby may be having difficulty digesting the extra iron in formula, discuss this with your pediatric care provider. You may also want to talk with your pediatric care provider about your baby's iron status and whether iron-fortified formula is right for your child.

Recently, formula companies have begun adding *long-chain polyunsaturated fats* to formula. The companies claim that these fats (which are present in human milk) will increase visual development and intelligence in children who consume them. There is little evidence that the supplements added to formula are effective. Breast-fed babies score higher on all measurements of visual acuity (sharpness) and indicators of intelligence than babies who receive these formulas.[16] The same companies are now marketing the fats for use by pregnant and nursing women, again with little evidence that using these supplements has positive effects on the baby. It is wise for pregnant and nursing mothers to consume foods containing these fats (including cold-water fish, meat, and eggs).

Powder, Concentrate, or Ready-to-Feed?

Formula comes in three forms: ready-to-feed, concentrated, and powder. These differ in cost and preparation. It's important to mix any type of formula properly so that your baby gets the right nutrients. Do not dilute formula to make it last longer, as this can lead to malnutrition for your baby. When choosing formula to buy, examine cans or bottles for seal, expiration date, broken packaging, and defects.

The least expensive form of formula is *powder*. A measured amount of the powder is mixed with two ounces of boiled water for feeding. You can mix one bottle at a time or several and keep the additional bottles in the refrigerator. It is important to mix the powder in the proportions indicated on the can. Powdered formula is not sterile. Once you mix up a bottle, it should be refrigerated. Clean the scoop or measuring spoon carefully before returning it to the can of formula.

A more expensive type of formula is *concentrate*, which comes in a can and must be mixed with equal parts of boiled water. It is very concentrated and is not the same as ready-to-feed, though the two look alike. If used undiluted (that is, not mixed with water), concentrated formula puts stress on the baby's kidneys and digestive system and can lead to kidney or digestive problems. Once you have added water, refrigerate the bottle to slow bacteria growth.

The most expensive type of formula is *ready-to-feed*. You can get ready-to-feed formula in bottles; it is already prepared and needs only a nipple and warming. Ready-to-feed also comes in cans, which usually hold a twenty-four-hour supply and can simply be poured into a bottle, warmed, and given to the infant. Once opened, cans should be refrigerated.

Avoiding Excess Fluoride

The American Dental Association recommends that parents avoid using fluoridated water when reconstituting infant formula, because excessive fluoride exposure may affect babies' teeth as they are developing.[17] Fluoride intake above recommended levels during early childhood increases the chance of *dental fluorosis* (problems with the formation of tooth enamel). In the United States, fluorosis is generally a cosmetic condition that consists of white lines or spots on the teeth. Most people do not notice mild fluorosis.

Natural fluoride levels in water vary. Many communities increase the level of fluoride in drinking-water supplies to prevent tooth decay. You can ask your health care provider or local board of health if your community's water is fluoridated to the recommended level of about one part fluoride per one million parts water (1 ppm). Bottled fluoridated water is marketed as good for the teeth, but should not be used for infants.

To avoid excess fluoride intake by babies up to twelve months old who get most of their nutrition from formula, the dental association recommends either choosing ready-to-feed formula that does not need to be mixed with water or mixing liquid or powder concentrated formula with water that is fluoride free or low in fluoride. Acceptable water includes drinking water that is labeled "purified," "demineralized," "deionized," "distilled," or "reverse osmosis filtered."

HOW MUCH AND HOW OFTEN?

A newborn's stomach at birth is about the size of a large marble, and over the first weeks it will grow to the size of a Ping-Pong ball. A newborn is not able to drink large amounts of liquid, but rather to drink small amounts frequently. It is important to respond to the infant's cues that she or he is satisfied and not "force-feed" a specific amount just because it is in the bottle. Overfilling a baby's stomach can cause the baby to throw up.

Formula feedings may be as much as three to four hours apart. This is less often than early breast-feeding, because it takes longer for a baby to digest formula than to digest breast milk.

Infants who are getting enough formula and are well hydrated will sleep after feeding, in most cases. Your baby's lips, tongue, and mouth should be moist. Urine should be a very light yellow and smell like ammonia. Another sign of good hydration is that your baby wets a diaper six times a day (although this is not always easy to see, especially if feces is mixed with the urine). If a diaper is dark yellow or looks like it is coated with "brick dust," these are signs that the baby is not hydrated well enough. The feces of formula-fed infants are less watery than those of breast-fed infants, but should not be hard to pass. The color will progress from dark green, in the first day or two, to yellow, and then to the familiar brownish color.

FORMULA MARKETING

When you are given formula by a doctor or nurse, you might think it has been selected because it is of better quality than other brands. After leaving the hospital, you might keep on buying the same product, believing that it must be the best, or at least knowing that it is familiar and has worked for you so far.

Formula companies count on—and profit by—just such thinking. Companies provide hospitals with free formula in order to increase brand recognition and influence new mothers' choice of formula. (Hospitals generally have rotating contracts, so they give out different company brands at different times.) Similarly, the Special Supplemental Program for Women, Infants, and Children (WIC) also gets formula through contractual agreements with the companies, which provide rebates to WIC as financial incentives. (WIC uses the rebate money to fund breast-feeding promotion programs.) Women are most likely to continue using whichever brand the hospital or other facility provides. Hospitals provide ready-to-feed formula in small bottles, which is the most expensive form to purchase no matter what brand you use.

Other marketing campaigns also try to influence parents' choices. The media are saturated with ads about infant formula, and baby magazines sign parents up to receive "gift" supplies of formula when the baby is born. However, as noted earlier, there is little difference between standard formulas made by different companies.

BOTTLE-FEEDING BREAST MILK OR FORMULA

CHOOSING THE RIGHT BOTTLE

Bottle and nipple options are available in a dizzying array in most stores. Before your baby is born, you may want to research different products and ask other mothers for their opinions. Ahead of time, purchase a few small bottles and newborn-size nipples, but once your baby is born, make sure to observe her or his feeding patterns closely. Does your baby have a hard time getting milk from one kind of nipple, or seem fussy or gassy after feedings? Many babies show a preference for one kind of bottle or nipple.

It is important to keep feeding supplies clean. Wash all bottles, nipples, and nipple rings well with soap and hot water, cleaning inside the nipples with a nipple brush. Bottles also can be sterilized in the top rack of a dishwasher or in boiling water, but this is not considered necessary.

HOW TO BOTTLE-FEED

Formula or breast milk should be warmed to room temperature before being offered to your baby. The best way to do this is to fill a pot or bowl with hot water and let the bottle stand in the water until it is at room temperature, shaking it periodically to disperse the warmed fluid evenly. Microwaving infant formula is not recommended. Microwaving creates pockets of steam in the mixture. Even if you shake the bottle after taking it out of the microwave, pockets of steam may remain and can burn the baby's mouth or digestive tract.

Once you've made sure that the formula or breast milk in the bottle is at a safe temperature, hold your baby close, coo, and make eye contact. You can bottle-feed your baby while holding the baby against your breast or bare skin, rocking in a chair, or sitting in bed or on a couch. It's a good idea to alternate the arm with which you hold your baby, so the baby's eyes get practice focusing on your face from both sides.

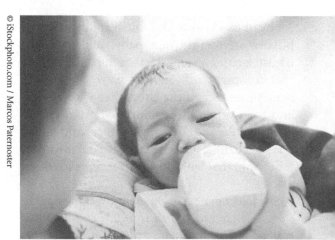

© iStockphoto.com / Marcos Paternoster

Angle the bottle so that the opening of the nipple inside the bottle is covered with formula, to prevent your baby from ingesting air. To do this, you will have to hold the bottle at increasingly high angles as the amount of liquid inside decreases. It is helpful to burp the baby after every couple of ounces, to allow the release of air that has been swallowed. If your baby seems to be gulping or struggling, try a different type of nipple on the bottle.

Avoid propping a bottle in an infant's mouth while she or he is sitting in an infant seat. A newborn cannot move away from the bottle if the liquid is coming out too fast and can choke. Leaving an infant with a bottle propped in her or his mouth for long periods of time also increases the risk of tooth decay.

Feeding is an important time for socializing with your baby. Stroke your baby and talk with her or him during feedings.

Bottles can deliver liquid faster than the breast. Therefore, if you plan to feed a breast-fed infant breast milk or supplemental formula by bottle, it is recommended that you wait until your baby is an established feeder (generally at six weeks or so) before you start.

CONCLUSION

Many of us envision childbirth ending with the blissful moment when baby, pulled to the breast, latches on and starts to nurse. Getting to that moment of mother-baby connection sometimes takes more effort than we expected, and for women in certain circumstances it is not possible. But for most mothers and babies it is the healthiest way to launch a nurturing relationship that will continue for years to come.

I now look back upon my breast-feeding days as so full of pleasure, with so much cuddling and closeness. There were also plenty of laughs during the last few months of nursing, when my almost two-and-a-half-year-old daughter began to "argue" with me—sometimes in public—about why she needed to nurse at that very moment. Friends of mine had babies who abruptly stopped nursing at nine months or one year— they just seemed to lose interest overnight. For some mothers, it was fine, but others had wanted the breast-feeding to continue. I was hoping that my daughter would just someday lose interest on her own around the age of two, but that didn't happen. So I started to wean her gradually, and she adjusted fine over a few months. But I'm sure that thoughts about nursing lingered on for years. Even at the age of five, she looked up at me one day and asked impishly, "Mommy, don't you want me to check to see if your breasts still have any milk?"

NOTES

1. S. Ip, M. Chung, G. Raman, P. Chew, N. Magula, D. DeVine, T. Trikalinos, J. Lau. "Breastfeeding and Maternal and Infant Health Outcomes in Developed Countries." Evidence Report/TechnologyAssessment No. 153 (Prepared by Tufts-New England Medical Center Evidence-based Practice Center, under Contract No. 290-02-0022). AHRQ Publication No. 07-E007. Rockville, MD: Agency for Healthcare Research and Quality. April 2007.
2. S. Ip, M. Chung, G. Raman, P. Chew, N. Magula, D. DeVine, T. Trikalinos, J. Lau. "Breastfeeding and Maternal and Infant Health Outcomes in Developed Countries." Evidence Report/TechnologyAssessment No. 153 (Prepared by Tufts-New England Medical Center Evidence-based Practice Center, under Contract No. 290-02-0022). AHRQ Publication No. 07-E007. Rockville, MD: Agency for Healthcare Research and Quality. April 2007.
3. L. M. Gartner, J. Morton, et al. American Academy of Pediatrics Section on Breastfeeding, "Breastfeeding and the Use of Human Milk," *Pediatrics* 115, no. 2 (February 2005): 496–506; accessed at http://aappolicy.aappublications.org/cgi/content/full/pediatrics;115/2/496.

4. Michael S. Kramer and Ritsuko Kakuma, "The Optimal Duration of Exclusive Breastfeeding: A Systematic Review," World Health Organization (2002), accessed on January 30, 2007 at www.who.int/nutrition/publications/optimal_duration_of_exc_bfeeding_review_eng.pdf.

5. Gartner et al., "Breastfeeding and the Use of Human Milk," accessed at http://aappolicy.aappublications.org/cgi/content/full/pediatrics;115/2/496.

6. J. Mercer, D. A. Erickson-Owens, B. Graves, and M. Mumford Haley, "Evidence-Based Practices for the Fetal to Newborn Transition," *Journal of Midwifery & Women's Health* 52, no. 3 (May–June 2007): 262–272.

7. Ross Mothers Survey, "Breastfeeding Trends Through 2000," Ross Products Division, Abbott Laboratories, accessed at www.ross.com/aboutross/survey.pdf on January 30, 2007.

8. Centers for Disease Control and Prevention, "Table 3: Any and Exclusive Breastfeeding Rates by Age, 2005," accessed at www.cdc.gov/breastfeeding/data/NIS_data/2005/age.htm on February 22, 2007.

9. Tanya M. Phares, Brian Morrow, Amy Lansky, Wanda D. Barfield, Cheryl B. Prince, et al., "Surveillance for Disparities in Maternal Health-Related Behaviors—Selected States, Pregnancy Risk Assessment Monitoring System (PRAMS), 2000–2001," U.S. Department of Health and Human Services, Centers for Disease Control and Prevention; accessed on February 1, 2007 at www.cdc.gov/mmwR/preview/mmwrhtml/ss5304a1.htm.

10. Baby-Friendly USA, "The Ten Steps to Successful Breastfeeding," accessed at www.babyfriendlyusa.org/eng/10steps.html on February 20, 2007.

11. L. Righard and M. Alade, "Effect of Delivery Room Routines on Success of First Breast-Feed," *Lancet* 336, no. 8,723 (November 1990): 1,105–1,107.

12. G. A. Tommaselli, M. Guida, S. Palomba, et al., "Using Complete Breastfeeding and Lactational Amenorrhoea as Birth Spacing Methods," *Contraception* 6 (2000): 253–257. See also J. Ingram, L. Hunt, M. Woolridge, et al., "The Association of Progesterone, Infant Formula Use, and Pacifier Use with the Return of Menstruation in Breastfeeding Women: A Prospective Cohort Study," *European Journal of Obstetrics & Gynecology and Reproductive Biology* 114 (2004): 197–202.

13. Baylor College of Medicine, "Contraception During Breastfeeding," *The Contraception Report* 13, no. 4 (January 2003), accessed at www.contraceptiononline.org/contrareport/article01.cfm?art=231 on March 6. 2007.

14. Katherine R. Shealy, Ruowei Li, Sandra Benton-Davis, and Laurence M. Grummer-Strawn, *The CDC Guide to Breastfeeding Interventions*, U.S. Department of Health and Human Services; accessed at www.cdc.gov/breastfeeding/pdf/breastfeeding_interventions.pdf on January 29, 2007.

15. Brian L. Strom, Rita Schinnar, Ekhard E. Ziegler, Kurt T. Barnhart, Mary D. Sammel, et al., "Exposure to Soy-Based Formula in Infancy and Endocrinology and Reproductive Outcomes in Young Adulthood," *Journal of the American Medical Association* 286, no. 7 (2001): 807–814. See also Russell J. Merritt and Belinda H. Jenks, "Safety of Soy-Based Infant Formulas Containing Isoflavones: The Clinical Evidence," *Journal of Nutrition* 134 (2004): 1,220–1,224, accessed at http://jn.nutrition.org/cgi/content/full/134/5/1220S on January 25, 2007.

16. K. Simmer, "Longchain Polyunsaturated Fatty Acid Supplementation in Infants Born at Term," *Cochrane Database of Systematic Reviews* 2001, Issue 4. Art. No.: CD000376. D01: 10.1002/14651858.CD000376.

17. Stacie Crozier, "ADA Offers Interim Guidance on Infant Formula and Fluoride," American Dental Association, November 9, 2006; accessed at http://ada.org/prof/resources/pubs/adanews/adanewsarticle.asp?articleid=2212 on November 30, 2006.

CHAPTER 16

Life as a New Mother

Becoming a mother marks a profound shift in a woman's life and personal identity. The days, weeks, and months after we give birth are full of change: We are learning to care for a new baby; recovering physically; navigating shifts in our relationships with our partners, friends, and family; and figuring out who we are as mothers.

New mothers have a tremendous range of experiences. Many of us find that being a mother brings deep pleasure, intimacy, growth, and insight. Birth and breast-feeding give us a new respect for our bodies. Caring for and cuddling our babies, we discover new dimensions to loving.

All three of my postpartum experiences have been among the sweetest times of my life. I felt centered and essentially satisfied in a way I have never felt before or since. Being with my babies gave me such incredible joy.

At the same time, almost all women experience some difficulties navigating the changes new motherhood brings.

During those early weeks, sometimes I wasn't sure where the baby ended and I began. I felt that I has lost my old self and was too tired, physically and emotionally, to find her again. But I was also discovering a new part of myself that I hadn't known about before: unexpectedly intense feelings for my new baby, a resurgence of love for my mother, connection with other women. I went from despair to overwhelming feelings of tenderness, all within the space of an hour.

EARLY ADJUSTMENT

Changing the diaper of a kicking infant or breast-feeding in public is not an innate skill or the product of inner knowledge that surfaces once your baby arrives.

THE BABY BLUES

As a new mother, you may feel more vulnerable, weepy, amazed, incredulous, or scared—or you may experience all these feelings. It is normal to feel overwhelmed, irritable, anxious, emotional, or tearful, especially in the first few weeks. This may be distressing to you and those around you, but the experience of so-called baby blues is very common. The baby blues usually run their course within a week or two. However, some women feel overwhelmed, depressed, or anxious off and on throughout the first year (see "Postpartum Mood Disorders," page 286). One important way you can prepare for this volatile period is to expect it and to line up a support team (see "Getting Support," page 282).

Each is an ability that is honed through experience. Similarly, you may not fall in love with your baby instantly, but instead discover that your bond strengthens over time.

Some women find the learning curve of early motherhood easy to master; others find it challenging. Many find it a relief to hear that motherhood isn't something a person necessarily has to be good at all at once or all the time. Whether learning on the job comes easily or is more hard-won, our competence as mothers generally grows along with our babies.

During the first few months after giving birth, we learn what it means to have a baby in our lives. Our babies eat and sleep at unpredictable times, and we find ourselves "on call" around the clock. For some of us, meeting these practical demands is tough; others find the change is not as dramatic as we anticipated. One new mother, who has a disability and uses a wheelchair, says of her transition to motherhood:

I never full appreciated having a "perma-lap" [permanent lap] until my son's first year of life. We rolled daily through our neighborhood with my son tucked up against my chest on his "boppy" (nursing pillow). He could (and did) nurse any-

time, whether I was in motion or not. My past experience of living for eight months in a rehabilitation center to relearn how to navigate my "new" body twenty years before prepared me in unexpected ways for the major adjustment of life with a baby.

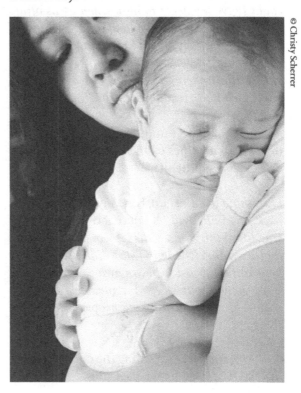

© Christy Scherrer

PHYSICAL RECOVERY

While you are adjusting to your new role as a mother, your body is recovering from the tremendous physical changes from pregnancy and birth. Typically it takes about three months (the "fourth trimester," as it is sometimes called) to recover physically. This period may be longer if you have had a particularly difficult birth or shorter if childbirth occurred without many challenges. (For detailed information, see Chapter 14, "Your Physical Recovery and Your Newborn.")

Many women find the adjustment more challenging.

I had a really hard time emotionally after the birth of my first child. He had lots of problems right after birth, and we didn't know if he would make it. I remember crying constantly. We almost lost this child that we wanted so desperately. How could I give my heart to him, when I was afraid I'd lose him? It took me a long time to let myself love him, but then I loved him so much. With my second child, it was very different. I had such an easy birth, and my daughter was a wonderful baby. I felt like a traitor to my son.

The fatigue—and sometimes despondency—that comes from sleep deprivation can be especially difficult.

I just thought, "I'm laid-back, my husband's laid-back, the baby will be laid-back." I don't know why I had this fantasy that it would just happen that way. But [the baby] just didn't sleep for so long and I was just so blown away by how hard it is to go without sleep. I remember sitting in moms' groups and thinking people are tortured this way.

Some of us, anticipating the difficulties, are instead surprised by the pleasures.

I had heard about the negatives—the fatigue, the loneliness, loss of self. But nobody told me about the wonderful parts: holding my baby close to me, seeing her first smile, watching her grow and become more responsive day by day. How can I describe the way I felt when she stroked my breast while nursing or looked into my eyes or arched her eyebrows like an opera singer? This was the deepest connection I'd felt to anybody. Sometimes the intensity almost frightened me. For the first time I cared about somebody else more than myself, and I would do anything to nurture and protect her.

How we feel in the early weeks and months of motherhood can be influenced by many factors, including our physical recovery from being pregnant and giving birth, our feelings about the birth, the health of our babies and how "easy" they are, how ready we feel to become a mother, our financial resources, the other demands we face, and the amount and kind of support we get from people around us.

GETTING SUPPORT

Flight attendants on airplanes explain that in the event of an emergency, when oxygen is needed, passengers with children should first

TIPS FOR THE FIRST WEEKS

- **Ask for help.** As much as possible, get family and friends to clean, cook, and take over your other responsibilities, so that you are free to focus on your baby and your recovery.
- **Sleep or rest when the baby sleeps.** Respecting your need to sleep and rest is one of the most important ways to recover, heal, and ease the stress of life with a newborn.
- **Nurture yourself with good food.** Eating well and staying well hydrated are important ways to recover from giving birth and have the energy to meet the demands of being a new parent.
- **Take time to relax and make time for some physical activity.** Rest and relaxation, balanced with gentle activities like talking a walk, can add to your sense of physical and emotional well-being.
- **Talk to other new mothers about your experience**—and listen to what they have to say about theirs. Hearing other people's stories can help normalize what's happening and ease isolation.
- **Remember that you have added a whole new twenty-four-hours-a-day, seven-days-a-week job to your life.** Be patient and gentle with yourself as you adjust. As you get to know your baby better and become more confident, it will get easier.

secure their own masks before fitting oxygen masks on their children. This is a lesson we can apply to the turbulence of our experience with motherhood: We cannot properly care for our children unless we are properly cared for ourselves.

As new mothers, we may focus on our babies to the exclusion of ourselves. We may feel ashamed to ask for help, or not realize that help is needed, or not even realize that asking for help is acceptable or possible. Some mothers may believe that involvement of a partner or support from family members means we aren't good enough. Our culture idealizes mothers who are eternally self-sacrificing. But help and support are crucial, and being attentive to your own needs can boost your ability to meet your child's needs.

Because I am single and have a disability, I could not and cannot get away with trying to be a supermom. I knew then and know even more clearly now that it does indeed take a village. I have relied heavily on my community of friends, some family, and a key group of child care providers. I am reminded how people enjoy being part of an emerging family, that isolation is the bane of parenthood, and that letting others help is a gift to everyone, especially the child. Asking for help has brought friends closer to me and my son in a more intimate way. I am grateful for that.

Mothering is hard work, and new mothers need many different kinds of care: practical help, emotional support, financial support, nurturing, and guidance. Unfortunately, it can be hard to find the care and community we

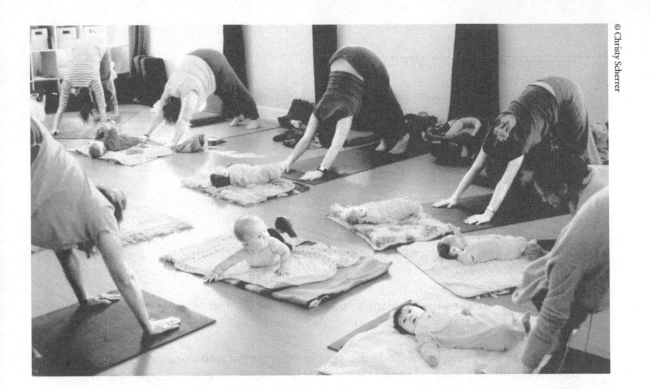

need. Our society provides little concrete help, whether in terms of paid maternity or paternity leave, subsidized child care, or other forms of support. In addition, aspects of our culture, such as families living far apart rather than in intergenerational households and neighbors often not knowing one another, make it likely that we are alone with our babies for long stretches of time. Independence and self-reliance are often prized in the United States.

This may be the first time since you were a child yourself that you need to ask for help. You may feel pressured to return to your previous life and act like nothing has happened, but the reality is that having a child is a major life shift. Acknowledge this and allow yourself to rely on others for help.

Asking for emotional support is also crucial. Loneliness and isolation can be very stressful and frightening, and in the midst of that kind of experience, our impulse may be to bur-

row farther down into it. As one mother of two put it:

My husband didn't feel like a failure when I was having trouble breast-feeding. My husband wasn't the one up all night crying hysterically. He was very supportive, but . . . the isolation that I felt postpartum actually had nothing to do with family proximity and the amount of help. It was the pure personal isolation that happens at that three-thirty-in-the-morning feeding when you're totally alone and everyone else is asleep, and you're bleeding and cramping, or in pain. It's very lonely, that place. And it's hard to even figure out what's going on for yourself, to even know what support you want.

When we feel helpless or lost or ashamed or confused, talking about what we're feeling may seem like the wrong idea. But often telling someone—your partner, a family member, a close friend, or your midwife, physician, or therapist—how you feel can help ease the stress and isolation that so often characterize new motherhood.

[My partner] was working hard all the time and feeling stressed out about his new responsibilities as sole financial provider for the family. We argued a lot. There were times when I couldn't even believe I had a baby with him! . . . I remember saying, "No one told me about all this!" to a friend, and she told me that she thought the same thing after she had her first baby. Then I realized the more I talked to other mothers, the better I felt. I was not alone! One of my friends gave me Sheila Kitzinger's book The Year After Childbirth. *I read it cover to cover. . . .*

I made a point to go over to the house of a friend who also had children a couple times a week. Getting out of the house and with other moms really helped. My partner and I started going to a really great therapist. Just taking the time to focus on our relationship felt so good. In a short time, we were communicating well again and our therapist told us that many new parents go through this. . . . If I could give one piece (or two!) of advice to a new mama, it would be to get together with other like-minded mamas often, and be patient with yourself. You are doing a great job!

WAYS TO GET SUPPORT

You can find support for yourself and your family in different ways. Many of us turn to family and friends or parenting, breast-feeding, or new-mother support groups both in our neighborhoods, cities, or towns and online. Others draw on the help of paid caregivers.

Family and Friends

Talking to your partner, your family, and close friends ahead of time about what you think you

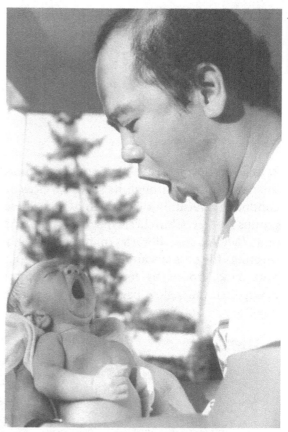

© Judith E. Halek

might need once the baby arrives helps set the stage for support. It is hard to know exactly what your needs will be, but having a support group of willing family members and friends is a good place to begin. Even if you didn't make plans in advance, turn to these people for help once the baby is born. It might also be helpful to talk with other women about what they thought was most helpful when they first became mothers.

As much as possible, ask for concrete help. Sometimes you are not even sure what you need when friends ask what they can do for you. Saying yes to small things—your partner offering to be with the baby and/or watch your other children while you sleep; friends who ask if they can bring you food, watch your kids, or clean your house—helps you to recuperate and to learn what kind of help is actually useful to you. Practicing saying yes can also help you realize when to say no—for instance, to people who offer things you don't really want or need or whose company drains you.

Parenting Support Groups

Your local hospital may offer support groups for new mothers through its social services or childbirth education department. Often these groups are free. Churches, synagogues, YWCAs and YMCAs, and libraries may host weekly meetings for mothers and new babies. You can find these groups by looking in your local newspaper, the yellow pages of the telephone directory, or online, or by asking friends, neighbors, or other new mothers. If you take a childbirth class, the instructors may have a list of community resources. Postpartum Support International offers information about the emotional adjustments that often occur in the postpartum period and can connect you with local support groups and area coordinators. You can reach them at 1-800-944-4PPD (1-800-944-4773) or 805-967-7636, and online at www.postpartum.net. La Leche League International also has local groups specifically designed to support breast-feeding mothers. You can reach them at 1-800-LALECHE (1-800-525-3243) or 847-519-7730, or visit www.lalecheleague.org.

If you have access to the Internet, there are many websites devoted exclusively to the experience of new mothers. Some sites offer online

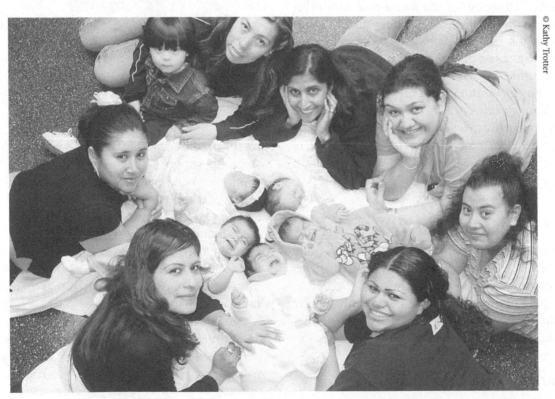

© Kathy Trotter

You may enjoy having a support group of women who are all entering motherhood at the same time that you are. Centering Pregnancy classes like this one are one way of finding such a group.

FEELINGS ABOUT THE BIRTH

We relive the births of our children many times during the days, weeks, months, and years afterward. Looking back upon your birth experience may call up a wide range of emotions. You may feel fulfilled, ecstatic, and immensely close to your baby and your loved ones, especially if you felt supported and respected throughout the process. You may feel joy, wonder, and a great sense of accomplishment.

Or, if unexpected complications occurred, you may experience a range of feelings, from a bewildering mix of disappointment and joy to feeling quite traumatized. It is not uncommon to apologize for having wanted more ("It doesn't matter—after all, my baby is healthy and that's all that counts") or to feel sad or guilty about not having had the birth you dreamed of and prepared for. Worst of all, you may blame yourself—"My body just didn't work right"—instead of recognizing that you did not get the support that might have resulted in a different outcome, or that labor and birth are unpredictable. You might also find yourself angry at your care providers if you think they did not meet your needs or provide the kind of care you expected.

We had planned a birth with no intervention, and I had an emergency cesarean instead. Even though I was relieved that everything was okay and thrilled with my baby, I had the nagging sense that I had failed somehow. Later I got over feeling that it was my fault, but I still felt cheated out of the birth experience we had hoped and planned for. Sometimes I still can't help feeling a little jealous when I hear women talk about their wonderful birth experiences.

It is normal to have doubts, regret, grief, or anger rising to the surface over time. Talk with your partner, good friends, or a counselor for comfort, understanding, and support. Women's support groups and Internet chat rooms may also be helpful.

If you are dissatisfied and want to learn more about what happened, ask to see the birth records. Check them against your memories. Ask your midwife or physician to review your records with you. Talk to her or him and others who attended your labor. You might find it helpful to write a letter to your provider, describing your experience and how your needs could have been better met. Some of us, motivated by our negative experiences, become involved in work to improve the current maternity care system. (For more information, see Chapter 17, "Advocating for Better Maternity Care.")

EMOTIONAL CHALLENGES

If you are experiencing any of the following problems for longer than two weeks, you may be experiencing a postpartum mood disorder such as postpartum depression or anxiety/panic disorder. Although many of us may experience one or two of the warning signs below at various times, experiencing a combination of them for an extended period may indicate a deeper problem. If the feelings are severe and get in the way of your daily life, don't wait to get help. Warning signs include:

- feelings of inadequacy, worthlessness, or guilt, especially failure at motherhood
- loss of interest or pleasure in activities that used to bring pleasure
- excessive anxiety over the baby's health or, the opposite, lack of interest in the baby
- inability to care for yourself or your baby
- restlessness, irritability, or excessive crying
- changes in appetite, such as forgetting to eat or overeating
- changes in sleep, such as waking in the night, having racing thoughts, and not being able to go back to sleep
- difficulty concentrating, remembering, or making decisions
- hopelessness and profound sadness
- uncontrollable mood swings, including feelings of rage or anger
- feeling overwhelmed or unable to cope
- fear of being alone

If you are experiencing one or more of the following symptoms, contact your health care provider immediately:

- unusual headaches, chest pains, heart palpitations, numbness, hyperventilation, panic
- fear or recurrent thoughts of harming the baby or yourself
- scary thoughts about the baby getting hurt (different from thoughts of you being the one to hurt the baby)
- compulsive behaviors such as washing your hands hundreds of times a day or constantly checking to see if your baby is breathing
- recurrent thoughts of death/suicide; feeling that the baby would be better off without you
- hallucinations

support groups for new moms, while other Internet resources, such as personal blogs, offer real women's stories about their day-to-day experience of motherhood. If you do not have a computer at home, find out if your local library or community center has one you can use. (For more information and a list of suggested online resources, see "Resources," page 325, or visit www.ourbodiesourselves.org/childbirth.)

Social Service Organizations

Your local family services agency, public health department, community health center, mental health agency, or hospital providing maternity services may offer counseling in a group or individual setting, often for a sliding fee.

Paid Caregivers

A postpartum doula, a caregiver whose role is to "mother the mother," can help with everything from providing breast-feeding support to caring for your baby day or night to making sure you are fed and well rested. Some doulas charge an hourly or flat rate, while others offer a sliding scale. To find a certified doula in your area, you can call Doulas of North America at 1-888-788-DONA (1-888-788-3662) or visit the organization's website at www.dona.org; or you can contact the International Childbirth Education Association at 952-854-8660 or online at www.icea.org/usdoula.htm. (For more information about doulas, see page 33.) Other people who offer paid care include private lactation consultants, private psychotherapists, night nannies, child care providers, and people who run businesses preparing meals.

POSTPARTUM MOOD DISORDERS

Most women experience some ups and downs in our moods in the first weeks after giving birth. But for some new mothers, these "baby blues" don't go away, or we experience new and troubling feelings. These postpartum difficulties, termed *postpartum mood disorders*, include depression (sometimes mixed with anxiety), anxiety/panic disorder, obsessive-compulsive disorder, post-traumatic stress syndrome, and, rarely, psychosis. Estimates vary, but it appears that ten to fifteen of every one hundred women experience a postpartum mood disorder.

Many women who experience postpartum difficulties, afraid of being labeled a "bad" mother or "insane," don't tell anyone about our feelings. The stigma attached to mental illness can make it difficult or shameful to reach out to others. But postpartum mood disorders are treatable, and it is important, both for our own sake and for the sake of our families, to seek help.

BABY BLUES OR POSTPARTUM DEPRESSION?

In the period following childbirth, many women feel irritable, moody, weepy, and overwhelmed. As noted on page 281, these "baby blues" are very common. They usually occur in the first two weeks and can last for days or a few weeks. Though you will have times of feeling down, you will also find yourself able to be consoled.

In contrast, postpartum depression is not short-lived, and it often includes more severe symptoms, including hopelessness, suicidal ideas, sleep and eating disturbances, an inability to experience pleasure or to be comforted, and social withdrawal. A woman experiencing postpartum depression may be unable or unwilling to care for her baby or perform the daily

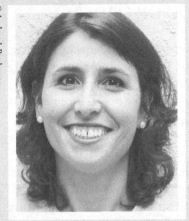

"Admitting that something is wrong is not a sign of weakness."

Elise Luce Kraemer

When I was suffering with postpartum depression (PPD), I could not care for myself or my newborn daughter. I could sleep only two to three hours in any twenty-four-hour cycle, had trouble eating, and developed a stutter. I was constantly frightened and my cognitive function was impaired. I felt myself slipping deeper and deeper into darkness.

After a few false starts in trying to get help, I was steered to a therapist by my daughter's pediatrician. [The therapist] explained to me and to my husband that I would get better eventually, but that my condition was serious and required serious attention, including therapy and medication. With time, effort, and support, everything began to change for the better. I feel so lucky to have received excellent care. Despite my rough start, I experienced a full recovery and I am now a confident mother of two daughters.

As someone who experienced PPD and recovery firsthand, it's important to me to reach out to other women. There is a lot of pressure to be a perfect and happy mom right from delivery. But admitting that something is wrong is not a sign of weakness. To the contrary, it shows that you are willing to do what it takes to be a great parent. If you are having symptoms, get help. If anyone minimizes what you are experiencing, they are not helping you; look elsewhere. For some women with mild PPD, a partner who can shoulder much of the burden of a newborn, understanding and helpful friends and relatives, and contact with women who have experienced PPD may suffice. Other women will require professional help, even with the best social support network. It is critical for women with PPD to get the right kind of care. Unfortunately, often a woman with PPD has to be an advocate for her own care when she is most vulnerable. That's one reason I now try to be vocal about my own experience.

activities of her life. Postpartum depression is the most common postpartum mood disorder. It can start any time in the first year after giving birth.

I know that I don't exude excitement and joy but I don't know how to process what I am feeling. I just want to have one really good cry and let it all out but I'm ashamed to. I'm afraid that if I start crying I won't be able to stop. There's so much love going on around me and all I feel like doing is screaming until my head explodes. I don't know how to share any of this with anyone, so I cry alone when I get a chance; just a few minutes here and there.

OTHER POSTPARTUM MOOD DISORDERS

Some women who have emotional difficulties in the months after giving birth do not experience a clear-cut depression but instead suffer from a variety of other postpartum mood disorders. Some women feel intense anxiety, fear, or panic, and experience symptoms such as rapid breathing, an accelerated heart rate, hot or cold flashes, chest pain, and shaking or dizziness. These are symptoms of an *anxiety/panic disorder*. Others may have recurrent frightening thoughts about ourselves or our babies, or may be compulsive about some behaviors, such as hand washing. These are symptoms of an *obsessive-compulsive disorder*. Others may experience a combination of depression with anxiety/panic disorder or obsessive-compulsive disorder.

Sometimes women who felt mistreated or powerless during the birth as a result of a distressing experience in the past develop post-traumatic stress responses. Women may experience symptoms such as intrusive thoughts, nightmares, agitation, avoidance behaviors, or even panic (for more information see page 104). A very small percentage of women will experience what is referred to as *postpartum psychosis*, a serious but rare illness affecting one to two of every one thousand new mothers. Women with postpartum psychosis may experience hallucinations and delusions and other symptoms including insomnia, agitation, and bizarre feelings and behavior. Postpartum psychosis generally develops within one to four weeks after giving birth.

WHO IS AT RISK?

Any woman can get a postpartum mood disorder. The hormonal changes that occur during pregnancy and birth appear to play a strong role in the development of these problems.

However, certain factors are associated with a greater likelihood of experiencing a postpartum mood disorder. These include severe or ongoing postpartum pain; health problems in the mother or baby; a "high-needs" baby; relationship, financial, or other major stresses; isolation; and a lack of social support. Ongoing sleep deprivation is also a risk factor for postpartum mood disorders.

Women who experience postpartum mood disorders are more likely to have a history of depression or other mental health issues; physical, emotional, or sexual abuse; substance abuse; or severe premenstrual syndrome. Adolescent mothers experience postpartum depression at a higher rate than the general population.

GETTING HELP

The exhaustion and feeling of being overwhelmed that many new mothers have can exacerbate any depression and anxiety we feel. If you are experiencing a postpartum mood disorder, try to ask for as much practical and emotional support as you can. If you have a partner—or other support people—available, ask him or her to share household chores and nighttime feeding duties. Do only as much as you can, and don't blame yourself for leaving things undone. (For other ideas on practical help and self-care, see "Tips for the First Weeks," page 283.)

Isolation can perpetuate depression and anxiety, so try to find at least one family member or friend with whom you can honestly share your feelings and your experience of motherhood. Meeting with a new mothers' group can be a great way to connect with others and feel less alone. Many support groups and online chat rooms focus specifically on helping women who experience postpartum depression. (See "Getting Support," page 282.)

Sometimes, however, the support and help of friends and family is not enough to get you through this period. If this is true for you, seek out a social worker, psychologist, or psychiatrist who is knowledgeable about postpartum mood disorders.

TREATMENT

The good news is that postpartum mood disorders often respond well to treatment. The two basic types of treatment offered by mental health professionals for postpartum depression and anxiety disorders are "talk therapy" and medication. Talk therapy involves regular discussions with a psychologist, social worker, or other therapist. Drug treatment for postpartum depression and anxiety disorders can include antidepressant medication, anti-anxiety medication, and sleep medication.

In the rare event that you experience postpartum psychosis, you will likely need to be hospitalized and treated with medications until you are stabilized.

Therapy

Therapy sessions can help you experience, express, and understand your feelings more fully. They can also help you explore possible solutions for postpartum challenges and learn better ways to communicate your needs and get them met. Therapists can direct you to other community supports for new mothers and families. A good therapist will monitor and advise you, providing support as well as guidance on when medication may be needed. If necessary, she or he can connect you with a psychiatrist or clinical nurse specialist who can prescribe medication.

When seeking help for postpartum mood disorders, it is best to see a therapist or medical provider who is knowledgeable about these problems. Finding a health care provider with training in postpartum depression, posttraumatic stress disorder, and/or perinatal mood disorders is critical, as some health care providers have inadequate or outdated knowledge. Postpartum Support International maintains a list of qualified practitioners throughout the United States and internationally. (For contact information, see "Where to Get Help," page 292.) It may take some trial and error to find the right therapist for you; the key is that you have a good rapport and feel that your therapist is trustworthy and respects you.

Medications

Antidepressant medications known as *selective serotonin reuptake inhibitors* (SSRIs) are commonly prescribed for postpartum mood disorders. SSRI medications include Prozac, Zoloft, Paxil, Luvox, Celexa, and Lexapro. Wellbutrin, Remeron, and Effexor are also widely prescribed; while these drugs are not SSRIs, they act on the brain in similar ways. All of these drugs are considered "second-generation" antidepressants because they have largely replaced the older antidepressants (known as *tricyclics*).

These drugs can be helpful for women with postpartum depression and anxiety, particularly when they are used in combination with talk therapy. However, there is some controversy over their effectiveness.[1] In addition, antidepressants (like other medicines) can produce negative effects, such as sleep, digestive, and sexual problems, and, rarely, more serious effects. Because of this, they should be taken only while under the care of a psychiatrist, psychiatric nurse, or other licensed professional who will monitor you regularly.

Some mothers experiencing postpartum depression recover without using medication, thereby avoiding the potential adverse effects, but other women may be in such crisis that talk therapy without medication would not be enough. (For more information on the potential benefits and harms of antidepressant medications, see "Depression During Pregnancy," page 101.)

If you are breast-feeding, be sure to tell your provider. While the second-generation antidepressants do pass into breast milk, the short-term negative effects on babies, if any, appear to be transient. Additional research, particularly on the long-term safety of antidepressants for breast-fed babies, is needed. To learn more about the effects of medication on breast milk, work with a provider who is knowledgeable about medications and breast-feeding and consult Thomas Hale's book *Medications and Mothers' Milk*. (For more information, see "Resources on Medications and Breast-Feeding," page 263.)

Deciding whether to take an antidepressant medication can be difficult. Depression can make bonding with your baby difficult, and it puts you at risk of relationship difficulties with your baby, which can affect the baby's overall development. On the other hand, antidepressants may have adverse effects, may not work, or may be incompatible with breast-feeding. Medication decisions should be guided by your preferences, the severity of your illness, the risks of the medicines in question, and the known risks of depression for you and your baby.

If you decide to take antidepressants, keep in mind that many psychotropic medicines can take several weeks before they have an effect, and often you have to try several before finding one that works for you. Be assertive with your health care provider if you have concerns or questions. If any medication you are taking seems to be making you feel more frightened, despondent, suicidal, or violent, inform your doctor, who can monitor you as you slowly go off the medication.

SEXUALITY

After childbirth, some of us experience increased sexual desire. Many new moms, however, feel less interested in sex, at least for a while. Some women choose to forgo sexual activity almost entirely during the postpartum period and focus instead on bonding as a family. Others miss being as sexual as we were before.

Often a woman and her partner experience mismatched levels of desire.

All that first year, our old forms of go-to-it sexuality were just too much. I was too tired and I'd fall asleep in the first five minutes, leaving Jack

WHEN CAN I HAVE SEX AGAIN?

Most health care providers suggest waiting four to six weeks, or until your perineum has healed and discharge has stopped, before engaging in vaginal or anal penetration. (This is true whether you gave birth vaginally or by cesarean section.) Before this, your cervix is still dilated (more open than usual), leaving you vulnerable to infection. Making love without penetration, snuggling, and solo sex (masturbation) are all okay as soon as you're interested and feel ready.

frustrated, even angry. Other times I've have the nursing and holding of the baby on my mind and intercourse seemed rough and crude. Also, I think that by the end of the day I had had a lot of skin-to-skin rubbing and touching and didn't feel sexually hungry at all. But Jack hadn't had much at all. The unevenness was driving us nuts.

How we feel sexually is affected by many factors, from our physical recovery to the strength of our relationship. Many of us need time to adjust to our new role as "Mother." Sleep deprivation and shifts in hormone levels can decrease our sexual desire. Our emotions are also key ingredients in how we respond sexually. Depression (and some drugs used to treat it) can negatively affect libido (see "Postpartum Mood Disorders," page 286).

Understanding the physical and emotional changes you are experiencing can help ease the transition, as can talking with other moms and looking critically at society's mixed messages about sex and motherhood. Sharing your concerns openly and honestly with your partner, asking for help, and maintaining a sense of humor can also help you feel comfortable with your sexuality.

RELATIONSHIP ISSUES

Frustration about a number of issues can be a roadblock to good sex when there's a new baby in the house. Anger or resentment about housework, role confusion, differing parenting styles, frequency of sex, not having enough time alone, and many other issues can lead to a lack of closeness, which often results in a limited sex life. If contact with your baby fulfills your desire for physical intimacy, your partner may feel jealous or left out.

When I nursed at night, the sight of me holding my full breast to this sleepy little baby used to drive Les nuts. When I'd get back into bed, he'd be wild to make love, fast and hard. It got to be quite a thing because I'd come back to bed feeling mild and sleepy. Les wanted to screw and I wanted to snuggle. We fought over it a lot.

Talking about your differences and setting aside special time to reconnect emotionally with your partner can lead to rediscovering physical intimacy together. Using "I statements" ("I feel ——— when you ———") to share your concerns and listening without judgment or blame can open the door to a healthy discussion, as well as to the bedroom.

After months and months of snarling, we just had to invent "middle ways" of being physical with one another. I think I picked it up from watching each of us with the baby—the nuzzling and snuggling that goes on with no expectation of orgasm, just affection.

PHYSICAL CONSIDERATIONS

Once your bleeding and discharge have stopped (generally four to six weeks after giving birth), it's fine to resume lovemaking that includes penetration.

Vaginal Discomfort

Many new mothers experience vaginal pain or a pulling sensation at the perineum, particularly if we have had stitches, when first resuming penetrative sex. Decreased estrogen levels may cause vaginal tissues to become thin and sensitive and lead to decreased lubrication, even when we are sexually aroused.

Sharing how you feel with your partner, taking things slowly, and using lots of water-based lubricant can help lead you back to pleasurable lovemaking. Experiment with different positions. Sometimes the pulling is less when the new mother is on top. Starting with finger penetration before intercourse may help you adjust to the changes and reduce anxiety.

Scar tissue from sutures will soften and perineal discomfort will likely ease within two to six months. Vaginal dryness is linked to changing hormone levels, especially when breast-feeding, and will likely ease with weaning. If either problem persists after you have stopped breast-feeding, and over-the-counter lubricants don't work, estrogen cream may be prescribed. (If you are breast-feeding, you may want to avoid estrogen, as it can reduce your milk supply.)

After vaginal birth, your vagina may feel stretched and less sensitive than before. Your pelvic floor muscles have been through a workout during childbirth. Kegel exercises (see page 38) can help strengthen your muscles and enhance sexual pleasure.

Abdominal Pain

If you had a cesarean birth, certain sexual positions may cause or increase abdominal pain. You may want to experiment with different positions, or delay sex until you have healed more.

Changes in Our Breasts

Many women find that our breasts are either more or less sensitive while we are nursing. Some of us with heightened sensation enjoy this, while others prefer that our breasts be entirely "off limits" for anything but breast-feeding, due to tenderness, feeling "touched out" from nursing all day, or difficulty separating the breast function of nursing from our sexuality.

If you are breast-feeding, your breasts may leak or spray during orgasm. Some of us enjoy this experience, while others find it unsettling. If it's a problem, you can wear a bra with nursing pads while making love.

Some women experience sexual arousal while nursing. This is a normal sensation and is related to the release of oxytocin, which is associated with both orgasm and breast milk letdown reflex.

Nursing mothers have higher levels of prolactin and lower levels of estrogen, which may result in less frequent or less intense desire.

While some women find that breast-feeding reduces our overall sexual drive, most of us find that sexual drive returns when we wean. However, many women who nurse have a strong sex drive, and many mothers who have never breast-fed still have a lowered sex drive after becoming mothers.

There were times when I got into bed, gave my husband a peck on the cheek, and leaned back onto my pillow relishing the prospect of some sleep. Sex was the last thing on my mind, and usually I conked out in minutes. But he would sometimes gently stroke my body in a few choice spots, and before I knew it, I actually felt aroused and suddenly interested in making love. Where that energy came from I still can't fathom.

BIRTH CONTROL

If you are having sex with a man, it's important to think about family planning before you are fertile again. If you do not breast-feed, your periods will likely resume four to six weeks after you give birth. This means that you may ovulate (release an egg from the ovary) as soon as twenty-five days after delivery and could become pregnant again even before your period starts again. If you are breast-feeding, your return to fertility will be delayed, but you can get pregnant even if you don't have regular periods.

When deciding on a birth control method, you face special considerations as a new mother. Some methods of birth control should not be used by nursing mothers; some methods need to be altered due to changes in the uterus, cervix, and vagina after childbirth; and some are less effective once a woman has given birth. The information listed below discusses only the aspects of birth control that are different for new mothers. For a full discussion of the efficacy, benefits, and potential harms of all birth control methods, see the birth control chapter of *Our Bodies, Ourselves.*

BARRIER METHODS
Condoms

Condoms (male or female) can be used as soon as you are ready to have intercourse. Using lubricated condoms or adding water-soluble lubricant may ease the discomfort from vaginal dryness that accompanies breast-feeding or from still-healing tears or episiotomies.

Diaphragms

Diaphragms should be fitted or refitted at about six weeks after giving birth or later, once the cervix, uterus, and vagina have returned to normal. To provide adequate protection, diaphragms should be used with contraceptive cream or gel.

Cervical Shields and the Vaginal Sponge

Cervical shields (Lea's Shield and FemCap) and vaginal sponges (Today) can be used starting six weeks after giving birth. However, the FemCap and the sponge are far less effective for women who have given birth than for women who have never given birth.[2]

The FemCap comes in different sizes, and if this is your first baby, you will need to get the larger size. Lea's Shield is a one-size-fits-all device and doesn't need to be refitted.

INTRAUTERINE DEVICE (IUD)

You can have an IUD safely inserted in your uterus six to eight weeks after giving birth, when the uterus has returned more or less to prepregnancy dimensions.

COMBINED ESTROGEN + PROGESTIN METHODS (THE PILL, PATCH, AND RING)

Combined hormonal contraceptives generally should not be used by breast-feeding mothers, as they reduce a woman's milk supply and may alter the composition of breast milk.[3] For these reasons, progestin-only pills are usually recommended over the combined hormonal methods for breast-feeding women. (For more information, see "Progestin-Only Methods," below.)

If you are not breast-feeding, you can use any of the combined birth control methods beginning three weeks after you give birth. The three-week wait is important, as combined hormonal methods contain synthetic estrogen, which increases the risk of blood clots. This risk is also elevated during pregnancy but returns to nonpregnant levels three weeks after a woman gives birth.

PROGESTIN-ONLY METHODS (MINI-PILLS, INJECTABLES, IMPLANT)

There are no known safety problems for new mothers, including breast-feeding mothers, using progestin-only methods (such as Mini-Pills, the injectables Depo-Provera and depo-subQ provera 104, and the implant Implanon). Progestin-only methods can interfere with the initiation of breast-feeding and have a significant impact on milk production in some women, so you may want to wait until you are six weeks postpartum and breast-feeding is well-established before beginning these methods. Once lactation is established, progestin does not appear to interfere with breast-feeding for most women.

EMERGENCY CONTRACEPTION (EC)

Plan B (consisting of progestin-only EC pills) is considered safe for use three weeks after giving birth. Women who are breast-feeding may want to avoid Plan B before six weeks postpartum, as it can, like other progestin-only methods, interfere with early breast-feeding.

FERTILITY AWARENESS METHOD (FAM)

The fertility awareness method is often difficult to use in the months after birth, particularly if you are breast-feeding. A method that can be effective for breast-feeding mothers is the lactational amenorrhea method (LAM), which can be used for the first six months of your baby's life. (For more information, see "Breast-Feeding as Birth Control," page 267.)

STERILIZATION

If you do not want more children, female sterilization (*tubal ligation,* or "getting your tubes tied") can be performed within forty-eight hours after vaginal delivery, during cesarean delivery, or six or more weeks after giving birth. A newer form of female sterilization does not require surgery and involves the insertion of a soft, flexible device (known by the trade name Essure) into each fallopian tube. This form of sterilization can be performed six or more weeks postpartum. You and your partner may also want to discuss vasectomy, as male sterilization is simpler and less risky than female sterilization.

BEING A MOTHER TODAY

Through the Internet, books, and parenting magazines, mothers today have more access to one another's stories and ideas about mothering than our foremothers did. Thanks to the voices of those brave enough to share our experiences with postpartum mood disorders, we have a fuller picture of the emotional landscape of motherhood. And thanks to changing attitudes, women can more easily pursue "nontraditional" options, from deciding to be a single mother or a co-parent with a female partner to continuing a career after having kids.

But the myth of the "supermom" who is perpetually cheerful, all-knowing, and self-sacrificing lives on, and it's hard to resist. We—both as individuals and as a society—still have certain expectations about what it means to be a mother.

Everyone's like, "This is the best time of your life, aren't you so happy?" There's no room to say no. . . . You're not allowed to have the negative emotions. You love and hate your child so much, all together, all at once.

It's important to be able to talk about how it feels trying to live up to these expectations. Traditionally, though, mothers have been expected to talk only about the positive, and voicing our frustrations with some of the more difficult moments can be tough. We expose not only our ambivalence, but our vulnerability.

I was afraid I wouldn't be a good mother, or would forget to feed him, or change him. I was afraid he wouldn't like me. I was afraid of everything in the world, and yet was so happy at the same time. It was the strangest feeling in the world. I still sometimes feel that way, and think that every mother does at some point. We doubt ourselves all the time, and really need to just relax and go with it, because chances are we're doing a really good job.

"MOMMY WARS" AND "OPTING OUT"

I'm a single mom. My son's father has just disappeared. My main support is my family, but it comes with a cost. My mom and aunt seem to feel they can tell me how to parent, especially since they are providing me with free babysitting while I work at the grocery store. I really wish I didn't have to work, but I have no choice. I would much rather be home with my son, because I just love being his mother.

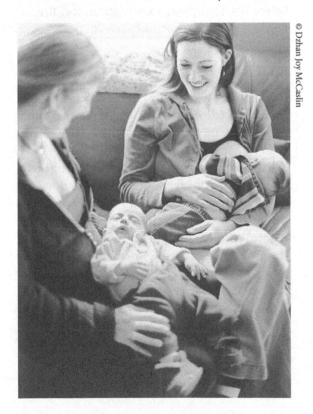

© Dzhan Joy McCaslin

In addition to feeling the pressure to be a supermom, many mothers are also conflicted about balancing work and family. Those of us who work outside the home often contend with the stress of arranging for full-time child care and may feel guilt and judgment about the choices we are making. Those of us who stop working to care for children may be frustrated by the loss of identity and advancement opportunities that often comes with leaving the workforce.

My brain is melting and coming out my ears. I feel like everything I was trained to do, all my hopes and aspirations, are frozen in time. My husband goes about his life and his job and then gets to come home and be a great daddy. [Sometimes] he says things like "You seem really touchy today," and all of a sudden I'm like, "Did you pee by yourself today? Did you go to the bathroom alone? That's how I'm rating the quality of my days right now."

For many women, working is not optional; it is a financial necessity. For other women, the cost of child care may make staying home a financially sensible choice. Some women make great financial sacrifices to stay home. These are complex decisions based on our values, priorities, and needs. In 2004, according to the U.S. Census Report, 55 percent of women with infants were in the labor force.[4] About seven of every ten employed mothers with children younger than three years old work full time. One-third of these mothers return to work within three months after birth and two-thirds return within six months.[5]

The media-driven talk of the "mommy wars" polarizes mothers into two camps: those who work outside the home and those who stay at home to care for our children. In reality, many of us cycle in and out of these roles. Too often, public discourse either praises working

mothers for our multitasking abilities or condemns us for neglecting our children; similarly, it often praises stay-at-home moms for being devoted to our children or condemns us for giving up so much of our identity and career potential for motherhood. Many mothers feel judged about our decisions, whether we are working outside the home or being the primary caregiver for our children.

While our society idealizes motherhood, our government provides little concrete support for children and families. Unlike most other industrialized countries, the United States has no guaranteed paid family leave, no guaranteed health care, and little affordable high-quality child care. Day care is often vilified in the media as an unacceptable substitute for mother care; it is blamed for causing everything from "aggression" to emotional and intellectual delays to lack of maternal-child attachment. But Caryl Rivers, coauthor of *She Works, He Works: How Two-Income Families Are Happy, Healthy and Thriving*, among other titles, counters that the same 2001 National Institute of Child Health and Human Development report used to bolster scare-mongering warnings about the impact of day care on children showed that, in fact, infants in day care were securely attached to their mothers. She also notes that children throughout history have been cared for by multiple caretakers, and that "fifty years of scientific evidence finds that the children of working mothers show few differences in emotional or intellectual development from the children of at-home mothers."[6] (For more information on the state of motherhood in the United States, please see Chapter 18, "Advocating for Mothers and Families.")

We need public policies that value and support families and caregivers, who are mostly women. Yet even without such necessary public commitments, and in the midst of mixed cultural messages, mothers are finding what works best for ourselves, our families, and our children.

Whenever I feel guilty or start worrying that I'm doing it wrong, I remind myself that in the end, it usually turns out okay. Because a huge part of our kids' emotional and physical health as adults is due to what kind of parents we are. But an even huger part is because of the kids themselves: their temperaments, abilities, intelligence, etc. And their teachers and peers also play a big role. There's no One True Path to successful motherhood.

NOTES

1. L. Jones and M. Stone, "Clinical Review: Relationship Between Antidepressant Drugs and Adult Suicidality," Food and Drug Administration, Center for Drug Evaluation and Research, accessed at www.fda.gov/ohrms/dockets/ac/06/briefing/2006-4272b1-index.htm, on November 16, 2006, p. 41.

2. Robert Hatcher, *Contraceptive Technology, 18th rev. ed.* (New York: Ardent Media, 2004), 226.

3. Ruth A. Lawrence and Robert M. Lawrence, *Breastfeeding: A Guide for the Medical Profession, 5th ed.* (St. Louis: Mosby, 1999), 665.

4. U.S. Census Bureau, "Fertility of American Women: June 2004," page 7, fig. 2: "Labor Force Participation Rates for Mothers with a Birth in the Last Year: 1976–2004," accessed at www.census.gov/prod/2005pubs/p20-555.pdf on June 22, 2006.

5. Katherine R. Shealy, Ruower Li, Sandra Benton-Davis, and Laurence M. Grummer-Strawn, *The CDC Guide to Breastfeeding Interventions,* "Support for Breastfeeding in the Workplace," page 7, U.S. Department of Health and Human Services, accessed at www.cdc.gov/breastfeeding/pdf/breastfeeding_interventions.pdf on June 22, 2006.

6. Caryl Rivers, "Day Care Report Launches Misinformed Hysteria," Women's eNews, run date April 21, 2001; accessed at www.womensenews.org/article.cfm?aid=524 on June 22, 2006.

Knowledge
Is Power

CHAPTER 17

Advocating for Better Maternity Care

Over the past century, childbirth has become safer for mothers and babies in the United States, thanks to improvements in sanitation, the discovery of antibiotics, advances in medical technology, and other positive developments. From 1900 to 1999, the risk of a baby dying during birth or in the first year of life plummeted from 1 in 10 to less than 1 in 100 in the United States.[1] The risk of a mother dying from pregnancy-related complications or childbirth decreased even more dramatically, from 850 deaths in every 100,000 births to less than 8 in every 100,000 births.[2] In addition, changes in the later twentieth century, such as childbirth education and encouraging women's partners or other close friends and family members to be present during labor and birth, have helped many women better understand the process of childbirth and enjoy more support through it. Women in the United States today have more childbearing options than our foremothers did and have healthier outcomes overall.

Yet despite this progress, mothers and babies still face many challenges. Today, the United States has unacceptably high rates of infant and maternal mortality compared to other industrialized countries. Many women do not have access to high-quality health care because of poverty, lack of insurance, insurers' requirements, racial discrimination, language barriers, or lack of local options. In addition, our government provides little concrete support for mothers and families: Unlike most other industrialized countries, the United States has no guaranteed paid family leave, no guaranteed health care, and little affordable high-quality child care. (For more information, see Chapter 18, "Advocating for Mothers and Families.")

The health care provided to women during pregnancy, childbirth, and the early postpartum period—what is known as *maternity care*—is also in need of improvement. Far too often, maternity care practices are not based on the best scientific research on safety and effectiveness. Many individuals and organizations throughout the United States are working to reform maternity care, reduce economic and racial disparities, and increase women's access to high-quality care. Some are featured in this chapter; others are listed in "Resources," starting on page 325.

MATERNITY CARE TODAY

Many elements of the care most women receive during pregnancy and childbirth in the United States are not based on the most reliable research on what is safe and effective. Procedures that are useful—and sometimes even lifesaving—when applied to women and babies with specific high-risk conditions are often extended liberally to other women and babies—"just in case." Such unnecessary medical interventions are not helpful and can even be harmful.

One procedure that is badly overused is episiotomy (cutting the perineum in order to make the opening to the vagina bigger). While episiotomy can help when the baby is very large or when the baby needs to come out immediately, its use should be limited to clear cases of need because it increases the likelihood of serious tears into or through the anal muscle.[3] Other overused interventions include continuous electronic fetal heart rate monitoring (see page 174), induction of labor (see page 146), and cesarean section.

Overuse of obstetric interventions is a widespread problem. A national survey of mothers who gave birth in hospitals in 2005 found that nearly all women experienced some combination of interventions that can interfere with the normal progression of birth.[4] Most of the women surveyed had continuous electronic fetal heart rate monitoring, urinary catheterization, administration of intravenous fluids, and epidural or spinal analgesia. One in two re-

ceived synthetic oxytocin to either start her labor or make her contractions stronger and more frequent, and slightly more than three in ten had a cesarean section. Most women also experienced practices that may do more harm than good, such as not eating or drinking anything during labor and lying on their backs during labor and while giving birth. The United States' C-section rate is more than twice the maximum rate recommended by the World Health Organization; this means that more mothers and babies are exposed to the negative effects of surgical birth. (For more information on C-sections, see Chapter 13, "Cesarean Births.)

While such procedures are *overused*, other practices that improve birth outcomes and increase women's satisfaction are widely *underused*. These practices include receiving continuous one-on-one support during labor; being able to change positions, get out of bed, and walk during labor; and using comfort measures such as massage, warm baths, and birthing balls. The same national survey mentioned above found that of every one hundred women giving birth in a hospital, only three were attended by a doula (a trained labor companion), only four used a shower to help cope with labor pain, and only six relaxed in a tub or pool of warm water during labor.[5]

We need to turn these numbers around. Medical procedures that are potentially harmful should be used only when needed, and practices that are known to improve outcomes should be made widely available.

Most health systems struggle to ensure that people receive evidence-based care. It is difficult for busy health care professionals to keep up with and interpret a large and ever-growing body of studies. Even when providers understand lessons from the best available research, it is often hard to change established beliefs and

EVIDENCE-BASED MATERNITY CARE[6]

"Evidence-based maternity care" uses the best research about the safety and effectiveness of specific tests, treatments, and other interventions to help guide maternity care decisions. This should be standard care for everyone, but it is not.

A rigorous systematic review of original studies, conducted according to established guidelines for research, gives the best possible answers to questions about beneficial and harmful effects of specific health interventions. A systematic review involves a thorough search for the best available studies on a specific topic. Only relevant and better-quality studies are included in the review. When possible, researchers reach a conclusion by combining data from the included studies using statistical techniques called "meta-analysis." Systematic review procedures help limit the bias and error that can easily distort results of single studies and of more conventional reviews of research. They allow us to draw much more accurate and confident conclusions.*

* The Cochrane Collaboration is an international group that prepares and updates systematic reviews of the best research about the safety and effectiveness of health and medical interventions. Abstracts of its reviews on pregnancy and childbirth are available online at www.cochrane.org/reviews/en/subtopics/87 .html. The full reviews are available only for a fee.

routines. Many groups have a role in ensuring that mothers and babies receive high-quality care. These include health care providers and women ourselves, as well as policy makers, payers, administrators, educators, researchers, and journalists.

WHY IS MATERNITY CARE LIKE THIS?

Why are some medical interventions still being overused in the United States today, despite the evidence against them? And why aren't approaches that are known to be helpful offered to all women? Advocates for improving maternity care point to the following roadblocks to change.

OBSTETRICAL TRAINING AND THE MEDICAL SYSTEM

Obstetricians provide care for the vast majority of pregnant women in the United States. Obstetrics is a surgical specialty, and doctors training to become obstetricians learn, among other things, to perform cesarean sections, apply forceps, and cut and repair episiotomies. They generally receive less instruction in the natural progression of childbirth or in birth techniques that minimize perineal tearing. The focus is on external management rather than on facilitating a woman's own capacities for labor. In many training programs, obstetricians are not even required to sit with a healthy woman throughout her labor or observe one birth without any interventions. This training leads obstetricians to be far more comfortable managing childbirth with medication and technological interventions than without.

The widespread use of epidurals also has transformed childbirth in the United States. While epidurals are a very effective form of pain relief during labor, they sometimes have adverse effects and can alter the natural progression of labor. A woman who has an epidural is usually restricted in her movements and for safety reasons must be monitored continuously by electronic fetal monitoring (EFM). The restricted movement and muscle relaxation caused by the epidural can cause babies who are facing backward to stay that way, which results in a longer second stage of labor and a higher incidence of forceps and vacuum deliveries. Use of epidurals also can lead to less effective pushing. (For more information on epidurals, see page 208.)

The use of continuous EFM has also changed childbirth. Continuous fetal heart rate monitoring is used nearly universally in hospitals. Because the fetal heart rate patterns seen when the heart rate is continuously recorded are sometimes difficult to interpret, EFM has increased the number of labors considered "complicated" or "risky." The widespread routine use of EFM has led doctors to overdiagnose complications, too narrowly define what is normal, and treat deviations from those norms as evidence that something is wrong.[7] For women who do not have labor interventions such as epidurals that make continuous monitoring necessary, intermittent monitoring appears to be as effective as continuous monitoring at detecting true problems, and is not associated with an increased risk of cesarean birth or of vaginal birth assisted by vacuum extraction or forceps. (For more information on fetal monitoring, see page 174.)

Epidurals and EFM have changed the kind of nursing care women receive. In the past, personal one-on-one care was the hallmark of obstetrical nursing. Today, for a variety of reasons, including nursing shortages, budgetary constraints, and less training in the natural progression of birth, labor nurses increasingly rely on continuous electronic fetal monitoring to help them care for more than one woman at a time. Therefore, fewer laboring women have access to this vital one-on-one support.

ECONOMIC INCENTIVES

Surgical interventions can save doctors time and money. Many payment systems offer a single or fixed fee to doctors regardless of whether a baby is born vaginally or by cesarean, and others offer a larger fee for a cesarean. Therefore, those doctors who patiently support natural labor, which starts at unpredictable hours and generally requires more time, are penalized financially.[8] Some systems provide increased payment for a cesarean section, making planned surgery the most cost-efficient and time-saving scenario for doctors. Inducing labor instead of waiting for it to start on its own also helps doctors control their hours. Elective cesarean sections and scheduled induction of labor help hospitals make nursing staff schedules more predictable and shift more of health care providers' work to convenient weekday hours.

FEAR OF LAWSUITS

If something goes wrong, doctors may be blamed for *not* doing something, but rarely are they blamed *for* doing something that is not necessary. For example, malpractice lawsuits for not performing a cesarean section are much more common than lawsuits for doing one when it wasn't necessary. To avoid litigation, many doctors and some midwives feel compelled to do "too much" rather than be accused of doing "too little." Market forces, pharmaceutical advertising, and other medical industry marketing practices may also contribute to a drive to "do something" even when observation and emotional support would be better for mother and baby than an additional test or procedure.

A RUSHED, RISK-AVERSE SOCIETY

The desire to eliminate pain and control outcomes may cause both health care providers and expectant parents to embrace unneeded and potentially harmful procedures. U.S. society today has an aversion to risk that contributes to a climate of doubt in which all labors are treated as potential problems, and healthy women with low-risk pregnancies receive treatments that were designed for use by women with high-risk pregnancies.

In addition, women sometimes are not allowed sufficient time for labor to progress and a vaginal birth to occur. Women's own expectations can contribute to rushing labor.

THE LANGUAGE OF "CHOICE"

Labor and birth approaches are sometimes presented as equivalent "choices" without full, accurate information about their potential consequences. For example, elective cesareans (cesarean sections done without a medical need) are increasingly presented by the media and some doctors in a misleading fashion— as a "reasonable" option for healthy pregnant women. (For more information, see "Maternal Request," page 43.)

ASSISTED REPRODUCTIVE TECHNOLOGIES AND OLDER MOTHERS

The use of assisted reproductive technologies is leading to more births by older women and more multiple births. In vitro fertilization has increased the number of births of twins, triplets, and other multiples, and such babies are often delivered by cesarean section.*

Whether we have used assisted reproductive technologies or not, those of us who get pregnant when we are older are more likely to have medical conditions such as high blood pressure or diabetes that can make pregnancy more complicated. Women over age forty have higher rates of medical interventions, including cesarean sections. Nevertheless it is important not to assume that your pregnancy is "high-risk" and requires interventions simply because of your age; the majority of women over forty have healthy, uncomplicated pregnancies.

ADVOCATING FOR CHANGE

Often motivated by personal experiences, some of us have become involved in groups that are working to change birth practices in the United States. Such advocates are addressing a range of problems, from the overuse of unhelpful medical interventions, to the lack of continuous care available to laboring women, to rules that prevent women who have had previous cesarean

* Such complications could be reduced by implanting only one embryo rather than two or more, but that is not standard procedure in the United States. In the UK, new guidelines that call for implanting only one embryo (rather than two or more) will reduce the number of such multiple births and their associated complications as well. If a woman has only one embryo implanted each cycle, it may take her more tries (and therefore more time) to become pregnant.

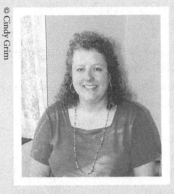

© Cindy Grim

My first reaction was, "Not in my state!"
Barbara Stratton

More than three hundred hospitals in the United States do not allow women to choose to have a vaginal birth if they have previously had a cesarean section, despite the facts that the option is very low-risk and that cesareans carry their own set of dangers. As a woman with a previous cesarean myself, I feel strongly that all women should be given information on the risks and benefits of vaginal birth after cesarean (referred to as VBAC) and allowed to make their own decisions.*

In Maryland, where I live, Frederick Memorial Hospital announced a ban on VBACs in August of 2004. My first reaction was, "Not in my state!" Birth activist Robin O'Brien and I quickly co-organized a rally that was held in November of that year. We began at a park near the hospital, then marched around the hospital itself while chanting and carrying signs. The event attracted a lot of local media attention. I contacted *The New York Times,* which published a front-page story on the nationwide problem of the bans.[9] A day after that article hit, the chief obstetrician at Frederick Memorial was invited on the *Today* show to debate the president of the International Cesarean Awareness Network (known as ICAN). *USA Today* and *The Washington Post* eventually did lengthy stories on the issue as well.[10]

After the rally, I continued to apply pressure to the Frederick hospital through the media and government agencies. In August of 2006, Frederick Memorial Hospital reversed its ban, citing "community pressure" as the reason. Now, individual doctors can decide whether to offer VBAC, and most do. Within a week of the reversal, we had our first VBAC there and the mom was ecstatic.

Since the rally, I have been working to reverse the bans nationwide. I helped lobby the National Organization for Women to pass a nationwide resolution in support of reversing the bans. (The resolution can be viewed on NOW's website at www.now.org/issues/reproductive/vbac.html.) I also wrote an article for *Midwifery Today* magazine titled "50 Ways to Protest a VBAC Denial."

One of the most promising approaches to reversing the bans involves having women file complaints through the Medicaid system and then appealing any negative decisions all the way up to the federal level. If successful, the approach would force all hospitals nationwide that receive Medicaid funding (as most do) to reverse their bans.

* For more information about VBACs, see page 233.

sections from trying to give birth to subsequent children vaginally.

The efforts of grassroots advocacy groups have helped alter some hospital rules and routines for the better, although such attempts to create change often meet with resistance. Sometimes, though, concern for hospitals' financial health may motivate changes that also protect women's and babies' health. For example, some hospitals concerned about soaring liability-insurance costs for birth units are reducing common practices that are unnecessary and are sometimes harmful to both mothers and infants.[11] These positive efforts include discouraging the induction of birth before 39 weeks, unless medically necessary. Physicians sometimes induce labor to fit their own schedules or mothers' desires, but research shows that giving birth even a few days early is associated with higher rates of emergency cesareans, admissions to neonatal intensive care with respiratory distress and other problems, and longer-term health issues for children. In another example, some hospital programs are trying to ensure better teamwork because research has demonstrated that communication breakdowns are at the root of most adverse events reported in obstetrics units.[12]

Ideally, such initiatives will reduce risks and complications for mothers and babies, in addition to reducing hospital costs. Unfortunately, these changes are not the norm, despite what the best evidence shows.

RIGHTS OF WOMEN DURING PREGNANCY AND BIRTH

No matter what situations you face when you are pregnant and in labor, understanding your rights as a childbearing woman is key to making good decisions and being better able to act on them. In the United States today, essential health care is not guaranteed for all women and infants, nor are scientific data about the best maternity care practices consistently applied in maternity care services. More important, women are not routinely given clear, complete information about the benefits and risks of drugs, tests, or treatments. And often we are unaware of our legal right to make health care choices for ourselves and our babies.

The statement below is excerpted and adapted from Childbirth Connection, a nonprofit group based in New York City that works to improve maternity care for all U.S. women and our families. The statement outlines a set of basic rights for childbearing women, applying widely accepted human rights to the specific situation of maternity care. Most of these rights are granted to women in the United States by law, yet they are not always honored.*

* For the full text of this statement, see Childbirth Connection's "Rights of Childbearing Women" at www .childbirthconnection.org/rights.

(continued)

EVERY WOMAN HAS THE RIGHT TO:

- Choose her birth setting from the full range of safe options available in her community, on the basis of complete, objective information about the benefits, harms, and costs of these options.
- Receive information about the professional identity and qualifications of those involved in her care, and know when any are trainees.
- Communicate with caregivers, receive all care in privacy (which may involve excluding nonessential personnel), and have all personal information treated according to standards of confidentiality.
- Receive full advance information about harms and benefits of all reasonably available methods for relieving pain during labor and birth, including methods that do not require the use of drugs. She has the right to choose which methods will be used and to change her mind at any time.
- Accept or refuse procedures, drugs, tests, and treatments, and have her choices honored. She has the right to change her mind.
- Leave her maternity caregiver and select another if she becomes dissatisfied with the care.
- Be informed if her caregivers wish to enroll her or her infant in a research study. She should receive full information about all known and possible benefits and harms of participation, and she has the right to decide whether to participate, free from coercion and without negative consequences.
- Have unrestricted access to all available records about her pregnancy, her labor, and her infant; obtain a full copy of them; and receive help in understanding them, if necessary.
- Receive maternity care that is appropriate to her cultural and religious background, and receive information in a language in which she can communicate.
- Enjoy freedom of movement during labor, unencumbered by tubes, wires, or other apparatuses. She also has the right to give birth in the position of her choosing.

These rights may sound like a utopian ideal, yet in many countries some or all of them are routinely recognized and enforced. While women in the United States (especially educated, articulate women with good health insurance) sometimes can demand the recognition of these rights, most U.S. women find that the wider social, political, and economic organization of health care, parenting, and the workplace make it difficult or impossible to consistently exercise these rights.

RACIAL AND ECONOMIC DISPARITIES

The United States has the highest rate of infant mortality among affluent nations, and higher rates of maternal mortality than all but five economically industrialized countries.[13] Not all mothers are equally vulnerable. Mothers and babies of color—especially African-American and Native American mothers and babies—are at higher risk for poor health outcomes, and women of color are less likely to receive adequate prenatal care than white women.[14]

The most well-documented and persistent racial disparity in this country is the difference in birth outcomes between African-American and white women. African-American newborns die at more than twice the rate that white newborns do. Urban Hispanic and African-American mothers are 145 percent more likely to experience an infant's death before the first birthday.[15] The reasons for this disparity include but are not limited to differences in the mother's pre-existing health conditions and access to good prenatal care and treatment for pre-existing conditions.[16] Preterm birth (before 37 weeks) and low birth weight (less than five pounds) account for many of the extra deaths among black babies, and are also associated with increased rates of childhood illnesses and disabilities.

Racial disparities in health outcomes are complex, and they persist even when education and income are the same. They are based on many factors that have not been fully explained. For example, African-American women smoke less than white women,[17] which would be expected to result in black infants being born at a low weight less often than white babies; but in reality, African-American babies are born at low weights more often. In addition, although African-American women are seeking prenatal health care in significantly greater numbers than ten or twenty years ago, this has had only a limited effect in reducing low birth weight or premature birth.[18] Preterm birth is a function not only of medical problems emerging during pregnancy, but also of social and environmental factors that influence a woman's health, behaviors, and access to preventive services and health care.[19] For example, women who report having experienced more racial discrimination are more likely to have preterm births and low-birth-weight babies.[20] Much more research is needed to fully understand the causes of disparate health outcomes.

Still, we can create change based on what we do know. Enhanced prenatal care is one strategy that may reduce infant deaths, although it alone will not eliminate the racial and ethnic gap. Prenatal care does little to reduce very low birth weight and occurs too late to influence women's health at conception. Currently the federal government is interested in developing and implementing pre-conception care models.

One model advocacy program for women of color during the childbearing years is the Boston Healthy Start Initiative, first funded by the U.S. Department of Health and Human Services (HHS) in 1984. The Boston Healthy Start Initiative has played a central role in mobilizing and motivating African-American and Latina women from the Boston neighborhoods with the highest rates of infant mortality to seek early prenatal and reproductive health care. The babies of women involved in the program have survived at higher rates than were seen before, according to a Boston Healthy Start report.[21]

In 1991, HHS launched the federal Healthy Start Initiative by funding fifteen urban and rural sites in communities with infant mortality rates that were 1.5 to 2.5 times the national average. The program now involves about one

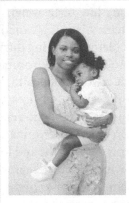

© Werner A. Meier

"Mother's Milk Club was part support group, part scientific discussion."

Jameca Johnson

My daughter was born at 25 weeks and weighed one pound, fifteen ounces. I was only seventeen, and I was nervous enough just to be a mother, but my fears of inadequacy as a parent were compounded by my worries over her condition.

I pumped my breast milk for my baby eight to ten times a day, and came to the hospital to hold her "kangaroo" (skin-to-skin on my chest) every day. I was the only one in my family to breast-feed since I don't know how long ago. Family members who didn't understand breast-feeding soon became believers when they saw Jamia coming home before her due date two and a half months later, weighing five pounds, seven ounces.

I was a single mom at first because her father (also seventeen) didn't accept responsibility. I found out later that he was just scared and couldn't deal with seeing a baby just about the size of his hand. With encouragement, he turned out to be a great father.

I loved breast-feeding Mia. It was a special time when I could drop whatever I was doing and feed her and look into her eyes. I continued pumping when I went back to work at McDonald's and at school for my GED. I never planned to, but I went over three and a half years breast-feeding her. Gradually, she weaned when she was ready.

I wouldn't have had this wonderful experience if it hadn't been for Dr. Paula Meier and the Mother's Milk Club that meets for lunch in Rush's Special Care Nursery (the neonatal intensive care unit, or NICU). Mother's Milk Club was part support group, part scientific discussion of articles and studies that showed the benefits of breast milk for premature babies. Even after Jamia went home, we attended Milk Club together.

I shared my experiences with the new moms and tried to give them some hope that one day their little ones would grow to be fat and healthy like my daughter did. For about four years, I volunteered at Rush and made home visits to the moms of newly discharged babies who needed help troubleshooting breast-feeding. Then I was hired to work in the NICU as a breast-feeding peer counselor.

I am in my third year of college, studying nursing, and Paula is working with me to gain admission and tuition [for me] at Rush University all the way up to my doctorate degree if I so choose. I also just recently married my child's father. I look forward to having more children, but that will have to wait.

I love my job. I enjoy helping moms during this difficult time in their lives. It's most rewarding to see babies come back big and healthy and know that I had a small part in that.

hundred different federally funded projects that develop community-based approaches to reducing infant mortality and improving the health and well-being of women, children, and families. One study in a peer-reviewed journal found that the program was modestly successful in enrolling women with factors associated with higher-risk pregnancies (younger, poorer women); the study also found that women in the program were more likely to rate their prenatal care highly than similar women not enrolled.[22] A report of the Florida Healthy Start Initiative said that the statewide infant mortality dropped 20 percent from 1992, when the initiative started, to 2004, while the national rate of infant mortality stayed almost level during the same time period.[23]

Significant work is also being accomplished by National Advocates for Pregnant Women (NAPW), a nonprofit organization that aims to reduce differences in women's access to high-quality maternity care. The group advocates on behalf of all women, especially those who are most marginalized: women of color, low-income women, incarcerated women, and women who use drugs. It uses a variety of strategies, from educating and organizing on the local and national levels to filing lawsuits. (For more information, see www.advocatesfor pregnantwomen.org.)

BETTER HEALTH CARE FOR MOTHERS AND BABIES

Advocates are working to improve maternity care in the United States and support safer and healthier experiences during pregnancy, birth, and motherhood. They are also helping to ensure that all women have access to high-quality, culturally competent prenatal care as well as full information about and support for pursuing our birth options. Such efforts challenge the financial, legal, and other factors that reinforce the status quo.

One longtime women's health advocate reflects on the vision that inspires her work:

Hearing from many hundreds of women about their birthing experiences over the past few decades has reinforced for me the extraordinary value of the midwifery model of care. I still dream of a maternity care system more like that in the Netherlands, where midwives attend most of the births, collaborating closely with doctors as needed. Women there report higher satisfaction with their care, outcomes are excellent, and the use of expensive, sometimes invasive interventions is far less frequent than in the United States. At the very least, I hope that we reach the point where most birthing women will base their decisions on balanced, accurate information rather than misleading newspaper stories that, for example, herald "elective" cesareans as equally safe [compared] to planned vaginal births.

NOTES

1. U.S. Centers for Disease Control and Prevention, "Achievements in Public Health, 1900–1999: Healthier Mothers and Babies," *Morbidity and Mortality Weekly Report* 48, no. 38 (October 1, 1999): 849–858, accessed at www.cdc.gov/mmwr/preview/mmwr html/mm4838a2.htm on October 17, 2006.
2. Ibid.
3. Randomized controlled trials have demonstrated that women who have had a routine episiotomy experience more anal and rectal tears and no difference in pelvic floor relaxation or incontinence compared to women who are not cut. K. Hartmann, M. Viswanathan, R. Palmieri, G. Gartlehner, J. Thorp, and K. N. Lohr, "Outcomes of Routine Episiotomy: A Systematic Review," *JAMA* 293 (2005): 2,141–2,148.
4. Eugene R. Declercq, Carol Sakala, Maureen P. Corry, and S. Applebaum, "Executive Summary," in *Listening to Mothers II: Report of the Second National U.S.*

Survey of Women's Childbearing Experiences (New York: Childbirth Connection, 2006.)

5. Ibid.

6. Excerpted from Childbirth Connection, "What Is Evidence-Based Maternity Care?" available at www.childbirthconnection.org/article.asp?ck=10080.

7. J. T. Parer, T. King, S. Flanders, M. Fox, and S. J. Kilpatrick, "Fetal Acidemia and Electronic Fetal Heart Rate Patterns: Is There Evidence of an Association?" *Journal of Maternal-Fetal and Neonatal Medicine* 19, no. 5 (May 2006): 289–294.

8. Carol Sakala, "Letter from North America: An Uncontrolled Experiment: Elective Delivery Predominates in the United States," *Birth* 33, no 4 (December 2006).

9. Denise Grady, "Trying to Avoid 2nd Caesarean, Many Find Choice Isn't Theirs," *New York Times,* November 29, 2004.

10. Rita Rubin, "Study Backs Natural Birth after C-section," *USA Today,* June 30, 2006; Tom Graham, "VBAC to the Future? A Weekly Check on Health Care Costs and Coverage," *Washington Post,* December 21, 2004.

11. Laura Landro, "New Practices Reduce Childbirth Risks," *Wall Street Journal,* July 12, 2006.

12. Joint Commission on Accreditation of Health Care Organizations, *Sentinel Event Statistics 2006,* accessed at www.jointcommission.org/SentinelEvents/Statistics on November 27, 2006.

13. Organisation for Economic Co-operation and Development, *OECD Health Data 2004,* "Infant Mortality, Deaths per 1000 Live Births; Millennium Indicators: Maternal Mortality Ratio per 100,000 Live Births" (Paris: World Health Organization, UNICEF, 2003). Of OECD nations, only France, Korea, Luxembourg, Mexico, and Turkey had maternal mortality rates as high as or higher than those in the U.S. (2000).

14. In 2003, 31 percent of African-American and Latina mothers received substandard or inadequate prenatal care, compared to 20 percent of white mothers. U.S. Centers for Disease Control and Prevention, *National Vital Statistics Report* 54, no. 2 (September 8, 2005).

15. Carol J. Rowland Hogue and Cynthia Vasquez, "Toward a Strategic Approach for Reducing Disparities in Infant Mortality," *American Journal of Public Health* 92, no.4 (2002): 552–556. See also Cynthia J. Berg, Lynne S. Wilcox, and Philip J. Almanda, "The Prevalence of Socioeconomic and Behavioral Characteristics and Their Impact on Very Low Birth Weight in Black and White Infants in Georgia," *Maternal and Child Health Journal* 5, no. 2 (2001): 75–84.

16. Michael C. Lu and Neal Halfon, "Racial and Ethnic Disparities in Birth Outcomes: A Life-Course Perspective," *Maternal and Child Health Journal* 7, no. 1 (March 2003): 13–30.

17. Ibid.

18. Ibid.

19. L. V. Klerman, S. L. Ramey, R. L. Goldenberg, S. Marbury, J. Hou, et al., "A Randomized Trial of Augmented Prenatal Care for Multiple-Risk, Medicaid-Eligible African American Women," *American Journal of Public Health* 91, no. 1 (2001): 105–111. See also Vijaya K. Hogan and Cynthia D. Ferré, "The Social Context of Pregnancy for African American Women: Implications for the Study and Prevention of Adverse Perinatal Outcomes," *Maternal and Child Health Journal* 5, no. 2 (2001): 67–69; Jennifer F. Culhane, Virginia Rauh, Kelly F. McCollum, Vijaya K. Hogan, Kathy Agnew, et al., "Maternal Stress Is Associated with Bacterial Vaginosis in Human Pregnancy," *Maternal Child Health Journal* 5, no. 2 (2004): 127–134.

20. Sarah Mustillo, Nancy Krieger, Erica P. Gunderson, Stephen Sidney, Heather McCreath, and Catarina I. Kiefe, "Self-Reported Experiences of Racial Discrimination and Black–White Differences in Preterm and Low-Birthweight Deliveries: The CARDIA Study," *American Journal of Public Health* 94, no. 12 (December 2004): 2,125–2,131.

21. Urmi Bhaumik, "Boston Healthy Start Initiative: A Case Study of Community Empowerment," Boston Healthy Start Initiative, accessed at www.ids.ac.uk/ids/civsoc/final/usa/USA15.doc on February 22, 2007.

22. Marie C. McCormick, Lisa W. Deal, Barbara L. Devaney, Dexter Chu, Lorenzo Moreno, and Karen T. Raykovich, "The Impact on Clients of a Community-Based Infant Mortality Reduction Program: The National Healthy Start Program Survey of Postpartum Women," *American Journal of Public Health* 91, no. 12 (2001): 1,975–1,977.

23. The Florida Healthy Start Initiative, *Healthy Start Annual Report, 2005,* Florida Department of Health, 2005, accessed at www.doh.state.fl.us/family/mch/hs/hsreport2005.pdf on February 22, 2007.

CHAPTER 18

Advocating for Mothers and Families

Unlike other industrialized countries, the United States provides little support for parenting and working families. For example, the United States stands out as the only industrialized country without universal health care coverage for children and adults. The United States also is the only wealthy nation that does not guarantee paid maternity leave. While nearly two-thirds of the countries included in a recent global study provide at least fourteen weeks of paid childbirth leave to working women—and more than one-third provide paid paternity leave—the United States guarantees only twelve weeks of unpaid family and medical leave, and many workers are not eligible because our employers are not covered or we do not meet working-time requirements (see "Know Your Rights: The Family and Medical Leave Act (1993)," page 320).[1] Three-quarters of private sector workers in the United States do not have a single day of paid sick leave that can be used to care for a sick child, and one-half of U.S. workers have no paid sick days at all.[2] Although the American Academy of Pediatrics and the U.S. Department of Health and Human Services recommend six months of exclusive breast-feeding,[3] the United States has no federal law protecting a mother's right to breast-feed, or requiring employers to provide breast-feeding breaks or sanitary breast-pumping facilities for lactating workers. (For more information on breast-feeding and work, see page 270.) In fact, a recent analysis of family-friendly policies worldwide found that the United States is falling behind other high-income countries, as well as many moderate-income and low-income countries, in creating public policies to protect the health and well-being of parents and children.[4]

How the U.S. Compares on Parental Leave*

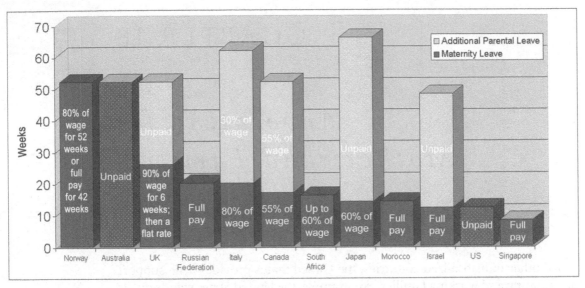

*This graph is based on information from the Clearing House on International Developments in Child, Youth and Family Policies at Columbia University, www.childpolicyintl.org, and "Maternity Leave Benefits," United Nations Statistics Division, available at http://unstats.un.org/unsd/demographic/products/indwm/ww2005/tab5c.htm.

Ever wonder how long your maternity leave would be if you lived in another part of the world? And whether it would be paid? This graph offers a sample of answers. The United States is one of only five countries out of the 173 surveyed in a recent study that does not guarantee some form of paid maternity leave; the other four countries are Lesotho, Liberia, Swaziland, and Papua New Guinea.[5]

PUTTING MOTHERS AND CHILDREN LAST

America's reluctance to invest in children and families has serious and potentially devastating consequences for new mothers and babies:

• U.S. mothers and children are more likely to be poor or extremely poor than mothers and children in other affluent nations. Single mothers are three times more likely to live in poverty than other non-elderly women in the United States, and are twice as likely to lack health insurance as married mothers.[6] Nearly one-third of children in single-mother families—and one-half of such children five years

old or younger—live below the official poverty line.[7]

• In 1971, the United States rejected legislation to make high-quality child care affordable and available to all families who want and need it. Today, low-income and working-poor families with children under five years old spend between 15 and 25 percent of their monthly household income on child care (while higher-income families spend less than 10 percent).[8]

• Working-time and labor regulations in the United States are more business-friendly than family-friendly and disadvantage workers who need time to care for children or family members with special needs. Two-thirds of new mothers report that they do not

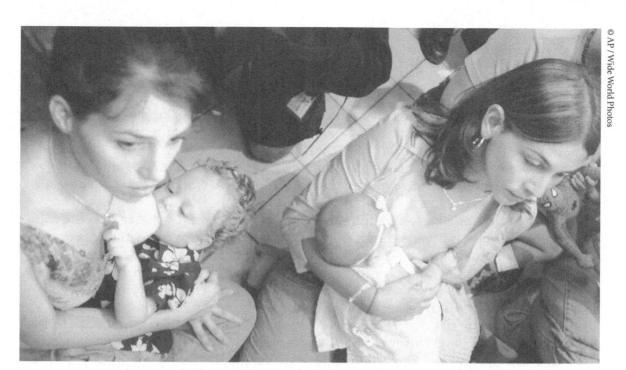

Dozens of mothers nurse their babies in protest on the floor of the Plaza de las Americas Mall in San Juan, Puerto Rico. The women rallied after a mother was asked to leave a store for nursing her baby. Similar protests have successfully changed policies and have led to a greater acceptance of public breast-feeding.

have enough job flexibility to meet their caregiving and personal needs. Those of us who are in the low-wage workforce are hit hardest by rules restricting when and how much time we can take off from work when our families need us, and are least likely to have outside help with caring for children and relatives with serious health problems or disabilities.[9]

MOTHERS IN THE WORKPLACE

Even financially secure mothers in the United States are at risk for unfair treatment in the workplace and future hardship. Gender bias is still common in our society and has a negative influence on women's wages and opportunities for job advancement. Although popular attitudes about women, work, and family have

changed over the last twenty-five years, one study found that two out of every five U.S. workers still believe it's better for fathers to concentrate on making money and for mothers to avoid paid employment when children are small.[10] For employed mothers, sex discrimination and rigid attitudes about men's and women's family roles amount to a double whammy. Mothers in white-collar jobs report they've been overlooked for promotions, pressured by employers to work more or fewer hours, or squeezed out of their careers altogether. Experts who study women in the workplace describe this well-known phenomenon as "hitting the maternal wall."[11] In nearly every U.S. state, it's even legal for employers to reject job applicants on the basis of parental status— a practice that's been called "maternal profiling."[12] Legal experts have identified a new

WHAT IS FAMILY RESPONSIBILITIES DISCRIMINATION?

Employment discrimination based on race, sex, religion, disability, and other personal characteristics is widely recognized as illegal and unfair. Employment law experts have recently identified another type of workplace discrimination. Family responsibilities discrimination, or FRD, is discrimination based solely on your status as a parent or caregiver. It can affect the pay, promotion, and job security of pregnant women, mothers and fathers of young children, and workers who take time off to care for aging parents.

FRD can be obvious—as when a supervisor tells a worker she can be a good worker or a good mother, but not both at the same time—or more subtle. For example, an employer may hold a mother to a more rigorous standard of attendance than other workers with similar job responsibilities, or may not consider a mother for promotion, even when she is highly qualified. Or, an employee who was previously recognized for excellence will get poor performance reviews after she has a child, even though the quality of her work hasn't changed. Fathers experience FRD, too. One new dad was informed that his wife would have to be "in a coma or dead" before his employer would give him time off to care for his infant daughter.

While sex discrimination is often a factor in FRD, motherhood itself appears to make women more vulnerable to unfair treatment in the workplace. When researchers at Cornell University conducted a study on mothers in the job market, they found that among equally skilled job applicants, mothers were less likely to be hired and were offered lower starting salaries than fathers, and than women without children.[13]

If you think you may have experienced FRD, contact the Center for Work-Life Law (1-800-981-9495 or www.uchastings.edu/?pid=3624) to find out more about family responsibilities discrimination, and how to take action if it's happening to you.

category of employment discrimination against workers with caregiving responsibilities, which they call "family responsibilities discrimination," or FRD (see "What Is Family Responsibilities Discrimination?" above).[14]

Nearly all working women in the United States are affected by the gender gap in pay. Today, full-time female workers earn just 76 cents for every dollar earned by full-time male workers. It doesn't matter if a woman has a high-earning salaried position or a lower-wage job; analysts who study the gender gap in earnings find that in almost every occupation, men are paid more than women for exactly the same work.[15] But an additional "motherhood penalty" takes an extra bite out of mothers' wages—decreasing moms' earnings by 5 to 7 percent for each child—while married fathers tend to have higher earnings than other male workers.[16] While researchers believe that gender bias is a contributing factor, the motherhood pay penalty—as well as its opposite, the "daddy bonus"—is mostly related to the fact that mothers spend fewer hours in the paid workforce and more time on unpaid family work than fathers do.[17] ("Unpaid family work" or "caregiving" includes caring for children and everything else people do to keep our homes and families comfortable, safe, and healthy.) Even when both parents in two-earner couples work similar hours and have similar earnings, women typically provide about two-thirds of the household's family work.[18] However, one-third of new mothers in the United States are not married, and many have full responsibility for both wage earning and caregiving. Outdated cultural attitudes, unsupportive social policies, and inflexible workplace practices can create substantial barriers to well-being for such moms and our families.

Today, between two-thirds and one-half of all American mothers manage family responsibilities by working less than full-time or remaining out of the paid workforce until children reach school age. Part-time work and periods of non-employment have a lasting effect on mothers' individual earnings and ability to move into higher-paying jobs, in part because business owners don't have to pay part-time employees the same hourly wages that full-time employees would get for doing the same job. Nor are employers required to give part-time employees the same paid benefits (prorated by hours of work), such as vacation time, health insurance, and retirement benefits, that they offer to full-time workers. The loss of income, benefits, and job experience during our childbearing and child-rearing years leaves American mothers especially at risk for financial insecurity if we are single, widowed, or divorced, if a spouse becomes unemployed or disabled, or if we retire.

The economic well-being and health outcomes of new mothers and babies are also affected by whether or not women have paid maternity leave. One recent study found that the earnings of first-time mothers who had taken paid maternity leave after the birth of their child were significantly higher than the earnings of mothers who had taken unpaid leave or had taken no maternity leave at all.[19] This effect was seen regardless of earnings, education, or job status. A separate study found that longer paid leaves and mothers' ability to work less than full-time for at least eighteen months following childbirth reduced infant mortality and improved children's developmental outcomes.[20] Yet in the United States, three-quarters of first-time mothers lack employer- or state-funded maternity leave.[21] Currently, California is the only U.S. state that provides paid parental leave, although paid-leave legislation has been approved in Washington State (to take effect in October 2009) and is being considered in several other states.*

Even without the benefit of paid leave, most American mothers take some time off when our babies are young. While seven out of ten mothers with children under eighteen work for pay and one-half are employed full-time, nearly one-half of mothers with babies younger than twelve months old are not employed, and only one in three works full-time.[22] Mothers who take a few months or a few years off from paid work sometimes feel isolated, overwhelmed, and frustrated because others (even loving partners or spouses) do not recognize or value the incredible amount of time, effort, and mental focus involved in caring for infants and toddlers. Although fathers today devote more time to housework and child care than dads of previous generations, men still face workplace and cultural pressures that conflict with equal participation in parenting. Because many Americans have fixed ideas about which kinds

* For information on state paid leave initiatives, see the National Partnership for Women and Families website, www.national partnership.org.

of activities should be rewarded as "real" work, the unpaid caregiving work mothers and fathers do—which is absolutely necessary to the health of the nation's families and the well-being of our society—is often taken for granted, or even counted as a "leisure" activity by some economists.

WE CAN DO BETTER!

Because our culture sets unrealistically high expectations for mothers, we sometimes try to take too much responsibility for problems caused by lawmakers' indifference to the hardships of women and families. For example, we often believe we would do a better job of coping with the demands of paid work and caregiving if we were more efficient workers, or more competent mothers. The truth is that new mothers in the United States need more and better support from the rest of society than we are getting.

In fact, a national survey found that 90 percent of American mothers feel the United States could do more to meet the needs of mothers

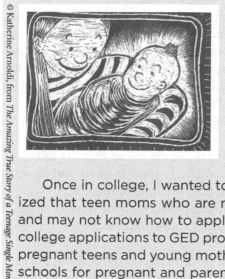

"I wanted to do for others what Jackie had done for me."

Katherine Arnoldi

After I became a mother as a teenager, I still wanted to go to college. But I did not know how to get there. I worked in a factory, saved my money, and ran into one bad thing after another until I met Jackie Ward, another teen mother, who told me the two words that changed my life forever: financial aid.

Once in college, I wanted to do for others what Jackie had done for me. I realized that teen moms who are not in high school miss out on guidance counseling and may not know how to apply to college, so I took financial aid applications and college applications to GED programs. The more I did, the more I learned about how pregnant teens and young mothers are discriminated against. Some are diverted to schools for pregnant and parenting teens when they would prefer another school. Some are moved from honors classes to special education. Some are told that their high school does not have insurance for them, when that is not true. All of these actions are against the law.

Hoping to encourage mothers to fight for their equal rights to education, I wrote and illustrated *The Amazing True Story of a Teenage Single Mom.* I worked with the Reproductive Rights Project at New York Civil Liberties Union to bring a class action lawsuit against the New York City Board of Education. The ongoing lawsuit was filed on behalf of teenage mothers who were denied equal rights by being coerced to leave their school or by not being allowed to enroll in the school of their choice.

Colleges, too, discriminate. For example, a college might say all first-year students have to live on campus, but make no accommodations for students who have children. Colleges need to add more family housing and provide more day care for students' children. Pregnant and parenting teens need to insist on their rights, with lawsuits if necessary. Also, like Jackie Ward, we all need to pass life-changing information along.*

* For a college guide for mothers, see www.katherinearnoldi.com.

and families.[23] This is not surprising; a 2006 report from Save the Children found that among wealthy Western nations, the United States is the worst place to be a mother.[24] Experts who study workplace issues and family life have devoted more than thirty years of research to identifying important gaps in U.S. family policy, and they consistently find that our nation comes up short in supporting caregivers and children. Based on the recommendations of people who care about the welfare of women and families, the following policies top the list of protections and benefits U.S. families urgently need:

- Universal health care for all children and adults.
- A minimum of twelve weeks of paid parental leave for the birth or adoption of a child, for both mothers and fathers and for same-sex partners.
- A minimum of seven days of paid sick leave per year for all workers that can be used to care for a sick family member or child.
- Federal protection for breast-feeding rights, in the workplace and wherever mothers and babies spend time.
- Excellent, affordable child care and eldercare for everyone who wants and needs it.
- Raising the federal minimum wage to a living wage, and making sure it increases when the cost of living increases.
- Welfare policies and regulations that provide more and better support for parental and paid caregiving in at-risk families, and effective programs to help women and families overcome poverty.
- The right for all workers to request flexible work hours and part-time work as our family and personal circumstances change.
- Equal pay rates and at least prorated benefits for part-time workers.
- Elimination of mandatory overtime and setting of an upper limit on weekly work hours to give parents and caregivers more control over our daily schedules and hours of work.
- Tax credits for family caregivers to defray some of the costs of unpaid caring work.
- Social Security benefits and disability coverage for non-employed caregivers.
- Revisions to family law so that the full value of unpaid family work is taken into account when parents separate or divorce.
- Counting unpaid caregiving work in national productivity measurements.

These policies stress collective support for families and children, and acknowledge the social and economic value of unpaid family work. On the basis of examples from other economically competitive countries, researchers know such policies work. Specifically, these programs and benefits reduce mothers' and children's poverty, improve maternal and infant health, and promote women's social and economic equality.

The goal of these policies is to create a solid "floor" for women and children by regulating

MOMSRISING

Fed up with how things are? Get involved! MomsRising (www.momsrising.org), a grassroots advocacy organization, offers an easy entry into the online world of citizen action. From the group's website you can learn more about the issues mothers confront, from discrimination in the workplace to the lack of paid maternity leave to the failure of policy makers to recognize the importance of caretaking. You can connect with other mothers, find out about MomsRising house parties and *The Motherhood Manifesto* book and film, sign petitions, and work to break the logjam that's been holding back family-friendly legislation for decades.

working conditions to make them less un- friendly to families and by reducing the un- equal costs of motherhood. But some mothers need more targeted protections and support in addition to the basic benefits listed above. These include those of us who have a disability or are mothers of children with disabilities, mothers with female partners, incarcerated mothers, mothers with mental illness or addic- tion, mothers who experience domestic vio- lence, and the growing numbers of us who have both child care and eldercare responsibilities. We and our families need access to a range of responsive social services to address our health and human needs, and more and better community-based programs to support our long-term well-being.

WHAT YOU CAN DO

Taking action for social change can be a great way to connect with other new mothers and advocate on issues that are vital to you. Many organizations and support groups provide in- formation and advocacy opportunities for mothers who want to make a difference.

Some organizations offer one-click Inter- net campaigns you can access from a home or library computer, as well as local, state, or re- gional chapters that you can join. Others offer in-depth information about policy issues and how workplace discrimination hurts pregnant and parenting women. Some groups offer face- to-face discussion and support with a special focus on motherhood as a social issue. There are many different ways to participate, and most groups fighting for a more family-friendly America welcome member volunteers. A list of some of these organizations is included in "Re- sources," at the back of this book (see the sec- tion "Advocating for Better Maternity Care and for Mothers and Families," beginning on page 335).

The hidden history of American progress is that mothers' collective activism has always been essential to improving social conditions for women, children, and families. From out- lawing child labor in the United States to lob- bying for the nation's first safe food and drug laws, from campaigning for public kindergar- tens to passing the Family Medical Leave Act of 1993, mothers have joined with other con- cerned citizens to create a more caring society. And when the time is right, you can make his- tory, too.

NOTES

1. Jody Heymann, Alison Earle, and Jeffrey Hayes, *The Work, Family, and Equity Index: How Does the United States Measure Up,* Global Project on Working Fami- lies, Institute for Health and Social Policy, McGill University, February 2007; available at www.mcgill .ca/files/ihsp/WFEI2007FEB.pdf.
2. Vicky Lovell, *No Time to Be Sick: Why Everyone Suf- fers When Workers Don't Have Paid Sick Leave,* Insti- tute for Women's Policy Research, May 2004; accessed at www.iwpr.org/Publications/pdf.htm on October 18, 2006.
3. American Academy of Pediatrics, "Policy Statement: Breastfeeding and the Use of Human Milk," *Pediatrics* 115, no. 2 (February 2005): 496–506. See also U.S. Department of Health and Human Services, *HHS Blueprint for Action on Breastfeeding* (Washington, DC: U.S. Department of Health and Human Services, Office on Women's Health, 2000).
4. Heymann et al., *Work, Family and Equity Index.*
5. Ibid.
6. Karen Christopher and Paula England, "Women's Poverty Relative to Men's in Affluent Nations: Single Motherhood and the State," *Research Summaries* 1, no. 1 (Joint Center for Poverty Research, 2000); Henry J. Kaiser Family Foundation, "Women's Health Insurance Coverage," July 2001.
7. U.S. Census Bureau, *Current Population Survey, 2005 Annual Social and Economic Supplement.*
8. U.S. Census Bureau, *Average Weekly Childcare Expen- ditures of Families with Employed Mothers,* winter 2002.

9. Jody Heymann, *The Widening Gap: Why America's Working Families Are in Jeopardy and What Can Be Done About It* (New York: Basic Books, 2000).

10. Families and Work Institute, *2002 National Study of the Changing Workforce*, 2003.

11. Joan C. Williams, *Unbending Gender: Why Family and Work Conflict and What to Do About It* (New York: Oxford University Press, 2000). See also Ann Crittenden, *The Price of Motherhood* (New York: Metropolitan Books, 2001).

12. Barbara Kate Repa, "State Laws Prohibiting Discrimination in Employment" [table], *Your Rights in the Workplace*, 7th ed. (Berkeley, CA: Nolo Press, 2005), 185–189.

13. Shelley Correll and Stephen Benard, "Getting a Job: Is There a Motherhood Penalty?" conference paper, American Sociological Association, August 12, 2005.

14. Center for WorkLife Law, UC Hastings College of the Law, "Current Law Prohibits Discrimination Based on Family Responsibilities and Gender Stereotyping," 2006.

15. Daniel Weinberg, "Evidence from Census 2000 About Earnings by Detailed Occupation for Men and Women," U.S. Census Bureau, May 2005.

16. Michelle J. Budig and Paula England, "The Wage Penalty for Motherhood," *American Sociological Review* 66, no. 2 (April 2000).

17. U.S. Department of Labor, Bureau of Labor Statistics, "The American Time Use Survey—First Results," September 2004.

18. U.S. Department of Labor, Bureau of Labor Statistics, "American Time Use Survey—First Results." See also W. Jean Yeung and John F. Sandberg, "Children's Time With Fathers in Intact Families," *Journal of Marriage and Family* 63, no. 1 (February 2001).

19. Heather Boushey, "Family-Friendly Policies: Boosting Mothers' Wages," Center for Economic Policy Research, April 2005.

20. Royal Economic Society, "Extending Paid Maternity Leave: Health Benefits for Children," *Economic Journal*, February 2005.

21. Boushey, "Family-Friendly Policies."

22. U.S. Census Bureau, "Fertility of American Women: June 2004," issued December 2005.

23. Martha Farrell Erickson and Enola Aird, "The Motherhood Study: Fresh Insights on Mothers' Attitudes and Concerns," commissioned by the Mothers' Council, sponsored by University of Minnesota, University of Connecticut, and Institute for American Values, May 2005.

24. Save the Children Foundation, "2006 Mother's Index Rankings," in "State of the World's Mothers 2006: Saving the Lives of Mothers and Newborns," May 2006.

Resources

Walk into any bookstore, and you will find shelves of books on pregnancy and childbirth. Search the Internet, and you'll find thousands of websites full of advice for pregnant women. Yet while a tremendous amount of information is available, its quality varies greatly. Finding information that is up-to-date, reliable, and grounded in a respect for the natural process of birth is often difficult.

The Childbirth Connection website (www.childbirthconnection.org) is one source that meets all three of these criteria. It provides extensive content on topics ranging from choosing a provider to vaginal births after cesarean section. With summaries of the best available research about the safety and effectiveness of women's options, and tips and tools for helping women make decisions, the website is an invaluable source of high-quality childbearing information.

The list below includes additional recommended resources on pregnancy, birth, and early motherhood. The resources are sorted into the following categories: General; Personal Experiences; Birth Companions and Birth Preparation Techniques; Taking Care of Yourself; Sexuality; Prenatal Testing and Disability; Special Concerns; Childbearing Loss; Cesarean Sections; Breast-Feeding; Life as a New Mother; Postpartum Mood Disorders; and Advocating for Better Maternity Care and for Mothers and Families.

For a more extensive list, as well as up-to-date information and resources on a wide range of women's health topics, visit the Our Bodies Ourselves website at www.ourbodiesourselves.org/childbirth.

GENERAL

Books and Article

Armstrong, Penny, and Sheryl Feldman. *A Wise Birth: Bringing Together the Best of Natural Childbirth with Modern Medicine.* 2nd ed. London: Pinter & Martin, 2006.

Davis, Elizabeth. *Heart & Hands: A Midwife's Guide to Pregnancy & Birth.* 4th ed. Berkeley, CA: Celestial Arts, 2004.

England, Pam, and Rob Horowitz. *Birthing from Within: An Extra-Ordinary Guide to Childbirth Preparation.* Albuquerque: Partera Press, 1998.

Gaskin, Ina May. *Ina May's Guide to Childbirth.* New York: Bantam Books, 2003.

——. *Spiritual Midwifery.* 4th ed. Summertown, TN: Book Publishing Company, 2002.

Goer, Henci. *The Thinking Woman's Guide to a Better Birth.* New York: Perigee Books, 1999.

Harper, Barbara. *Gentle Birth Choices: A Guide to Making Informed Decisions.* 3rd ed. Rochester, VT: Healing Arts Press, 2005.

Kitzinger, Sheila. *Birth Your Way: Choosing Birth at Home or in a Birth Center.* Rev. ed. London: Dorling Kindersley, 2002.

——. *The Complete Book of Pregnancy and Childbirth.* 4th ed. New York: Knopf, 2004.

——. *Rediscovering Birth.* New York: Atria, 2001.

Lothian, Judith, and Charlotte DeVries. *The Official Lamaze Guide: Giving Birth with Confidence.* Minnetonka, MN: Meadowbrook Press, 2005. Also available for download at www.lamaze.org/birth_confidence.

Rogers, Judith. *The Disabled Woman's Guide to Pregnancy and Birth.* New York: Demos Medical Publishing, 2006.

Simkin, Penny, and April Bolding. "Update on Nonpharmacological Approaches to Relieve Labor Pain and Prevent Suffering." *Journal of Midwifery & Women's Health* 49, no. 6 (2004): 489–504.

Simkin, Penny, Janet Whalley, and Ann Kepler. *Pregnancy, Childbirth and the Newborn, Revised and Updated: The Complete Guide.* Minnetonka, MN: Meadowbrook Press, 2003.

van der Ziel, Cornelia, and Jacqueline Tourville, *Big, Beautiful and Pregnant: Expert Advice and Comforting Wisdom for the Expecting Plus-Size Woman.* New York: Marlowe, 2006. Also available at www.bigbeautifulandpregnant.com.

Periodicals

Journal of Midwifery & Women's Health
240-485-1815
www.jmwh.org

Midwifery Today
800-743-0974 (orders only) or 541-344-7438
www.midwiferytoday.com

Audiovisual Materials

Jarmel, Marcia, and Ken Schneider. *Born in the USA.* DVD/VHS. 60 minutes. 2000. Available from PatchWorks Films, 663 Seventh Avenue, San Francisco, CA 94118; 415-387-5912; www.patchworksfilms.net.

Relaxation, Rhythm, Ritual: The 3 Rs of Childbirth. DVD/VHS. 15 minutes. 2003. Available from Penny Simkin, Inc., 1100 Twenty-third Avenue, East Seattle, WA 98112; 206-325-1419; www.pennysimkin.com.

Organizations

American Association of Birth Centers (AABC)
3123 Gottschall Road, Perkiomenville, PA 18074

215-234-8068
www.birthcenters.org

American College of Nurse-Midwives
8403 Colesville Road, Suite 1550,
    Silver Spring, MD 20910
240-485-1800
www.midwife.org

American College of Obstetricians and
    Gynecologists (ACOG)
409 Twelfth Street SW, PO Box 96920,
    Washington, DC 20090
202-638-5577
www.acog.org

Childbirth Connection
    (formerly Maternity Center Association)
281 Park Avenue South, 5th Floor,
    New York, NY 10010
212-777-5000
www.childbirthconnection.org

Midwives Alliance of North America (MANA)
375 Rockbridge Road, Suite 172–313,
    Lilburn, GA 30047
888-923-MANA (888-923-6262)
www.mana.org

North American Registry of Midwives
    (NARM)
5257 Rosestone Drive, Lilburn, GA 30047
888-842-4784
www.narm.org

Websites

American College of Obstetricians and
    Gynecologists
http://acog.org

Childbirth.org
www.childbirth.org

Childbirth Connection's Labor Pain Initiative
www.childbirthconnection.org/article.asp?
    ck10130&ClickedLink=0&area-34

Coalition for Improving Maternity Services
To access "Having a Baby? Ten Questions
    to Ask," see www.motherfriendly.org/
    resources/10Q.

myMidwife.org
www.mymidwife.org

PERSONAL EXPERIENCES

Books

Armstrong, Penny, and Sheryl Feldman. *A Midwife's Story.* London: Pinter & Martin 2007.

Limburg, Astrid, and Beatrijs Smulders (text), and Saski Van Ress (photos). *Women Giving Birth.* Translated by Olga Smulders. Berkeley, CA: Celestial Arts, 1993.

Lipper, Joanna. *Growing Up Fast.* New York: Picador, 2003.

Logan, Onnie Lee. *Motherwit: An Alabama Midwife's Story.* New York: Plume Books, 1991.

Menelli, Sheri. *Journey into Motherhood: Inspirational Stories of Natural Childbirth.* Carlsbad, CA: White Heart Publishing, 2004.

Schwegel, Janet, ed. *Adventures in Natural Childbirth: Tales from Women on the Joys, Fears, Pleasures, and Pains of Giving Birth Naturally.* New York: Marlowe, 2005.

Smith, Margaret Charles, and Linda Janet Holmes. *Listen to Me Good: The Life Story of an Alabama Midwife.* Columbus: Ohio State University Press, 1996.

Steingraber, Sandra. *Having Faith: An Ecologist's Journey to Motherhood.* Cambridge, MA: Perseus Publishing, 2001.

Thatcher-Ulrich, Laurel. *A Midwife's Tale: The Life of Martha Ballard, Based on Her Diary, 1785–1812.* New York: Knopf, 1990.

Vincent, Peggy. *Baby Catcher: Chronicles of a Modern Midwife.* New York: Scribner, 2002. Also available at www.babycatcher.net.

BIRTH COMPANIONS AND BIRTH PREPARATION TECHNIQUES

Books

Klaus, Marshall H., John H. Kennell, and Phyllis H. Klaus. *The Doula Book: How a Trained Labor Companion Can Help You Have a Shorter, Easier, and Healthier Birth.* Cambridge, MA: Perseus Publishing, 2002.

Odent, Michel, and Grantly Dick-Read. *Childbirth Without Fear: The Principles and Practice of Natural Childbirth.* London: Pinter & Martin, 2004.

Simkin, Penny. *The Birth Partner: Everything You Need to Know to Help a Woman Through Childbirth.* 2nd ed. Boston: Harvard Common Press, 2001.

Periodical

Special Delivery
www.alace.org/special_delivery.html

Audiovisual Material

Maraesa, Aminata. *Woman to Woman: Doula Assisted Childbirth.* DVD/VHS. 26 minutes. 2003. Available from Documentary Educational Resources, 101 Morse Street, Watertown, MA 02472; 800-569-6621 or 617-926-0491; docued@der.org.

Organizations

Childbirth and Postpartum Professionals Association (CAPPA)
PO Box 491448, Lawrenceville, GA 30049
888-MY-CAPPA (888-692-2772)
www.cappa.net

Doulas of North America (DONA)
PO Box 626, Jasper, IN 47547
888-788-DONA (888-788-3662)
www.dona.org

International Childbirth Education Association (ICEA)
PO Box 20048, Minneapolis, MN 54420
952-854-8660
www.icea.org

Lamaze Institute for Normal Birth
2025 M Street NW, Suite 800, Washington, DC 20036-3309
800-368-4404 or 202-367-1128
http://normalbirth.lamaze.org/institute

Websites

Birth Works
www.birthworks.org

Birthing from Within
www.birthingfromwithin.com

Bradley Method
www.bradleybirth.com

Mindfulness-Based Childbirth and Parenting Education Program
www.mindfulbirthing.org

HypnoBirthing
www.hypnobirthing.com

TAKING CARE OF YOURSELF

Books

Erick, Miriam. *Managing Morning Sickness*. Rev. ed. Boulder, CO: Bull Publishing, 2004.

Groenou, Aneema van. *The Active Woman's Guide to Pregnancy: Practical Advice for Getting Outdoors When Expecting*. Berkeley, CA: Ten Speed Press, 2004.

Lim, Robin. *Eating for Two: Recipes for Pregnant and Breastfeeding Women*. Berkeley, CA: Celestial Arts, 2004.

Noble, Elizabeth. *Essential Exercises for the Childbearing Year: A Guide to Health and Comfort Before and After Your Baby Is Born*. 4th ed. Harwich, MA: New Life Images, 2003.

Roberts, Holly. *Your Vegetarian Pregnancy: A Month-by-Month Guide to Health and Nutrition*. New York: Fireside / Simon & Schuster, 2003.

Romm, Aviva Jill. *The Natural Pregnancy Book: Herbs, Nutrition, and Other Holistic Choices*. Berkeley, CA: Celestial Arts, 2003.

Schettler, Ted, Gina Solomon, Marian Valenti, and Annette Huddle. *Generations at Risk: Reproductive Health and the Environment*. Cambridge: MIT Press, 2000.

Website

Motherisk.org
www.motherisk.org/index.jsp

SEXUALITY

Books

Raskin, Valerie D. *Great Sex for Moms: Ten Steps to Nurturing Passion While Raising Kids*. New York: Fireside / Simon & Schuster, 2002.

Raykeil, Heidi. *Confessions of a Naughty Mommy: How I Found My Lost Libido*. Emeryville, CA: Seal Press, 2005.

Winks, Cathy and Anne Semans. *Sexy Mamas: Keeping Your Sex Life Alive While Raising Kids*. Makawao, HI: Inner Ocean, 2004.

PRENATAL TESTING AND DISABILITY

Books

Adolphson, Tyler. *Beyond the Stares: A Personal Journal for Siblings of Children with Disabilities*. St. Louis, MO: Delta Gamma Center, 2004.

Bérubé, Michael. *Life as We Know It: A Father, a Family, and an Exceptional Child*. New York: Vintage Books, 1998.

Kingsley, Jason and Mitchell Levitz. *Count Us In: Growing Up with Down Syndrome*. San Diego, CA: Harvest / HBJ, 1994.

Pueschel, Siegfried, ed. *Adults with Down Syndrome*. Baltimore: Brookes Publishing, 2006.

——. *A Parent's Guide to Down Syndrome: Toward a Brighter Future*. Rev. ed. Baltimore: Brookes Publishing, 2001.

Rapp, Rayna. *Testing Women, Testing the Fetus: The Social Impact of Amniocentesis in America*. New York: Routledge, 2000.

Read, Janet. *Disability, the Family, and Society: Listening to Mothers*. Buckingham, England: Open University Press, 2000.

Rothman, Barbara Katz. *Recreating Motherhood: Ideology and Technology in a Patriarchal Society*. New Brunswick, NJ: Rutgers University Press, 2000.

Zuckoff, Mitchell. *Choosing Naia: A Family's Journey*. Boston: Beacon Press, 2003.

Organizations

The Arc of the United States
1010 Wayne Avenue, Suite 650, Silver Spring,
    MD 20910
301-565-3842
www.thearc.org

Family Voices, Inc.
2340 Alamo SE, Suite 102, Albuquerque,
    NM 87106
888-835-5669 or (505) 872-4774
www.familyvoices.org

Genetic Alliance, Inc.
4301 Connecticut Avenue NW, Suite 404,
    Washington, DC 20008-2369
202-966-5557
www.geneticalliance.org

Website

March of Dimes
www.marchofdimes.com/pnhec/4439_1206.asp

SPECIAL CONCERNS

Violence and Sexual Abuse

Book

Simkin, Penny, and Phyllis Klaus. *When Survivors Give Birth: Understanding and Healing the Effects of Early Sexual Abuse on Childbearing Women*. Seattle: Classic Day Publishing, 2004.

Hotlines

National Domestic Violence Hotline
    (English and Spanish)
PO Box 161810, Austin, TX 78716

800-799-SAFE (800-799-7233);
    TTY: 800-787-3224
www.ndvh.org

Rape, Abuse & Incest National Network
    (RAINN)
2000 L Street NW, Suite 406, Washington, DC
    20036
Hotline for survivors of sexual assault:
    800-656-HOPE (800-656-4673)
www.rainn.org

Lesbian Mothers

Book

Brill, Stephanie. *The New Essential Guide to Lesbian Conception, Pregnancy, and Birth*. Los Angeles: Alyson Books, 2006.

Diabetes

Books

Task Force of the American Diabetes Association Council on Pregnancy, Lois Jovanovic, editor in chief. *Diabetes & Pregnancy: What to Expect*. 4th ed. Alexandria, VA: American Diabetes Association, 2001.

Task Force of the American Diabetes Association Council on Pregnancy, Lois Jovanovic, editor in chief. *Gestational Diabetes: What to Expect*. 5th ed. Alexandria, VA: American Diabetes Association, 2005.

Organization

American Diabetes Association
1701 North Beauregard Street, Alexandria, VA
    22311
800-342-2383
www.diabetes.org/gestational-diabetes.jsp

Teens

Book

Arnoldi, Katherine. *The Amazing True Story of a Teenage Single Mom.* New York: Hyperion, 1998.

Website

GirlMom
www.girlmom.com

CHILDBEARING LOSS

Books and Article

Abbey, Amy L., ed. *Journeys: Stories of Pregnancy After Loss.* Boulder, CO: Woven Word Press, 2006.

Ash, Lorraine. *Life Touches Life: A Mother's Story of Stillbirth and Healing.* Troutdale, OR: New Sage Press, 2004.

Bennett, Nina. *Forgotten Tears: A Grandmother's Journey Through Grief.* Bangor, ME: Booklocker.com, 2005.

Berman, Michael R. *Parenthood Lost: Healing the Pain After Miscarriage, Stillbirth, and Infant Death.* Westport, CT: Bergin & Garvey, 2001.

Isle, Sherokee. *Empty Arms: Coping After Miscarriage, Stillbirth, and Infant Death.* Rev. ed. Maple Plain, MN: Wintergreen Press, 2000.

Kluger-Bell, Kim. *Unspeakable Losses, Healing from Miscarriage, Abortion, and Other Pregnancy Loss.* New York: HarperCollins, 2000.

Layne, Linda L. " 'A Women's Health Model for Pregnancy Loss': A Call for a New Standard of Care." *Feminist Studies* 32, no. 3 (2006).

———. *Motherhood Lost: A Feminist Account of Pregnancy Loss in America.* New York: Routledge, 2002.

Nelson, Tim. *A Guide for Fathers: When a Baby Dies.* Rev. ed., Tim Nelson, 2007.

Organizations

Center for Loss in Multiple Birth (CLIMB)
P.O. Box 91377, Anchorage AK 99509
907-222-5321
www.climb-support.org

Hygeia Foundation, Inc., and Institute for Perinatal Loss and Bereavement
413 Temple Street, New Haven CT 06511
800-893-9198
www.hygeia.org

MISS Foundation
PO Box 5333, Peoria, AZ 85385-5333
623-979-1000
www.missfoundation.org

Share Pregnancy Loss & Infant Support, Inc.
St. Joseph Health Center
300 First Capitol Drive, St. Charles, Missouri 63301-2893
800-821-6819 or 636-947-6164
www.nationalshareoffice.com

Wisconsin Stillbirth Service Program (WiSSP)
Waisman Center, Room 343, 1500 Highland Avenue, Madison, WI 53705-2280
www.wisc.edu/wissp

CESAREAN SECTIONS

Article

Childbirth Connection. "What Every Pregnant Woman Needs to Know About Cesarean Birth." Rev. ed. 2006. Also available for free download at www.childbirthconnection.org/article.asp?ck=10164.

Organization

International Cesarean Awareness Network (ICAN)
1304 Kingsdale Avenue, Redondo Beach, CA 90278
800-686-ICAN (800-686-4226)
www.ican-online.org

Website

VBAC.com
www.vbac.com

BREAST-FEEDING

Books

Behrmann, Barbara. *The Breastfeeding Café: Mothers Share the Joys, Challenges & Secrets of Nursing.* Ann Arbor: University of Michigan Press, 2005.

Berggren, Kirsten. *Working Without Weaning: A Working Mother's Guide to Breastfeeding.* Amarillo, TX: Hale Publishing, 2006.

Hale, Thomas W. *Medications and Mothers' Milk.* 12th ed. Amarillo, TX: Hale Publishing, 2006.

Hicks, Jennifer, comp. and ed. *Hirkani's Daughters: Women Who Scale Modern Mountains to Combine Breastfeeding and Working.* Schaumburg, IL: La Leche League International, 2005.

Huggins, Kathleen. *The Nursing Mother's Companion.* 5th ed. Boston: Harvard Common Press, 2005.

Kroeger, Mary, and Linda Smith. *Impact of Birth Practices on Breastfeeding: Protecting the Mother and Baby Continuum.* Boston: Jones & Bartlett Publishers, 2004.

La Leche League International. *The Womanly Art of Breastfeeding.* 7th rev. ed. New York: Plume, 2004.

Mohrbacher, Nancy, and Kathleen Kendall-Tackett. *Breastfeeding Made Simple: Seven Natural Laws for Nursing Mothers.* Oakland, CA: New Harbinger Publications, 2005.

Renfrew, Mary, Chloe Fisher, and Suzanne Arms. *Bestfeeding: How to Breastfeed Your Baby.* Berkeley, CA: Ten Speed Press, 2004.

Steiner, Andy. *Spilled Milk: Breastfeeding Adventures and Advice from Less-Than-Perfect Moms.* New York: Rodale, 2005.

Audiovisual Material

In Your Hands: The Best Start for Your Breastfed Baby. Video. 10 minutes. 2002. Available from Breastfeeding Center, Boston Medical Center, 850 Harrison Avenue ACC5, Boston, MA 02118-2393; 617-414-MILK (617-414-6455).

Organizations

International Lactation Consultant Association (ILCA)
1500 Sunday Drive, Suite 102, Raleigh, NC 27607
919-861-5577
www.ilca.org

La Leche League International
PO Box 4079, Schaumburg, IL 60168-4079
800-LALECHE (800-525-3243)
www.lalecheleague.org

MOMS (Making Our Milk Safe)
1125 High Street
Alameda, CA 94501
www.safemilk.org

Websites

The Breastfeeding Café
www.breastfeedingcafe.com

MotherRisk
www.motherisk.org/index.jsp

Common Sense Breastfeeding
www.wiessinger.baka.com/bfing

LactMed
http://toxnet.nlm.nih.gov/cgi-bin/sis/
   htmlgen?LACT

Mothers Overcoming Breastfeeding Issues
   (MOBI)
www.mobimotherhood.org

The National Women's Health Information
   Center
www.4women.gov/breastfeeding/index
   .cfm?page=home

World Alliance for Breastfeeding Action
www.waba.org.my

LIFE AS A NEW MOTHER

Books

Cockrell, Stacie, Cathy O'Neill, and Julia Stone. *Babyproofing Your Marriage: How to Laugh More, Argue Less, and Communicate Better as Your Family Grows.* New York: Harper-Collins, 2007.

Gore, Ariel. *The Hip Mama Survival Guide: Advice from the Trenches.* New York: Hyperion, 1998.

Gottman, John, and Julie Schwartz Gottman. *And Baby Makes Three: The Six-Step Plan for Preserving Marital Intimacy and Rekindling Romance After Baby Arrives.* New York: Crown, 2007.

Jordan, Pamela L., Scott M. Stanley, and Howard J. Markman. *Becoming Parents: How to Strengthen Your Marriage as Your Family Grows.* San Francisco: Jossey-Bass, 1999.

Karp, Harvey. *The Happiest Baby on the Block: The New Way to Calm Crying and Help Your Newborn Baby Sleep Longer.* New York: Bantam, 2003.

Kendall-Tackett, Kathleen. *The Hidden Feelings of Motherhood: Coping with Stress, Depression, and Burnout.* Oakland: New Harbinger Publications, 2001.

Klaus, Marshall, and Phyllis Klaus. *Your Amazing Newborn.* New York, NY: Perseus Books, 1998.

Lim, Robin. *After the Baby's Birth: A Woman's Way to Wellness: A Complete Guide for Postpartum Women.* Rev. ed. Berkeley: Celestial Arts, 2001.

Placksin, Sally. *Mothering the New Mother: Women's Feelings and Needs After Childbirth; A Support and Resource Guide.* 2nd ed. New York: Newmarket Press, 2000.

Romm, Aviva Jill. *Natural Health After Birth: The Complete Guide to Postpartum Wellness.* Rochester, VT: Healing Arts Press, 2002.

Singer, Katie. *The Garden of Fertility: A Guide to Charting Your Fertility Signals to Prevent or Achieve Pregnancy—Naturally—and to Gauge Your Reproductive Health.* New York: Avery, 2004. Also see www.gardenof fertility.com.

Periodicals, Including Online Magazines

Brain, Child: The Magazine for Thinking
   Mothers
888-304-6667
www.brainchildmag.com

Literary Mama
www.literarymama.com

Mamaphonic
www.mamaphonic.com

Mamazine
(Feminist web 'zine for mothers and the
    people who love them)
www.mamazine.com

Mommy, Too! Magazine
(Web and print magazine celebrating mothers
    of color)
www.mommytoo.com

Mothering Magazine
(Natural family living, attachment parent-
    ing, natural and eco-conscious child-
    rearing)
800-984-8116
www.mothering.com

Organizations

Circumcision Resource Center
PO Box 232, Boston, MA 02133
617-523-0088
www.circumcision.org

Fertility Awareness Network
PO Box 1190, New York, NY 10009
800-597-6267 or 212-475-4490
www.FertAware.com

Mocha Moms
PO Box 1995, Upper Marlboro, MD 20773
www.mochamoms.org

National Association of Mothers' Centers
1740 Old Jericho Turnpike, Jericho, NY 11753
877-939-6667
www.motherscenter.org

Planned Parenthood Federation of America
434 West Thirty-third Street, New York, NY
    10001
212-541-7800
www.plannedparenthood.org

Websites

Child Care Aware
www.childcareaware.org

Circumcision Information and Resource
    Pages (CIRP)
(Information and FAQs for parents and
    educators, and a virtual reference library)
www.cirp.org

Familydoctor.org
http://familydoctor.org

Hip Mama
www.hipmama.com

National Organization of Single Mothers
www.singlemothers.org

Postpartum Education for Parents (PEP)
www.sbpep.org

Rebel Dad
www.rebeldad.com

POSTPARTUM MOOD DISORDERS

Books

Beck, Cheryl T., and Jeanne W. Driscoll. *Post-
    partum Mood and Anxiety Disorders: A
    Clinician's Guide.* Sudbury, MA: Jones &
    Bartlett Publishers, 2005.
Bennett, Shoshana S., and Pec Indman. *Be-
    yond the Blues: A Guide to Understanding*

and Treating Prenatal and Postpartum Depression. San Jose, CA: Moodswings Press, 2006.

Kendall-Tackett, Kathleen. *Depression in New Mothers: Causes, Consequences, and Treatment Alternatives.* Binghamton, NY: Haworth Press, 2005.

Websites

Postpartumcouples.com
www.postpartumcouples.com

Resources on Depression in Mothers
www.granitescientific.com/
    depressionfrontpage.htm

Postpartum Support International
P.O. Box 60931, Santa Barbara, CA 93160
800-944-4773
www.postpartum.net

ADVOCATING FOR BETTER MATERNITY CARE AND FOR MOTHERS AND FAMILIES

Books

Annas, George J. *The Rights of Patients: The Authoritative ACLU Guide to the Rights of Patients.* 3rd ed. Carbondale: Southern Illinois University Press, 2004.

Barnett, Rosalind, and Caryl Rivers. *Same Difference: How Gender Myths Are Hurting Our Relationships, Our Children, and Our Jobs.* New York: Basic Books, 2004.

Blades, Joan, and Kristin Rowe-Finkbeiner. *The Motherhood Manifesto: What America's Moms Want—and What to Do About It.* New York: Nation Books, 2006.

Davis-Floyd, Robbie E., and Christine Barbara Johnson, eds. *Mainstreaming Midwives:*

The Politics of Change. New York: Routledge, 2006.

Douglas, Susan, and Meredith Michaels. *The Mommy Myth: The Idealization of Motherhood and How It Has Undermined Women.* New York: Free Press, 2004.

Hochschild, Arlie R., with Anne Machung. *The Second Shift.* New York: Penguin Books, 2003.

Institute of Medicine Committee on the Consequences of Uninsurance. *Insuring America's Health: Principles and Recommendations.* Washington, DC.: National Academies Press, 2004.

Kitzinger, Sheila. *Birth Crisis.* New York: Routledge, 2006.

———. *The Politics of Birth.* New York: Elsevier, 2005.

Minkler, Meredith, ed. *Community Organizing and Community Building for Health.* 2nd ed. New Brunswick, NJ: Rutgers University Press, 2004.

Perkins, Barbara Bridgman. *The Medical Delivery Business: Health Reform, Childbirth, and the Economic Order.* New Brunswick, NJ: Rutgers University Press, 2004.

Roberts, Dorothy. *Shattered Bonds: The Color of Child Welfare.* New York: Basic Books, 2003.

Silliman, Jael, Marlene Gerber Fried, Loretta Ross, and Elena Gutierrez. *Undivided Rights: Women of Color Organize for Reproductive Justice.* Cambridge, MA.: South End Press, 2004.

Audiovisual Materials

Carson, Christopher, and Suzanne Arms. *Birth: The Journey That Shapes Our Lives,* 3 one-hour episodes, 2006 (currently in production). Available from Reverie Productions, 866-738-3743; www.reverieproductions .com/htmls/100yearsofbirth.html.

The Motherhood Manifesto. DVD. Approximately 60 minutes. 2006. To find a screening or to purchase, see www.momsrising.org.

Organizations

Association for Research on Mothering (ARM)
726 Atkinson, York University, 4700 Keele Street, Toronto, ON M3J 1P3
416-736-2100, ext. 60366
www.yorku.ca/a

Citizens for Midwifery
PO Box 82227, Athens GA 30608-2227
888-CfM-4880 (888-236-4880)
www.cfmidwifery.org

Coalition for Improving Maternity Services (CIMS)
PO Box 2346, Ponte Vedra Beach, FL 32004
888-282-CIMS (888-282-2467) or 904-285-1613
www.motherfriendly.org

Dads & Daughters
2 West First Street, Suite 101, Duluth MN 55802
218-722-3942
www.dadsanddaughters.org

Foundation for the Advancement of Midwifery
1779 Wells Branch Parkway, #110B-284, Austin, TX 78728
877-594-9996
www.formidwifery.org

Legal Momentum Family Initiative
212-925-6635
www.legalmomentum.org/legalmomentum/programs/familyinitiative

MomsRising.org
202-371-1999
www.momsrising.org

Mothers & More
PO Box 31, Elmhurst, IL 60126
630-941-3553
www.mothersandmore.org

National Advocates for Pregnant Women
39 West Nineteenth Street, Suite 602, New York, NY 10011-4225
212-255-9252
www.advocatesforpregnantwomen.org

National Organization for Women (NOW)
1100 H Street NW, 3rd Floor, Washington, DC 20005
202-628-8NOW (202-628-8669)
www.now.org

National Partnership for Women & Families
1875 Connecticut Avenue NW, Suite 650, Washington, DC 20009
202-986-2600
www.nationalpartnership.org

National Women's Health Network
514 Tenth Street NW, Suite 400, Washington, DC 20004
202-628-7814 (for health information) or 202-347-1140 (office)
www.nwhn.org

National Women's Health Resource Center
157 Broad Street, Suite 315, Red Bank, NJ 07701
877-986-9472
www.healthywomen.org

National Women's Law Center
11 Dupont Circle NW, Suite 800, Washington, DC 20036

202-588-5180
www.nwlc.org

9to5, National Association of Working
  Women
207 East Buffalo Street, #211, Milwaukee, WI
  53202
414-274-0925
www.9to5.org

SisterSong
PO Box 311020, Atlanta, GA 31131
404-344-9629
www.sistersong.net

United States Equal Employment
  Opportunity Commission (EEOC)
National Contact Center: 1-800-669-4000
Job Survival Hotline: 1-800-522-0925
www.eeoc.gov

Websites

The Mothers Movement Online
www.mothersmovement.org

Women's eNews
www.womensenews.org

MORE ON THE WEB

This list includes recommended online resources available at the time of this book's printing. But new websites are launched every day, and web addresses often change. To find up-to-date links to websites, as well as updated lists of other recommended materials, visit www.ourbodiesourselves.org.

Authorship and Acknowledgments

THE EDITORIAL TEAM

Executive Editor: Heather Stephenson

Editor: Kiki Zeldes

Editorial Advisers: Elana Hayasaka, Neda Joury-Penders, Tekoa King, Lydia Mayer, Judy Norsigian, Cornelia van der Ziel

Graphics Editor: Elana Hayasaka

CHAPTER 1: APPROACHING BIRTH WITH CONFIDENCE

By the Editorial Team.
With thanks to: Maureen Corry, Henci Goer, Gary Richwald, Judith Rooks, Carol Sakala, and Amanda Buck Varella.

CHAPTER 2: CHOOSING YOUR HEALTH CARE PROVIDER AND BIRTH SETTING

By Leah Diskin and the Editorial Team.
With thanks to: Anne Brewster, Barbara Fildes, JoAnne Fischer, Marsha Jackson, Timothy Johnson, Jane Kilthei, Michael Klein, Kate McLachan, Christine Morton, Beri Meltzer Norman, Judith Rooks, Amanda Buck Varella, and Deanne Williams.

CHAPTER 3: PREPARING FOR CHILDBIRTH

By Lisa Noguchi and the Editorial Team.
With thanks to: Nancy Bardacke, April Bolding, José Gorrin-Peralta, and Christine Morton.

CHAPTER 4: YOUR DEVELOPING PREGNANCY AND PRENATAL CARE

By Laurine Korfine, with Linda Schutt and Barbara Behrmann and the Editorial Team. With thanks to: Beth Greenberg.

CHAPTER 5: TAKING CARE OF YOURSELF

By Sarah Cox and the Editorial Team.
With thanks to: Myron Allukian, Sarah Campbell, Beth Greenberg, Alice Horowitz, Audra Karp, Kay Perrin, Nadine Saubers, Naomi Stotland, and Amanda Buck Varella.

CHAPTER 6: RELATIONSHIPS, SEX, AND EMOTIONAL SUPPORT

By the Editorial Team, with Penny Simkin (effects of childhood sexual abuse), Heidi Raykeil (sexuality), Margaret Lazarus and Stacey Kabat (violence), and Kristin DeJohn.
With thanks to: Elia Abi-Jaoude, Warren Bell, Sarah Campbell, Michele Chausse, Robyn Churchill, Denise Crooks, Ralph Faggotter, Beth Greenberg, David Healy, Deborah Issokson, Sheila Kitzinger, Phyllis Klaus, Michael Klein, Peter Mansfield, Carol Nadelson, Malkah Notman, Kathleen O'Grady, Kay Perrin, Ros Powrie, Judith Rooks, Anthony Scialli, Nada Stotland, Amanda Buck Varella, Carole Warshaw, Beverly Whipple, James Wright, and Diony Young.

CHAPTER 7: PRENATAL TESTING

By Adrienne Asch and Taran Jefferies, with Janelle Taylor ("Ultrasound: Medical Test, Bonding Opportunity, or Consumer Entertainment?") and the Editorial Team.
With thanks to: Timothy Johnson, Patricia Lohr, Kelly Ormond, Ellen Perrin, Nancy Press, and Jon Weil.

CHAPTER 8: SPECIAL CONCERNS DURING PREGNANCY

By Sarah Cox, with Caitlin Rothermel and Lois Jovanoic (diabetes), Naomi Stotland (pre-eclampsia, preterm premature rupture of membranes), and the Editorial Team.
With thanks to: Michelle Borowski, Jill Clark, Martha Katz, Bruce Moore, Jean Ramsey, Jihad Slim, and Amanda Buck Varella.

CHAPTER 9: CHILDBEARING LOSSES

By Elizabeth Fabel and the Editorial Team, based on an earlier chapter by Our Bodies Ourselves.
With thanks to: LindaMae Lucas, Linda Layne, Catherine McKinley, and Heidi Raykeil.

CHAPTER 10: LABOR AND BIRTH

By Cheryl de Jong-Lambert and the Editorial Team, based on an earlier chapter by Our Bodies Ourselves.
With thanks to: Deborah Fiedler, Barbara Fildes, Faith Gibson, Judith Lothian, Cindy

Pierce, Amanda Buck Varella, and Deanne Williams.

CHAPTER 11:
COPING WITH PAIN

By Mayri Sagady Leslie and the Editorial Team.

With thanks to: Jill Antoine, April Bolding, Tina Cassidy, Robyn Churchill, Barbara Fildes, Michael Klein, Judy Luce, Nancy Oriol, Marcie Richardson, Gary Richwald, Mark Rosen, Carol Sakala, and Amanda Buck Varella.

CHAPTER 12: SPECIAL CONCERNS DURING LABOR AND BIRTH

By Naomi Stotland, with Jacqueline Lapidus and the Editorial Team.

With thanks to: Joanna Shulman and Elisabeth Winterkorn.

CHAPTER 13: CESAREAN BIRTHS

By Khady Diouf, with Alice Rothchild and the Editorial Team.

With thanks to: Mary Barger, Zobeida Bonilla, Eugene Declercq, Jeff Ecker, Barbara Fildes, Beth Greenberg, Marcie Richardson, and Carol Sakala.

CHAPTER 14: YOUR PHYSICAL RECOVERY AND YOUR NEWBORN

By Sayantani DasGupta and the Editorial Team.

With thanks to: Beth Greenberg, Polly Kornblith, Kathryn Kravetz, and James McKenna.

CHAPTER 15: FEEDING YOUR BABY

By Andy Steiner, with Cindy Turner-Maffei, Jan Weingrad Smith, and the Editorial Team.

With thanks to: Myron Allukian, Barbara Behrmann, Janet L. Engstrom, Suzanne Haynes, Alice Horowitz, Lynn Isenhart, Polly Kornblith, Miriam Labbok, Anne Merewood, Jan Weingrad Smith, Amanda Buck Varella, and Diana Zuckerman.

CHAPTER 16:
LIFE AS A NEW MOTHER

By Andrea Buchanan, with Heidi Raykeil (sexuality), Patricia Lohr (birth control), and the Editorial Team.

With thanks to: Elia Abi-Jaoude, Shoshana Bennett, Michele Chausse, Julie Feinland, David Healy, Deborah Issokson, Ann Keppler, Miriam Labbok, Bruce Moore, Patricia Murphy, Malkah Notman, Jean Ramsey, Judy Roth, Jennifer Runquist, Susan Sered, Geradine Simkins, Toni Weschler, and Ruth Wilf.

CHAPTER 17: ADVOCATING FOR BETTER MATERNITY CARE

By the Editorial Team, with Jo-Anna Rorie ("Racial and Economic Disparities").

With thanks to: Tai Antoine, Michael Klein, Gary Richwald, and Carol Sakala.

CHAPTER 18: ADVOCATING FOR MOTHERS AND FAMILIES

By Judith Stadtman Tucker and the Editorial Team.

With special thanks to: Tali Averbuch, Christine Morton, Susan Sered, and Amanda Buck Varella.

RESOURCES

By Cathryn Brubaker and the Editorial Team.

With thanks to: All the contributors to the book.

WITH THANKS TO:

Other Our Bodies Ourselves staff: Wendy Brovold, Ayesha Chatterjee, Sarah Light, Anne Sweeney, and Sally Whelan.

Our Bodies Ourselves consultants: Pam McCarthy and Marianne McPherson.

Our Bodies Ourselves interns: Alexis Felder, Ilana Glosser, Akilah Jefferson, Hyejo Jun, and Alyssa Tartaglione.

At Simon & Schuster: Cherise Davis, Lisa Healy, Michelle Howry, Meghan Stevenson, Ellen Silberman, Trish Todd, Chris Lloreda, Debbie Model, Marcia Burch, Sue Fleming, and Mark Gompertz.

Our Bodies Ourselves board members (2006): Shahira Ahmed, Anne Brewster, Marcia Browne, Sally Deane (past chair), Nancy Forsyth, Teresa Harrison, Myriam Hernandez-Jennings, Rema Iyer, Neda Joury-Penders, Mary (Bebe) Poor, Penelope Riseborough, Patricia Roche, Bonnie Shepard (past cochair), Donna Soodalter-Toman, and Amanda Buck Varella (chair).

Our Bodies Ourselves advisory board members: Marjorie Agosin, Hortensia Amaro, Byllye Avery, Joan Bavaria, Linda Ellerbee, Teresa Heinz, Cathy Inglese, Wanda Jones, Florence Ladd, Susan M. Love, Meizhu Lui, Ngina Lythcott, Evelyn Murphy, Cynthia Pearson, Vivian Pinn, Ellen Poss, Joan Rachlin, Isaac Schiff, and Gloria Steinem.

Founders of the Boston Women's Health Book Collective: Ruth Bell-Alexander, Pamela Berger, Paula Doress-Worters, Joan Ditzion, Vilunya Diskin, Paula Doress-Worters, Nancy Miriam Hawley, Elizabeth MacMahon-Herrera, Pamela Morgan, Judy Norsigian, Jane Pincus, Esther Rome (1945–1995), Wendy C. Sanford, Norma Swenson, and Sally Whelan.

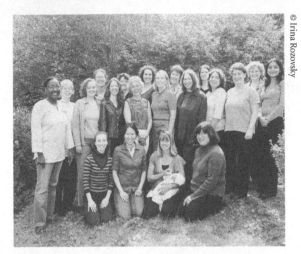

© Irina Rozovsky

Some members of the board, staff, founders, and consultants of Our Bodies Ourselves. Front row, left to right: Marianne McPherson, Elana Hayasaka, Anne Brewster holding daughter Hannah Weyerhaeuser, and Sally Deane. Second row: Shahira Ahmed, Sally Whelan, Heather Stephenson, Judy Norsigian, Marcia Brown, Joan Ditzion, Myriam Hernandez-Jennings, and Kiki Zeldes. Back row: Patricia Roche, Penelope Riseborough, Rachel A. Wilson, Neda Joury-Penders, Bonnie Shepard, Amanda Buck Varella, Nancy Forsyth, and Ayesha Chatterjee.

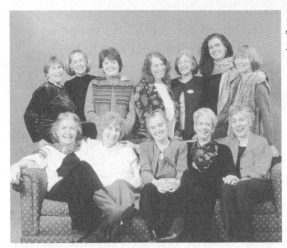

© Jörg Meyer

Founders of the Boston Women's Health Book Collective. Front row, seated left to right: Norma Swenson, Pamela Berger, Sally Whelan, Nancy Miriam Hawley, Judy Norsigian. Back row, left to right: Jane Pincus, Pamela Morgan, Vilunya Diskin, Joan Ditzion, Paula Doress-Worters, Elizabeth MacMahon-Herrera, Wendy C. Sanford. Not pictured: Ruth Bell-Alexander and Esther Rome (deceased).

About the Contributors

EXECUTIVE EDITOR

Heather Stephenson was the managing editor of the 2005 edition of *Our Bodies, Ourselves* and editor of *Our Bodies, Ourselves: Menopause*. She is the publisher at the Appalachian Mountain Club.

EDITOR

Kiki Zeldes was part of the editorial team for the 2005 edition of *Our Bodies, Ourselves* and for *Our Bodies, Ourselves: Menopause*. She develops content for and manages the Our Bodies Ourselves website, www.ourbodiesourselves.org.

EDITORIAL ADVISORS

Elana Hayasaka formerly worked on publications for Our Bodies Ourselves. A graduate of Wellesley College, she holds a master's degree in science and medical journalism from Boston University.

Neda Joury Penders, MPH, chairs the Public Policy Committee for Our Bodies Ourselves. Her experience includes women's health advocacy and work on legislative issues. She has consulted on numerous political campaigns. She is the mother of two young sons.

Tekoa L. King, CNM, MPH, is editor in chief of the *Journal of Midwifery & Women's Health* and an associate professor in the Department of Obstetrics, Gynecology, and Reproductive Sciences at the University of California at San Francisco.

Lydia Mayer, MD, MPH, is an obstetrician and medical ethicist. Her work focuses on community health and balancing social and personal ethics in healthcare.

Judy Norsigian is executive director of Our Bodies Ourselves. A cofounder of the Boston Women's Health Book Collective and coauthor of all Simon & Schuster editions of *Our Bodies, Ourselves*, she is a renowned speaker and writer on women's health.

Cornelia van der Ziel, MD, is an obstetrician-gynecologist who works at Harvard Vanguard Medical Associates in Cambridge and is a clinical instructor at Harvard Medical School. She coauthored *Big, Beautiful and Pregnant*, a book for plus-size women.

CONTRIBUTORS

Adrienne Asch is the director of the Center for Ethics at Yeshiva University. She is also professor of epidemiology and population health at Albert Einstein College of Medicine and the Edward and Robin Milstein Professor of Bioethics at Wurzweiler School of Social Work at Yeshiva University.

Katherine Arnoldi (www.katherinearnoldi .com), an activist for equal rights to education for teenage mothers, is the author of *The Amazing True Story of a Teenage Single Mom* and *All Things Are Labor*.

Barbara L. Behrmann, PhD, is the author of *The Breastfeeding Café: Mothers Share the Joys, Secrets & Challenges of Nursing*. She maintains a growing website at www.breastfeedingcafe .com and speaks throughout the United States and Canada on breast-feeding from a woman's perspective.

Cathryn Elise Brubaker, MA, is a doctoral candidate in sociology at the University of Massachusetts Amherst. Her dissertation concerns sex, gender-role orientation, and health-behavior engagement. She is also interested in comparative childbirth practices and strengthening the rights of midwives.

Andrea J. Buchanan is the author of *Mother Shock: Loving Every Other Minute of It* and editor of the anthologies *It's a Boy, It's a Girl* and *Literary Mama*. She is a founding editor of the online magazine *Literary Mama* (www.liter arymama.com).

Sarah Cox is the director of maternity services for St. Luke's Hospital in Boise, Idaho, and is a contributing editor for the *Journal of Midwifery & Women's Health*. She has worked in national and international health for over twenty-five years.

Sayantani DasGupta is a pediatrician at Columbia University and mother of two. Her books include *Her Own Medicine: A Woman's Journey from Student to Doctor* and *Stories of Illness and Healing: Women Write Their Bodies*.

Kristin DeJohn, an award-winning writer and television producer, has been honored by the American Medical Association and by American Women in Radio and Television. She is the mother of two young daughters.

Cheryl de Jong-Lambert is a senior development editor for Pearson Allyn & Bacon and an occasional freelance writer. She lives in Manhattan with her husband, William; son, Riley, age four; and daughter, Halina, who's sixteen months old.

Khady Diouf, MD, grew up in Dakar, Senegal, and is pursuing her training in obstetrics-gynecology in Boston. She hopes to focus her skills on working with women in underserved communities.

Leah Diskin is raising two daughters, and writing, from home. Her master's degree in anthropology is from Stanford University, where she focused on the social construction of gender. She is a daughter of an Our Bodies Ourselves founder.

Elizabeth Fabel has given birth to two beautiful daughters, one of whom died in infancy. She has a master's degree from the Harvard School of Public Health and is a senior technical adviser at EngenderHealth, an international nonprofit agency.

Taran Jefferies is a research fellow at the Centers for Disease Control and Prevention. She immersed herself in sociology and molecular biology at Wesleyan University, and decided to dedicate herself to public health issues with a master's degree from Harvard.

Lois Jovanovic, MD, is the chief scientific officer of the Sansum Diabetes Research Institute. She has written more than 250 articles on diabetes and obstetrics, as well as the American Diabetes Association publication *Medical Management of Pregnancy Complicated by Diabetes.*

Stacey Kabat is an Academy Award–winning human rights advocate. She has been recognized internationally for her work with battered women and children. Currently she works as a maternal child health nurse and lactation consultant in inner-city Boston.

Lauren Korfine is a home-birth mama, doula, birth activist, and lecturer in psychology and women's studies. She received her degrees from Cornell and Harvard, but her education from her three children. She lives in Ithaca, New York, with her family.

Jacqueline Lapidus is an editorial consultant with extensive experience in the fields of health care, business, and travel, as well as a poet and essayist. For ten years she taught the writing component of Current Topics in Medicine at Harvard Extension School.

Margaret Lazarus is an Academy Award–winning documentary filmmaker who, with Renner Wunderlich, has made many films about social justice for Cambridge Documentary Films. She is the author of the chapter about violence and abuse in the 2005 edition of *Our Bodies, Ourselves.*

Mayri Sagady Leslie is a certified nurse-midwife and faculty member at Georgetown University. She chairs the Coalition for Improving Maternity Services and is a leader with the International MotherBaby Childbirth Initiative, working to make mother-friendly maternity care a worldwide standard.

Patricia Lohr is an ob-gyn and a fellow in contraceptive research and family planning at Magee–Women's Hospital, University of Pittsburgh Medical Center. She agrees with Spike Milligan, who said, "Contraceptives should be used on every conceivable occasion."

Catherine McKinley is the author of *The Book of Sarahs: A Family in Parts.*

Lisa Noguchi conducts anti-HIV vaginal microbicide research at the University of Pittsburgh. She earned her master's degree in nurse-midwifery from the University of Pennsylvania and was formerly service director of St. Luke's Hospital Nurse-Midwifery Service in San Francisco's Mission District.

Heidi Raykeil is the author of the book *Confessions of a Naughty Mommy: How I Found My Lost Libido.* She is an editor and columnist at the online magazine *Literary Mama* (www.literarymama.com).

Judith P. Rooks is a midwife, epidemiologist, consultant, and writer focusing on maternal and child health, family planning, and midwifery. She is a past president of the American College of Nurse-Midwives and the author of *Midwifery and Childbirth in America*.

Alice Rothchild is an assistant professor of obstetrics, gynecology, and reproductive biology at Harvard Medical School. She has been honored with a community service award from the school and a Best of Boston's Women Doctors Award from *Boston* magazine.

Caitlin Rothermel is the editorial director of CADRE (the Council for the Advancement of Diabetes Research and Education). She is also a Seattle-based mom, wife, medical writer, and MPH candidate at the University of Washington.

Linda Schutt, BS, CM, CPM, has been a home-birth midwife since 1982. She is chairperson of the New York State Board of Midwifery and a preceptor for the National College of Midwifery. She has two sons, both born at home.

Penny Simkin is a childbirth educator, doula, and birth counselor who lectures and writes extensively on childbearing topics, including sexual abuse.

Andy Steiner is a freelance writer, author of *Spilled Milk: Breastfeeding Adventures and Advice from Less-Than-Perfect Moms*, and former senior editor at *Utne Reader*. She lives in St. Paul, Minnesota, with her husband and two daughters.

Naomi E. Stotland, MD, is assistant professor of obstetrics and gynecology at the University of California, San Francisco. Her research area is weight gain and nutrition during pregnancy. She and her husband have a three-year-old daughter.

Janelle S. Taylor teaches anthropology at the University of Washington. She has written numerous articles on the social, cultural, and political dimensions of obstetrical ultrasound, and is coeditor of the volume *Consuming Motherhood*. She has two children.

Judith Stadtman Tucker is a writer and advocate for mothers' and caregivers' rights. She is the founder and editor of The Mothers Movement Online (www.mothersmovement.org).

Cindy Turner-Maffei, MA, IBCLC, is national coordinator for Baby-Friendly USA, a faculty member of the Healthy Children Project, and an adjunct professor at the Union Institute & University. She is the author of several publications about breast-feeding.

Disclosures

Our Bodies Ourselves is a nonprofit group committed to providing fair and accurate health information. In the interest of maintaining its independence, Our Bodies Ourselves does not accept any funding from pharmaceutical companies. All contributors who wrote sections of this book were asked to disclose any financial interest or other relationship since January 1, 2001, with any manufacturers of products or providers of services that they have discussed in the book. The information they provided is listed below.

Lois Jovanovic has a financial interest, arrangement, or affiliation with the following corporate organizations, which offer her financial support or educational grants: Amylin, Bristol-Myers Squibb, Cygnus, DexCom, Eli Lilly & Company, Insulet, LifeScan, Medtronic MiniMed, MannKind, Merck & Company, Novo Nordisk, Pfizer, Roche Diagnostics, Sanofi-Aventis, SenSys, and Takeda.

Andy Steiner was employed from 2005 to 2006 as an online expert on www .sisterhoodsix.com, a website sponsored by Avent America, a manufacturer and distributor of breast pumps, milk storage containers, bottles, and other infant-feeding accessories.

Naomi Stotland has received honoraria twice from CBR, a cord blood company.

Index

Page numbers in *italics* refer to illustrations.

breast-feeding (*cont.*)
early patterns of, 260–62
effects of birth practices on, 252–53
engorgement and, 243, 265–66
establishing, 255–63
frequency of, 261, 268, 276
fully, 268
HIV and, 140, 142, 251, 252
latching on for, 256–59, *256, 258,*
  264, 265, 267
low milk supply and, 267–68
mastitis and, 266–67
medications and, 104, 210, 252–53,
  263, 293
mother's diet while, 263–64
mother's health and, 251
nipple shape and, *264*
oxytocin and, 262–63, 295
planning ahead for, 251, 253–54
of premature babies, 135, 136
in public, 251, 270, *317*
reasons not to, 251, 252
recommended length of, 251, 315
relationship issues and, 294
resources for, 332–33
retained placenta and, 217
rooming in and, 24, 244
sex and, 295–96
smoking and, 263–64
sore nipples and, 264–65
systemic medicine and, 207
of twins, 259–60, *259*
uterus and, 187, 262
weaning from, 270, 273, 295, 296
who can help with, 266
work and, 252, 263, 272, 315, 322
breast milk, 253, 264, 265, 266
bottle-feeding of, 277–78
coming in of, 260
formula compared with, 250–51,
  274, 275
hormonal contraceptives and, 267,
  297
let-down of, 263
low supply of, 267–68, 297
manual expressing of, 265, 268,
  270–72
pumping of, 266, 268, 270–72, 315
storage of, 272
breast pads, 267
breasts:
abscess of, 267
areola of, 50, 264, 265, 268, 271
colostrum produced by, 59, 188,
  254, 255, 260
engorgement of, 243, 265–66

implants, 268
increase in size of, *49,* 50
pain in, 104
surgery for, 267–68
tender or sore, 50, 52, 95, 243,
  264–65
see also nipples
breathing, breath:
contractions and, 170, 181
deep, 101
holding, pushing and, 181
music as aid to, 203
pain management and, 38,
  199–200
rapid, 291
shortness of, 59
SIDS and, 158
breathing techniques, 99
Lamaze, 35–36
patterned, 199–200
breech baby, 145–46, 221–22, 225,
  227, 234
butorphanol (Stadol), 206
buttocks, 78
B vitamins, 64, 68
folate/folic acid, 65

caffeine, 66, 83–84
Cajuns, 115
calcium, 64, 66–67, 68, 72, 140
cramps prevented by, 80
California, parental leave in, 319
Canada, 98
cancer, 52, 112, 155, 251
radiation treatment for, 268
vitamin K in, 246
CAPPA (Childbirth and Postpartum
  Professional Association), 34, 37
carbohydrate intolerance, 138
carbohydrates, 175
simple vs. complex, 138
carbonated drinks, 71
carboprost tromethamine
  (Hemabate), 218
cardiovascular disease, 112
careers, identity changes and, 92
caregivers, 310
birth plans and, 11
see also doctors; doulas; health care
  providers; midwives; *specific*
  kinds of doctors
carpal tunnel syndrome, 78–80
home treatments for, 79–80
prevention of, 79
car seats, infant, 40, 249
car travel, 82

catheters, 214, 227, 229, 230, 231, 304
heparin lock, 233
cats, 88, 144
CBC (complete blood count), 52
CD players, battery-operated, 40
celebrities, pregnant, 55
Celexa, 103, 292
Census Report, U.S., 299
Center for Work-Life Law, 318
Centering Pregnancy, 17, *17, 286*
Centers for Disease Control and
  Prevention (CDC), 61, 141, 253
central nervous system, 103
cephalohematoma, 184
cerclage, 137
ceremonies, childbearing loss and,
  159
certified midwives (CMs), 18
certified nurse-midwives (CNMs), 18
certified professional midwives
  (CPMs), 18–19
cervical canal, 60
cervical cancer, 52
cervical polyps, 133
cervical ripening, 147
cervical shields (FemCap; Lea's
  Shield), 296
cervix, *49,* 54, 99
abnormalities of, 153
birth control and, 296
breech baby and, 145
dilation of, 99, 134, 154, 165, 166,
  166, 167, 171, 173, 177, 179, 180,
  181, 184, 204, 214, 215, 217, 218,
  294
effacement of, 167
incompetent (cervical
  insufficiency), 99, 136–37
labor induction and, 11
in latent phase, 168, 171
length of, 134
multiples and, 131, 132
paracervical blocks and, 208, 210
placenta previa and, 99, 133–34,
  217, 225, 228
post-miscarriage closing of, 154
sewing close of (cerclage), 137
sexual intercourse and, 133
softening of, 60, 147, 148, 167
tearing of, 217, 218
cesarean sections (C-sections), 19, 20,
  22, 27, 32, 140, 184, 185, 211,
  221, 224–36
back labor and, 215
bleeding and, 217, 228
breast-feeding and, 228–31, 250

moxibustion, 145
MRI (magnetic resonance imagining), 222
mucus, 186
mucus discharge, 167, 168
mucus plug, *49,* 60, 99, 165, 167, 218
multiple babies, 23, 130–32, 307
    C-sections and, 22, 131, 225, 307
    helpful suggestions and, 131
    identical, 130–31
    nonidentical (fraternal), *130,* 131
    premature, 158
    reduction of, 132
    see also twins
multiple gestation pregnancy, 156
multiple marker screening, 53, 117
multivitamin supplements, 67, 140, 243
muscular dystrophy, 115, 122
music, 59, 203, 230

nalbuphine, 206
nannies, night, 289
naps, 50, 81, 135, 170
narcotics (opioids), 38, 191, 205–8, 212*n*
    C-sections and, 229, 230, 231, 242
National Academy of Sciences, 66
National Advocates for Pregnant Women (NAPW), 313
National Domestic Violence Hotline, 106
National Institute of Child Health and Human Development, 299
National Marrow Donor Program, 42
National Organization for Women, 308
National Organization of Mothers of Twins Clubs (NOMOTC), 260
National Partnership for Women and Families, 319*n*
Native Americans, 82, 138, 311
    childbearing loss of, 158
natural childbirth, 18, 192, 210–11, 215, 236
    birth plans and, 37
    in hospitals, 24–25
nausea, 50, 52, 63, 231
    coping with, 66, 71–72
    depression and, 102
    prenatal vitamins and, 66, 68, 71
    in transition phase, 168, 180
neck, 78, 144, 201
    massage of, 201
    pain in, 155, 241

needle sharing, 143
neonatal herpes, 143
neonatal intensive care units (NICU), 220, 309, 312
"nesting collection," 167
nesting impulse, 167
neural tube defects, 117, 118
    folate/folic acid and, 65, 67
    surgery for, 121
    see also anencephaly; spina bifida
neurological disease, 226
newborns, *see* babies
new mothers, life as, 280–300
    baby blues and, 243, 281, 289–91
    birth control and, 296–97
    disabled, 281, 283
    early adjustment to, 280–82
    emotional challenges of, 288
    feelings about the birth and, 287
    lack of social help for, 284
    mommy wars and, 298–300
    postpartum mood disorders and,
        see postpartum depression;
        postpartum mood disorders
    resources for, 333–34
    sexuality and, 293–96
    supermom myth and, 298–99
    support for, 281–86, 289, 291, 292
    tips for first weeks of, 283
    work and, 316–17, 319
new mothers' groups, 291
New York Civil Liberties Union, Reproductive Rights Project at, 321
New York Times, 308
NICU (neonatal intensive care units), 220, 309, 312
nightmares, 104
nipples:
    babies' locating of, 255, 256
    hand-expression and, 271
    latching on to, 256–57, *256*
    leaky, 265
    shape of, *265*
    sore, 250, 261, 264–65
    sore, prevention of, 256
    stimulation of, 99, 148, 179, 215, 262
    washing of, 254
nipples, for bottle-feeding, 277
nitrous oxide, 205–6
NOMOTC (National Organization of Mothers of Twins Clubs), 260
nonsteroidal anti-inflammatory drugs (NSAIDs), 231, 267

non-stress test, 146, 147
North America, decline of breast-feeding in, 253
Northern Europeans, prenatal testing and, 115
Norway, 253
Nubain, 191, 206
numbness, 78, 288
nurse-anesthetists, 208
nurse-midwife programs, closing of, 14
nurse-midwives, 16, 24
    certified (CNMs), 18
nurse-practitioners, 246–47
nurses, 32, 37, 219, 220, 235, 246
    breast-feeding and, 257, 259, 271
    labor and delivery, 19, 22, 306
    postpartum, 231, 244
    psychiatric, 292
    shortage of, 306
    "smoke breaks" of, 50
    visiting, 232
nursing bras, 40, 251, 254, 266, 295
nursing pads, 265, 295
nutritionists, diabetes and, 138, 139
nystatin, 265

obesity, 138
O'Brien, Robin, 308
obsessive-compulsive disorder, 289, 291
obstetrician-gynecologists (ob-gyns), 19, 22, 266
obstetricians, obstetrics, 13, 31, 135, 170, 191, 205, 265
    breech baby and, 146
    C-sections and, 230–31
    decline of specialization in, 14
    episiotomies and, 183
    interventions of, 10
    need for, 16
    training of, 305–6
    VBACs and, 235
Odent, Michel, 131
omega-3 fatty acids, 64, 67, 69
omega-6 fatty acids, 64, 67
open mind, maintaining of, 10
operative vaginal births, defined, 11
    see also forceps; vacuum extractors
ophthalmologists, 139
opiates, 84
opioids, *see* narcotics
optometrists, 139
oral sex, 97
orgasm, 95, 97, 148, 262, 295
os, *49*

spina bifida, 65, 112, 115, 122
  screening for, 117, 118
spinal canal, *49,* 208
spinal cord defects, fetal, 53
spinal headache, 210, 241
spinals, 208–9, 210, 304
  for C-sections, 227, 229, 230
spirituality, birthing and, 36
sports bras, 95
spotting, 132, 133, 153
squatting, 76, 195
squatting bars, 177
SSRIs, *see* selective serotonin reuptake
  inhibitors
Stadol, 206
stairs, walking up and down, 232
stem cells, in cord blood, 41
sterile water injections, 204
sterilization, 297
steroids, 135, 136
stillbirths, 69, 84, 157
stillness, pain relief and, 200
stomach, *49,* 55, 175
stool, of babies, 261–62, 275, 276
stories, childbirth, 55–56, 100
Stratton, Barbara, 308
stress management, 101, 103
Sublimaze, 206
substance abuse, 48, 103, 153, 291
  alcohol, 48, 69, 82, 85, 103, 106
  drugs, 48, 84, 85, 106
  partners with, 8
sucking reflex, 51, 188
sudden infant death syndrome
  (SIDS), 83, 158, 244–45, 251
suffering vs. pain, 191–93
suicidal thoughts, 101, 288, 289
suicide, 103
supermom, myth of, 298–99
supplemental nursing system, 273
supplements:
  calcium, 64, 66–67
  folic acid, 48, 65, 67
  formula as, 273
  herbs as, 87
  iron, 66
  multivitamin, 67, 140, 243
  vitamin D, 67
support, 8–12, 32–34, 204, 223
  in active phase, 173
  after the birth, 40
  for breast-feeding, 259–60, 264
  challenges in finding, 34
  childbearing loss and, 151, 153,
    154, 220
  continuous, 32

during C-sections, 230
from doulas, *see* doulas
emotional well-being and,
  99–100
from family, 11, 32, 223, 283,
  285–86, 290, 291, 303
from friends, 11, 32, 40, 154, 283,
  285–86, 290, 291, 303
during labor, 9, 11, 32, 38, 42–43
for new mothers, 281–86, *286,* 289,
  291, 292
from paid caregivers, 289
from partners, 32, 283, 284, 290,
  291, 303
during pregnancy, 8, 10, 12
in recovery phase, 242–43,
  248–49
relationship changes and, 93
sexual abuse aftereffects and, 105
from social service organizations,
  289
teenage pregnancies and, 129
support groups:
  bereavement, 151, 220
  parenting, 286, 289
  for postpartum depression, 291
surgery:
  breast, 267–68
  for neural tube defects, 121
  pelvic, 155
  uterine, 225
  see also cesarean sections
Swaziland, *316*
Sweden, 253
swelling, 56, 57, 59, 78, 80, 248
  air travel and, 82
  exercise and, 73
  of gums, 73
  see also specific body parts
swimming, 74, 78, 99–100, 131
swimsuits, 40
swollen glands, 144
swordfish, 69
symphysis, *49*
syphilis, 52
systematic review, 305
systemic medicine, 205–7
  advantages and disadvantages of,
    207
  nitrous oxide, 205–6

t'ai chi, 101
talk therapy, 292
tampons, 240
tax credits, 322
Tay-Sachs disease, 115, 116, 121

tearfulness, 101
tearing, 218–19
  of anus, 219, 304, 313*n*
  of cervix, 217, 218
  of perineum, 183, 218–19
  of rectum, 219, 313*n*
  of vagina, 183, 210, 217, 218,
    296
teenage pregnancies, 16, 128–29, 312,
  321
  Centering Pregnancy and, 17
  postpartum depression of, 291
  resources for, 331
telephone calls, intrusive, 243
telephone numbers:
  800, 264, 266, 286, 293
  of family and friends, 40
temperature instability, 243
tennis balls, 40, 199
TENS (transcutaneous electrical
  nerve stimulation), 204
Ten Steps of the Mother-Friendly
  Childbirth Initiative, 23
Ten Steps to Successful Breastfeeding,
  254–55
tests:
  of baby's well-being, 146, 147
  hepatitis, 143
  for HIV, 140–41, 142
  after miscarriage, 154
tests, prenatal, 20, 52, 53, 109–27
  choosing, 120
  concerns about, 110
  to confirm pregnancy, 51, 53
  continuing the pregnancy and, 123,
    125
  counseling and, 122, 124, 125
  decision making about, 110,
    125–27
  ethical and social questions raised
    by, 110, 114, 119
  for Group B streptococcus,
    54, 61
  information gained from,
    109–10
  information not available from,
    111, 112–13
  multiple births and, 132
  for older mothers, 130
  paying for, 123
  questions to consider about, 111
  resources for, 329–30
  responding to results of, 123–25
  Rhesus status (Rh screening test),
    52, 57
  types of, 114–20

work:
   putting mothers and children last
     and, 316–20
   rest at, 50, 81
   safety and, 8, 81, 107
   self-care and, 80, 81
World Health Organization, 251, 254,
   304
worthlessness, feelings of, 101,
   288

wrists, exercising of, 80
wrist splints, supportive, 80

xiphoid cartilage, *49*
X-linked inheritance, 115
X-rays, dental, 73

Y chromosomes, 115
Year After Childbirth, The (Kitzinger),
   285

yeast infection, 133,
   264–65
yelling, *195*, 203
yoga, 75, 99–100, 101,
   131
yogurt, 66, 71, 72, 274

zinc, 68
Zoloft, 103, 292
Zyban, 83

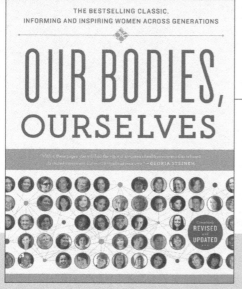
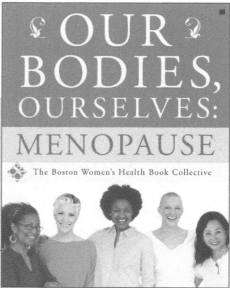